Holistic London

*The London Guide to
Mind, Body & Spirit*

Kate Brady
Mike Considine

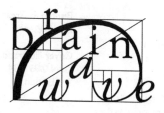

Brainwave • London

Acknowledgements

Book reviews

Brian Wade of Changes Bookshop for reviews in the Psychotherapy Section
David Redstone and staff at Watkins Bookshop for reviews in Body and Spirit section

Writers

Will Parfitt for the section on Qabalah
Richard Mowbray for the section on Primal Integration

Production team

Heather Jameson, Amanda Barkwith, Mike Considine

Other help

Thanks also to: The Institute of Complementary Medicine, Malcolm Stern, William Bloom, Stephanie Collins and Guy Dauncey for information.

Disclaimer

While every effort has been made to provide accurate information, the publishers do not assume and hereby disclaim any liability to any party for omissions in this book.

Inclusion in this book is not intended in any way as a recommendation or endorsement of individuals, organisations or therapies and is not an indication of the quality of therapy, medicine or instruction given by any of the individuals or organisations included.

Further copies of this book

These can be obtained from Brainwave, BCM Brainwave, London WC1N 3XX. Please send £12.95 plus £1.95 post and packing (£6 overseas). Or phone Brainwave on (0181) 677 8000

Published by Brainwave
BCM Brainwave
London WC1N 3XX (full address)

© **Brainwave 1995**

Printed in Great Britain by BPC Wheatons Ltd, Exeter.

Cover illustration by Mike Considine
ISBN 0 9513347 7 8
3rd Edition.

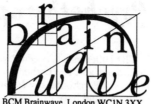

BCM Brainwave, London WC1N 3XX
(0181) 677 8000
serving holistic business

Who are we?

Brainwave is a publisher and marketing specialist serving the Holistic health/New Age field. We serve publishers of books, audio and visual tapes, product suppliers and holistic health centres.

Mailing Lists

If you need to send your brochure/ leaflet to individuals or organisations in the holistic health/ New Age field, we have a range of mailing lists on offer. Our laser printed address labels are high quality at a very affordable price.

Guidebooks

We publish two guidebooks aimed at the public who are interested in the holistic health/New Age field. This book *Holistic London*, now in it's third edition is packed with information on psychotherapy, alternative medicine and spiritual centres in the capital, as well as a list of resources including bookshops and products. It's an easy to use guidebook which has stood the test of time and is the only book of its kind for London. *The Whole Person Catalogue* is destined to be the definitive nationwide guide to this growing field.

Mail Order

We sell a wide range of books, tapes, videos and holistic products. Phone or write for a free colour brochure.

Trade Directory

We publish the *Holistic Marketing Directory*, which is aimed at holistic businesses. It's an essential handbook with comprehensive details of marketing outlets such as retailers, wholesalers, mailing lists, magazines, mail order catalogues etc as well as a wealth of listings on organisations that can help you promote yourself.

Practitioner Services

As well as this book which seeks to link clients to practitioners, we publish the Holistic London Guide, which is a free guide for the public aimed at helping them find a therapist, centre, course, event or product. The guide is sent free to referral agents and distributed widely throughout the London area. It is the ideal and most cost effective way finding new clients.

Psychotherapy

Introduction

What is Psychotherapy? **1**; The Difference between Psychotherapy and Counselling **1**; The Difference between Psychology and Psychotherapy **1**; Approaches to Psychotherapy **2**; The Varieties of Psychotherapy **4**; Does Psychotherapy Work? **5**; Styles of the Therapist **5**; Who Should have Psychotherapy? **6**; How to Choose a Particular Psychotherapy **7**; How to Choose a Therapist **7**; Individual Therapy Versus Group Therapy **9**; Does the Sex of the Therapist Matter? **10**; Too Old for Therapy? **10**; Cost **10**; What the Different Centres are Like **11**

Training in Psychotherapy

Why Train in Psychotherapy? **11**; Which School of Psychotherapy to Train In? **11**; The Training Programmes **11**; Accreditation and 1996 **13**; Can I get Work When Trained? **14**; Entry Requirements **14**; Cost of Training **14**

The Psychotherapies

Other Psychotherapies

Other Trainings

Body Therapies

Introduction

Training in Body Therapies

Body Approaches

Other Body Approaches

Other trainings

Spirit

Introduction
What is Spiritual? **175**; The Difference between Religion and Spirituality **175**; The Search for a New Spirituality **175**; East meets West **176**; Gurus & spiritual teachers **177**; Cults **178**; Different Types of Groups **178**; What they do **179**; Spiritual Groups in London **181**; Spirituality versus Psychology **181**; The 'New Age' **182**

Meditation 183

The Traditions

Modern Teachers 195

Other Groups 197

Resources

Communication

Learning

Services

Food

London Getaway

Events

Help

Products

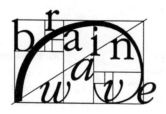

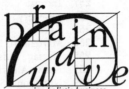

INTRODUCTION TO PSYCHOTHERAPY

What is Psychotherapy?

Psychotherapy is a term used to denote a variety of methods in dealing with emotional problems. There are many different types of psychotherapy, and each of these therapies may differ considerably from one another. What they all have in common is they all try to help the client in changing. In each of their own ways they will enable the client to better understand his or her self, feelings and relationships with others and help to explore new ways of behaving. It may involve the client re-enacting old conflicts within the therapy but with a resulting different outcome so that the client finds new ways of dealing with, and resolving those conflicts. Most of the therapies can be seen as a teaching in the art of therapy so that when the client leaves the therapy he or she will be able to continue his or her own analysis.

In general usage the word psychotherapy is confined to what goes on between a therapist and a client, though this limited definition leaves out self-help and help that can be offered by lay people - and the magnitude of this help should not be underestimated. The advantage of seeing a therapist is that the client will have the space to deal with his or her concerns with someone who has an armoury of strategies in helping.

The Difference between Psychotherapy and Counselling

Counselling used within this book refers to psychotherapeutic counselling rather than other types of counselling such as career or financial counselling. A caption on an Oxfam billboard advertisement many years ago read 'Give a man a fish and you feed him for a day. Teach a man to fish and you feed him for a lifetime'. Analogously counselling is usually an approach which helps the client with a problem, whereas psychotherapy is aimed at helping the client to help himself with his own problems. After receiving psychotherapy the client should be able to manage the daily tasks of living without getting tied up in destructive or mundane patterns of behaviour or negative feelings. Counselling is usually much shorter and involves less personal change on the part of the client. Counselling usually revolves around a specific problem while psychotherapy may not do so. However, having said that, there is still a great overlap between counselling and psychotherapy.

The Difference between Psychology and Psychotherapy

Psychology is the study of human behaviour. It is primarily a science. The domain of psychology is large and covers such things as perception, intelligence, conditioning, the nervous system, and the behaviour of people in groups, to name but a few. Psychotherapy is only one aspect of psychology. Psychologists enter the jobs market within a specialised field, either as industrial psychologists, educational psychologists, experimental psychologists, social psychologists or clinical psychologists. Clinical psychologists have more experience of psychotherapy than their fellows as they apply their knowledge of psychology to dealing with emotional and behavioural problems. They work in different settings throughout the National Health Service, especially in mental hospitals and institutions for people with a mental handicap. Psychotherapists, on the whole, have much more varied backgrounds. Whilst some are clinical psychologists, others are psychiatrists and social workers, and there are many who have a teaching and management background.

Approaches to Psychotherapy

There are four main approaches to psychotherapy: psychoanalytic, humanistic, cognitive and behavioural. The psychoanalytic approach developed by Sigmund Freud explains behaviour in terms of the interplay between the conscious and unconscious mind of an individual. Freud believed that innate instincts, especially the sex and aggressive instincts, are often disapproved of in our society and are driven out of the individual's awareness, but remain in the unconscious affecting behaviour. Glimpses of the unconscious are to be had from dreams, slips of the tongue, mannerisms, some symptoms of mental illness and some artistic endeavours. Most psychoanalysts prefer to speak in terms of levels of awareness rather than a conscious-unconscious divide.

The second approach is humanistic or phenomenological. The ideas of the humanistic psychologists are similar to, and draw upon, the writings of the existentialists. Emphasis is placed on how individuals subjectively experience the world, and what sense they make of it. The humanistic psychologists are concerned with the inner life of individuals and how they experience themselves and others. They are interested in concepts of self-esteem, feelings, authenticity, self awareness and consciousness.

Thirdly there is the cognitive approach. This approach argues that we are constantly processing information in selective and organised ways, such as when planning and solving problems. We make sense of the world using particular views and assumptions which have been conditioned by our previous experience. By consciously adopting another point of view, we can change our behaviour.

Fourthly there is the behavioural approach, sometimes known as Stimulus/

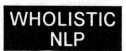

Response Psychology. This approach is based on 'learning theory' which grew from experiments with animals. Behaviourists emphasise how the environment 'conditions' people to behave in certain ways and that people modify their behaviour to suit the surroundings. Punishment and reward are the stick and the carrot for this process. For instance if a child is punished for succeeding and rewarded for failing then the child will learn to fail; or we might say the child has been conditioned to fail. Since behaviour was learned, behaviourists argue that undesirable behaviour could be unlearned and be replaced by more desirable forms of behaviour.

The Varieties of Psychotherapy

Most therapists practise one of the four approaches (or a combination of these approaches) described above. There are, however, literally hundreds of different types or 'schools' of psychotherapy which come under the four basic approaches. Each of these schools has its own theories about why people behave the way they do and on how to treat emotional problems. These different types of psychotherapy may differ dramatically from one another, even though the

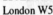

desired aims of the therapies may well be the same.

In this book we describe the major schools of psychotherapy, enabling the reader to steer through the minefield. The less well known psychotherapies are catalogued at the end of this section.

Does Psychotherapy Work?

Nobody knows if any one psychotherapy is better than another. This is partly because a great deal of research has yet to be carried out before any satisfactory conclusions can be drawn, and partly because the effectiveness of psychotherapy depends on the particular circumstances of the client and upon the unique quality of any therapeutic relationship. This is one reason why therapists tend to draw upon other psychotherapeutic approaches in their work. A transactional analysis therapist, for instance, may at times use a psychoanalytic approach, or some technique he or she has borrowed from another school of psychotherapy.

Styles of the Therapist

Any label the therapist gives herself may not accurately describe what she

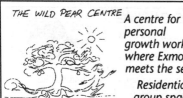

does. Two gestalt therapists, for instance, may operate in completely different ways. One may tend to ask the group to try out lots of exercises, whereas the other may not do this at all. One therapist may be very warm and protective of the group members whereas the other may be cold and reserved. This is partly due to the character of the therapist, but it is also because no psychotherapeutic approach can ever fully determine a therapist's behaviour.

Who Should have Psychotherapy?

Most people can benefit from psychotherapy. Some people are put off therapy because they think it is just for people who are mad, or that it is an admission of weakness and of not being able to cope, or that it is something that New Yorkers spend a great deal of time and money having without ever really getting anywhere. Therapy is usually intended both as a way of healing and a method of personal growth. It is meant to help those with conflicts and problems, as well as those who are simply dissatisfied with themselves and their lives, who feel blank, bored or want more out of themselves and their relationships. Sometimes people in this last category feel drawn to psychotherapy, but worry that if they go to see a therapist, he or she will think they are 'malingering' because they are not desperate or in crisis. In fact many therapies concentrate a great deal on the idea of growth, and that therapy is too good to be limited just to those whose problems severely restrict their lives.

The most important thing is perhaps that you make the choice to do it. While this is not irrevocable, and leaves room for experimentation, it is important that you do not feel pushed into doing it by someone else, or that you know it would be a good idea but do not really feel very enthusiastic. If you do not feel it is your decision then you may just feel resentful so that the whole process may not work for you. Sometimes people who are doing therapy may try and push partners, friends or relatives into therapy because they want them to change. Unfortunately this kind of pressure can turn the decision into a kind of power struggle, and make it very difficult for the person considering therapy to feel that they can make the decision of their own free will.

How to Choose a Particular Psychotherapy
This book explains many of the different psychotherapies on offer. If any particular approach appeals to you, further reading will give you more information, though this will be theoretical. To get an experience of therapy, many of the centres listed run weekend workshops which will enable you to get a taste of the therapy in action in a group setting. If you want to get an idea of what a particular approach is like in one to one sessions, then introductory sessions with a psychotherapist who uses the approach might be indicated.

How to Choose a Therapist
The title 'psychotherapist' is not regulated by law and at present in this country there is no licensing procedure. This means that anyone can set themselves up as a psychotherapist, even if they have no formal training in psychotherapy. So it is possible that you might choose a therapist who has not undergone adequate training. However, having said that, in our experience those therapists who are

poor at their job don't last long in the marketplace, and soon retire.

If you have decided that a particular therapy appeals to you then there are a number of ways of finding a psychotherapist. Look up that therapy in this book and you will find the organisations that practise them listed, together with training organisations. It is suggested that you contact one of the training organisations if one is listed. They usually keep a register of practitioners they have trained and will be able to refer you to one. Training organisations are a reliable way of finding a therapist because they are likely to recommend only those who they think have reached a certain standard, and who and subscribe to their code of ethics. If no training organisation is listed, then choose one of the centres which practice the therapy and contact them. They are listed under the description of the therapy. It's worth asking either the training organisation or centre to send you a brochure of what they offer. This will enable you to browse through their literature before making any commitment.

If you do not know which type of therapy you want and you do not feel you can make that decision then you can contact an umbrella organisation, such as the *Association for Humanistic Psychology Practitioners (AHPP), the United Kingdom Council for Psychotherapy (UKCP), the British Psychoanalytic Society (BPS)* or the *British Association for Counselling (BAC)*. All are listed at the back of this book with some details about them. A new independent organisation who will refer you to a therapist is Neal's Yard Agency in Covent Garden. You can browse round their shop, look at the leaflets on display and at biographies of practitioners they have on their records.

Having found a psychotherapist, it is advisable to have a few introductory sessions before embarking on a long-term commitment. It is important to find a therapist with whom you can have a good working relationship. Carl Rogers, a well-known figure in the field of counselling and psychotherapy, suggests that clients gain positive benefits from psychotherapy if the therapist is perceived by the client to be warm and caring, authentic and honest, and understanding of the way the client sees the world. If you perceive your therapist to have these qualities, and if you are learning about yourself in the therapy, then he or she may be the right therapist for you.

Individual Therapy Versus Group Therapy

Individual psychotherapy is the most common form of psychotherapy. The advantage of this type of approach is that the client and the therapist can focus on the client's particular problems for the entire session. Individual therapy also has the advantage that confidential information can be discussed without fear of public criticism. It is also useful in that the client has the opportunity to develop a close relationship with one person. This might be useful if the client has had difficulty in forming close relationships and finds the idea of groups frightening.

In individual therapy the client and therapist usually meet at least once a week for one hour. Some therapists prefer to work to the golden 50 minute hour, others may work for up to two hours. Often therapists insist on meeting for more than once a week and for psychoanalysis five times a week is the norm. Many therapists work outside of normal office hours to accommodate their clients.

The advantage of group therapy is that it allows others to give feedback on one person's behaviour, rather than the solitary feedback offered by the therapist in individual therapy. The therapist sees how you are interacting with other members of the group rather than simply listening to your reports. It may be that the therapist and the group members can offer some observations on your behaviour with others of which you may have been unaware. A further advantage of group therapy is that it enables you to understand how others may have similar problems and difficulties as yourself and so feel less alone.

Group therapy is usually conducted in small groups of between four and fourteen members with one psychotherapist present, though there are a number of exceptions to this. There may be more than one therapist; for instance in couple therapy the norm is two therapists. Sometimes the groups can be larger, and 'large group therapy' as it is called can involve over one hundred people in one group (the Introductory Course at the The Institute of Group Analysis runs a group of one hundred and forty members) though such large groups in therapy are rare.

The timeframe for the group may vary considerably between different groups and different therapies. The two most frequent formats are weekend workshops or once weekly evening workshops. Some of the other variations include meeting throughout the day for one, two, three or four weeks (these are usually residential and are sometimes known as intensives); 24 and 48 hour marathons (the members stay together for all of this period and get little sleep); meeting in the early morning before normal working hours; twice weekly evening groups; a combination of the aforementioned. Some people prefer to live in therapeutic communities where the boundary between therapy and everyday life can be blurred.

Does the Sex of the Therapist Matter?

Generally the sex of the therapist does not matter. Many people have difficulty in communicating with people of one or other gender. In this case they may find it too difficult to develop a relationship of trust with a therapist of this gender, and it might be best to choose a therapist of the sex with which they feel more comfortable. For example if a woman is scared of men it might be best if she chooses a female therapist, or if a man is angry at women he might do better choosing a male therapist. However it may not necessarily be the opposite sex which the client finds difficult. The individual might, after some therapy, switch to a therapist of the more problematic sex to work through any unresolved issues to do with that gender.

Too Old for Therapy?

Undergoing therapy requires that you be open to change and open to new feelings and experiences. This openness to what is new and novel in understanding oneself is not related to chronological age.

Cost

Psychotherapy is expensive, but the rates may vary enormously from practitioner to practitioner. Usually the more experienced a practitioner is the more he or she will charge. But don't think that if you pay more you will automatically get a better practitioner. It is best to hunt around for value for money. Some therapists offer discounts for the low waged.

What the Different Centres are Like

Psychotherapy centres can vary from a therapist working from a room at his or her own house to a bevy of practitioners and associated administrative staff accommodated in a six storey purpose-built block. The usual set-up is a handful of practitioners who have banded together to form a practice, and use a room in one of their houses, or hire rooms in a building in which to practise. It is therefore advisable if you are not familiar with the centre to ring beforehand to make an appointment rather than turn up on the doorstep. Do not be disconcerted if the centre does not turn out to be a prestigious building. The cost of running a prestigious building may well be reflected in the fees that are charged. What is important is the quality and training of the therapist.

TRAINING IN PSYCHOTHERAPY

Why Train in Psychotherapy?

Helping other people can be very rewarding. Training as a psychotherapist means that you will have the opportunity to work on your own growth and use what you have learnt to help others undergoing the same process. Some practical advantages of working as a therapist are that you are your own boss, you can earn a decent living, and, having trained, you may also be able to apply your skills in some other setting, such as education or social work. However, the work of a psychotherapist can also be very stressful. Sometimes it is hard to cut off emotionally from clients outside working hours. It may well not turn out to pay as well as you think it will. You may even end up finding that you cannot get enough clients to support yourself. You may need to work outside of the normal nine to five office hours, and this may well bite into your social life. Are you sure you want to do it?

Which School of Psychotherapy to Train In?

Before you apply for training in any psychotherapy you should have some experience of that psychotherapy yourself. In fact many training organisations make this a requirement. Rather than embark on a training programme for a therapy you have been involved in, it might be best to sample different psychotherapies before training, just to be sure that you are making the right decision.

The Training Programmes

A training programme should include (1) opportunity for the trainee to work on own personal material (2) observation of practitioners at work with their

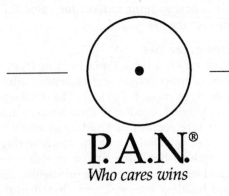

The P.A.N. Academy

The P.A.N. Academy is the first to conduct an all-encompassing, PanLife training programme especially for social and global pioneers.

The PanLife™ course is designed to help you develop yourself and your project to the maximum potential.

The training is rigorous, as each candidate is wholly prepared for leading and completing diverse projects on ever-expanding levels.

For interview, send a personal profile and SAE to:

The P.A.N. Academy,

P.O. Box 929, Wimbledon, London SW19 2AX.

The word PAN means "one complete whole" • The symbol ⊙ represents "one & infinity" clients/groups (3) adequate supervision when a trainee begins to see clients/ groups (4) personal experience of being a participant in a group if training is in group work, or of being a client in one to one sessions if the training is in individual therapy. A training programme in psychotherapy is usually at least three years long. Most are conducted on a part-time basis, utilising evenings and weekends, so that it is possible to hold a full-time job at the same time. It is best to be wary of trainings that are only short in duration. Whilst they may be called a 'training' they will not be able to offer you a full programme which will equip you for this profession. Trainings in counselling are usually shorter than therapy training.

However, bear in mind that these training programmes have not been independently assessed. This means that any graduation certificates or diplomas they award on completion of the training may, in the end, be recognised only by the institute itself. The value of the training rests upon whether or not the therapeutic community as a whole finds the institute to be reputable. If you know someone who is a psychologist, therapist, psychiatrist, social worker, counsellor or psychiatric nurse, they may be able to advise you about the reputation of the training institute.

Accreditation and 1996

At present there is no licencing procedure for counsellors or psychotherapists in this country. Many therapists have invested a lot of money in training, in the knowledge and fear that future legislation may exclude them from practising. Many potential trainees are wondering whether to invest their money in training for similar reasons. There has been a demand lately for controls on the practise of psychotherapy and for some type of licencing procedure to be introduced. What is the story so far, and what advice can be offered?

Rumours of some form of legislation have been around for some twenty years, none has materialised. It's unlikely that the present government, with its anti-regulatory stance will impose it on the profession, (builders for instance are not required to be licensed and there is a more pressing case that they should be controlled than therapists). A more likely scenerio is that the therapists themselves, under an umbrella organisation, will lobby for legislation. At present there are three organisations which have taken it upon themselves to monitor and approve training programmes, and it may be that singly or combined they will succeed in getting a bill passed in parliament. The three organisations are (1) The United Kingdom Council for Psychotherapy (2) The British Association for Counselling (3) The British Psychological Society. The UKCP monitors and approves psychotherapists and psychotherapy training programmes, the BAC monitors and approves counsellors and counselling training programmes and the BPS approves and monitors 'counselling psychologists' and degrees with a large element of counselling.

As a safeguard you are probably best training with an organisation which is registered with one of the three aforementioned bodies, not only because legislation might come, but these organisations monitor trainings and hence see that certain standards are set, and further, because the public may ask you whether you are 'UKCP' or 'BAC' approved.

Can I get Work When Trained?

Few psychotherapists are employed within the NHS, though there are many health service professionals who practice psychotherapy. The majority of psychotherapists work in the private sector and are thus self employed. Working for oneself can be perilous as one is at the mercy of market forces. Should the market be saturated with psychotherapists at any one time then there are less clients to go round and psychotherapists trying to set up a practice will find it especially difficult. Before you embark on a training programme you should be thinking about how you will get your clients when you have finished. Will the training institute supply you with clients? Will they supply you with enough clients? It is important that they will support you when you are initially setting up a practice, as this is a most difficult time. You should discuss these points with them. There are quite a few therapists now barely scratching out a living from the few clients they have on their books. Very few training institutes equip their trainees with knowledge of business practices, something every successful psychotherapist operating in the private sector must know.

Entry Requirements

Most centres do not require that you hold a degree to be accepted for training. Many of the centre organisers believe that a degree is not a good indicator of what makes a good therapist. There is no general agreement as to what makes a good therapist. Different institutes have their own criteria, based on their own idea of what qualities are needed in a therapist. Some prefer you to be medically trained, other centres think this might work against you. Some prefer you to be somewhat crazy (so that you will have some idea of mental suffering), others want the opposite. We indicate wherever possible the basic entry requirements of each training centre.

Cost of Training

Training is expensive and in some cases may run into five figures. There are not only fees for the course, but there may also be hidden costs, such as supervision fees and own required psychotherapy, which may be considerable and far in excess of the training fees. For instance if you are required to undergo personal therapy three times a week then this could amount to £3000 per year alone. We have tried to include all of these costs wherever possible. Do not forget to include VAT at 17.5% in your calculations when determining the total cost of training.

THE PSYCHOTHERAPIES

Art Therapy

People know intuitively that self expression is a way of healing oneself, whether it is through drawing, dancing, sculpting or building. Art therapy is one such means of seeking release and of understanding oneself. Its usefulness is not only for emotional release. An art therapist, through interpreting the meaning of the symbols produced, hopes to come to some understanding of the client, and to enable the client to make fresh discoveries about life and self.

The process of drawing, painting or modelling can help the client to objectify or detach themselves from feelings or problems that may seem otherwise too overwhelming to deal with. The contents of the unconscious can become visible in a very immediate way, and this method often by-passes the censoring process with which we obscure feelings and thoughts which disturb us.

Therapists of different persuasions use the medium of art. Their approach will differ depending on their school of thought. Art therapy is widely used in the humanistic psychologies, where there is more emphasis on interpretation by the client of his or her own productions. They may be interpreted in a Freudian or Jungian way if the art therapist subscribes to either of these frameworks.

Within the health service it is used mainly in psychiatric hospitals and day centres. It is especially effective with severely disturbed people who find it difficult to express their feelings verbally.

It may be used by psychotherapists practising within the NHS, or by specifically trained Art Therapists.

READING
Art As Therapy *by Dalley, T. (eds) RKP £5.95.* Subtitled 'An Introduction to the

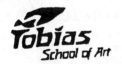

ABT

ASSOCIATION FOR ANALYTIC AND
BODYMIND THERAPY AND TRAINING
Director: Glyn Seaborn-Jones, Ph.D. Consultant in
Psychodynamics
AIM: To help remove the cause of unhappiness. We are
seven caring specialists, each with special skills. We offer:

- Hypnoprimary therapy
- Two year Diploma training
- Individual bodymind sessions
- Couple therapy
- Bodymind Self-expression and
  problem sharing group

Also Training in bodymind therapy, hypnotherapy and Self-
hypnotism and Hypnoprimary therapy. (0181) 883 5418

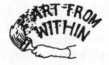

ART AND PSYCHOSYNTHESIS

A fascinating journey through your inner world
of image, sensation and feeling. A chance to
counter that "inner critic" and rediscover
sources of creative vitality. Lack of technical
ability could be an advantage.!

**Contact Avril Wigham, qualified art
therapist and psychosynthesis
counsellor on 0171 354 1603**

ART PSYCHOTHERAPY UNIT

Applications are invited for postgraduates,
commencing in Autumn 1995

- MA ART PSYCHOTHERAPY
- DIPLOMA IN ART PSYCHOTHERAPY
- DIPLOMA IN GROUP PSYCHOTHERAPY

From 1995 the Unit intends to offer an
MA in Group Psychotherapy.
For further details and application forms,
please send an A4 size envelope to:
Laura Barsi, Art Psychotherapy Unit,
Goldsmiths' College, University of
London, 23 St James', New Cross, London
SE14 6AD (0171) 919 7237

VOCATIONAL,
PART-TIME
courses

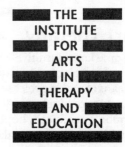

THE
INSTITUTE
FOR
ARTS
IN
THERAPY
AND
EDUCATION

- CERTIFICATE IN THERAPEUTIC AND
EDUCATIONAL APPLICATION OF THE ARTS
(Art, Dance, Drama, Music, Play, Poetry,
Psychodrama, Puppetry)
- DIPLOMA IN INTEGRATIVE ARTS
PSYCHOTHERAPY
- B.Phil.(Ed)/M.Ed. IN THE ARTS IN
EDUCATION AND THERAPY (University of
Exeter validation)
- CERTIFICATE IN THE EDUCATION OF THE
EMOTIONS
- CERTIFICATE IN THE EDUCATION OF THE
IMAGINATION

Application forms and further detail are
available from:
The Administrator
TERPSICHORE
70 CRANWICH ROAD
LONDON N16 5JD
0181 549 9583
NOW BOOKING

Brainwave now publishes a

Free Guide

for the public aimed at guiding them
through maze of therapists, centres,
events and products in London. The
Holistic London Guide is available at
selected venues throughout the
London area.

If you would like to advertise any service,
event or product, or if you would like
information on where to get a free copy
of the **Holistic London Guide,**
call 0181 677 8000

Use of Art as a Therapeutic Technique', this is a collection of articles by practitioners of various backgrounds showing the many ways art therapy is used. It covers work both inside institutions and outside in growth oriented situations. **The Inward Journey; Art as Therapy** by Keyes, M. Open Court 1984, £9.50. Based around Jungian and Gestalt approaches, this is a practical handbook, full of strategies using sculpture, painting, mandalas, music and myth, providing a useful insight into how art therapy can work for the individual.

CENTRES OFFERING ART THERAPY

Art from Within N5, Association of Jungian Analysts, Astro-Psychotherapeutic Practice W3, Bodywise E2, British Association for Social Psychiatry, Cabot Centre NW1, Centre for the Expressive Arts N8, Circle of Creative Arts Therapy N8, Graigian Community NW5, Healing Centre NW5, Highbury Centre N5, Imprint SW19, Institute For Arts In Therapy & Education N16, London Lighthouse W11, Pearl Healing Centre CR7, Person-Centred Art Therapy Centre NW11, Playspace NW1, St James Centre for Health and Healing W1V, Studio 8 BS3, Tobias School of Art RH19, Universitas Associates SM2, Violet Hill Studios NW8, Women and Health NW1.

TRAININGS IN ART THERAPY

Goldsmiths' College Title of Training: Diploma in Art Psychotherapy Duration: Two years full-time, three years part-time (2 days per week). Entry requirements: Degree in Art or Design or other relevant subject. One years work experience in NHS or Social Services or similar. Fees: Full-time £2,200 p.a., part-time £1,100 p.a. Not including personal therapy costs. Comments: Trainees required to be in therapy themselves throughout. The course emphasizes social context of therapy and cross cultural issues.

Tobias School of Art Title of Training: Artistic Therapy Training Duration: 3 years full time Entry requirements: Open to anyone with basic knowledge of anthroposophy, with an interest in colour and the artistic process. All applicants are interviewed. Fees: Refer to organisers Comments: Situated in a rural campus. This exciting course draws students from all five continents and is inspired by the work of Rudolf Steiner. Art therapy 'is a new approach to the whole human being, to be seen distinctly as a synthesising approach rather than analytical or diagnositc'.

Person-Centred Art Therapy Centre Title of Training: Person-centre art therapy course, leading to a certificate from Crawley College. Duration: Part time, three terms with 30 sessions of 2 hours per week, plus one whole day per term. Fees: £400.00 in total. Comments: In this course, learning is experiential and based on self/peer assessment and utilises the approach originated by Carl Rogers on the therapeutic use of art.

Institute For Arts In Therapy & Education *Title of Training:* 1) Certificate in the Therapeutic and Educational Application of the Arts *Duration:* Part time, 1 days per week for 1 year, plus 6 weekends. *Entry requirements:* Qualification in education, counselling or helping profession. Undergoing personal psychotherapy throughout training. *Fees:* Refer to organisers *Comments:* Course content consists of 75% practical and 25% theoretical. Practical element incorporates art, dance/movement, music, drama, puppetry, sandplay, psychodrama (experiential only), basic counselling, group process etc. Theoretical element incorporates Philosophy and Psychology of Art, Human Creativity and Imagination, The Arts Emotional Pain and Pleasure etc. Students may go onto the Diploma in Integrative Arts Therapy on receipt of this Certificate.

Assertion Training

Assertion training, which is sometimes known as assertiveness training, aims to help the client gain specific social skills in expressing feelings, thoughts, wishes and behaviours which allow her or him to stand up for their rights in particular situations. Because the focus is on particular change in behaviours, behaviour therapy has contributed much to this field, although humanistic psychology has also had its part to play.

The procedure of assertion training can be mapped under three headings. Firstly there is skills training, where verbal and non-verbal behaviours are taught and practised. This is mostly done in role play, where a situation requiring assertion is rehearsed and acted out. For example, a situation of returning faulty goods to a store may be enacted. The client is instructed on how to go about getting satisfaction, and the stage is set for the client to act as the irate customer with other members of the group playing the part of shopkeeper, manager and so on. Emphasis is placed on the difference between acting assertively and appearing aggressive. Homework may also be given and clients may be asked to keep a journal. Clients may be asked to assert themselves in situations outside the group and to report back on their endeavours.

Secondly, methods of reducing anxiety are taught. This may take the form of relaxation exercises, or of desensitisation. Desensitisation as used in assertion training is the process of learning to handle one's anxiety by taking the assertive role in easy stages, perhaps initially by fantasising about it and then taking on an easy assertiveness task, so that in this way the anxiety does not overwhelm. To some extent anxiety is reduced when a role play is satisfactorily completed.

Thirdly, values and beliefs about the rights of the individual in society are examined. This is particularly the case for groups within society such as women, children and ethnic minorities. The effects of social conditioning and the part it plays in people's perceptions of their own rights is considered.

In London there is a wealth of adult education classes on this subject. Consult *Floodlight* for a list of venues.

READING

A Woman in Your Own Right *by Dickson, A. Quartet 1982 £4.95.* Assertion is often confused with aggression. In this book the author dispels this myth and presents a full programme for developing a more fulfilling life by standing up for yourself. She deals with assertive approaches to sexuality, the workplace, money, personal criticism and more. Although aimed at women, the ideas are usable by men and she has applied the techniques in mixed sex situations. **Your Perfect Right; A Guide to Assertive Living** *by Alberti, R & Emmons, I. Impact Publications 1970 (revised 1989) £6.95.* The original book on assertion training and still one of the most comprehensive. It's written as a workbook to read and work through, using the exercises and practice situations. These are related to how one can incorporate the ideas into one's life.

CENTRES OFFERING ASSERTION TRAINING

Cabot Centre NW1, Centre for Personal & Professional Development N17, Centre for Stress Management SE3, Changes NW3, Clapham Common Clinic SW4, Hayes Hypnotherapy Centre UB4, Life Directions W1X, Ravenscroft Centre NW11, Redwood Women's Training Association M24, Refuah Shelaymah Natural Health Centre N16, Skills with People N5, Spiral W12, Women and Health NW1, Women Unlimited SW16.

TRAINING IN ASSERTION

Redwood Women's Training Association *Title of Training:* Assertiveness Training *Duration:* Part Time *Entry requirements:* Nothing formal, places allocated by interview. *Fees:* Refer to organisers *Comments:* All trainers hold a Redwood Diploma and have undergone extensive training and reached the high standards. All trainers are women although single sex courses for women or men are run as well as mixed sex courses.

Astrological Counselling

In astrological counselling the positions of the planets are believed to indicate the character and functioning of the individual's psyche.

The astrological counsellor will draw up the client's 'birth chart', which is a symbolic diagram of the positions of the planets at the time of birth. Through the interpretations of the chart the counsellor hopes to provide the client with insights into his or her own psychology. Events in the client's life may also be assessed by comparison between the position of planets at birth and their present position or at a time of major life events. Through interpretation of the symbolism of these, the counsellor aims to determine what psychological forces are at work and may suggest what action, if any, the client should take. The birthchart of the client may also be compared with a birthchart of a partner, to throw light on the workings of the relationship.

Astrological counselling can be distinguished from other forms of astrological birth chart interpretation because it focuses on issues broached by psychotherapy (such as how the 'shadow' of mother affects present relationships with men) rather than on character traits (such as being overgenerous). It attempts to find meaning and reveal patterns in life events rather than attempting to predict future events. The astrological counsellor will not only interpret, but also allow the client's own response to the material to emerge and become part of the counselling relationship.

Much astrological counselling has been influenced by the psychology of C G Jung (see Jungian Analysis in this section), who was interested in astrology, stating that it was 'the summation of all the psychological knowledge of antiquity'.

All but one of the research studies undertaken to confirm a connection between the planets and an individual's psyche have failed. This does not mean that astrological counselling does not work, but suggests the factors for therapeutic change lie outside that explained by its theory - though the same could be said for some other therapies.

CENTRES OFFERING ASTROLOGICAL COUNSELLING

Alternative Therapies Centre N16, Astro-Psychotherapeutic Practice W3, Cabot Centre NW1, Centre for Psychological Astrology NW3, Edgware Centre for Natural Health HA8, Institute of Structural Bodywork WD4, Lotus Healing Centre NW8, Neal's Yard Therapy Rooms WC2H, Silver Birch Centre NW10.

TRAINING IN ASTROLOGICAL COUNSELLING

Faculty of Astrological Studies *Title of Training:* Astrology *Duration:* Certificate: 1 year; Diploma: 2-3 years; Counselling within Astrology Course: 2 years.

Classes available in London. Correspondance course throughout the world. *Entry requirements:* None at Certificate level, Certificate or equivalent at Diploma level. Diploma or equivalent for Counselling within Astrology Course. *Fees:* Refer to organisers *Comments:* The Counselling course requires participants to be in personal therapy during the course. Acknowledged by the Advisory Panel for Astrological Education.

Autogenic Training

Autogenic training is a procedure which has many elements in common with biofeedback, relaxation training, hypnotherapy and some types of stress management, but at the same time adds some new elements of its own. It helps to induce a particular hypnotic state which is somewhere between full consciousness and sleep, and in which one has greater access to the unconscious. In this state repressed material can be accessed and then used for creative problem solving, or positive affirmations can be implanted in the unconscious. Once the technique is learned from the therapist it can be practised on one's own.

At the turn of the century Oscar Vokt found that his patients could hypnotise themselves once they had been initially hypnotised by him, and were then able to use this new-found method to relieve stress and induce relaxation. A few years later H. Schultz developed a series of formulaes to help patients to enter this state quickly.

The particular hypnotic state is induced by passive concentration. The client is asked to concentrate either on the breathing process, on differences between the right and left side of the body or on tensions within the body and to repeat such statements as 'I am calm and quiet'. The client is then given exercises inducing warmth and heaviness in various parts of the body. Once the client has reached a particular stage in the training, which may take many months and which may require practice several times a day, he is then given visual exercises, such as recalling incidents from the past, or recalling the face of someone known in vivid detail. If a pleasant incident is recalled it can be 'anchored' by crossing finger and thumb, so that in the future crossing finger and thumb can induce the pleasant feelings associated with the incident.

Unwanted behaviour patterns are changed when the client is open, in the hypnotic state, to ways of being and acting which are different from his or her normal stereotyped responses. The origins of the feelings associated with the behaviour pattern may also be explored. Self affirmations such as 'I am a loving and valuable person' are often used, especially to finish the session.

Autogenic training would seem best suited to those who have difficulty relaxing and who suffer from physical ailments induced by tension, such as headaches, ulcers, high blood pressure and colitis.

READING
Autogenic Therapy *by Luthe, W & Schultz, J. (Gruer & Stratton 1969)*. These are the original manuals produced by the originators of the method, unfortunately out of print (and extremely expensive when they were available). There are no easily available books on the subject, but is is worth checking out **The Silva Mind Control Method** *by Silva, H. (Grafton £3.99)* as he incorporated much autogenics into his work.

CENTRES OFFERING AUTOGENIC TRAINING
All Hallows House EC3R, Changes NW3, Hampton Holistic Centre for Homoeopath and Autogenic Training TW12, Heath Health Care NW3, Homoeopathic Centre W13, Natural Health Clinic HA3, Neal's Yard Therapy Rooms WC2H, Positive Health Centre.

Bioenergetics

Bioenergetics is a body-oriented psychotherapy. The term was introduced by Alexander Lowen who evolved this particular therapy based on the initial insights and theories of Wilhelm Reich. Lowen, an American, was analysed by Reich, and he developed Reich's work in two ways. He modified and evolved Reich's approach into his own particular school of therapy. He also wrote lucidly on the mind/body relationship, avoiding the psychoanalytic jargon which abounded in Reich's writings, and made it accessible to a larger number of people.

Much of the theory is based on Reich's original formulation that the body, mind and feelings are interrelated. The body reflects the person's character. A particular configuration of tensions within the body reflects the psychological make-up of the person. It is possible to diagnose someone's emotional constraints from looking at the tensions in their body, how they hold themselves and how they move.

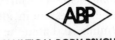

By working on areas of tension within the body it is possible to contact some underlying feelings. For example, if a client grinds his or her teeth at night and complains about difficulty expressing anger, the therapist may massage or knead the jaw muscles and surrounding area which is likely to provoke this underlying rage.

Much of the therapy is taken up by doing exercises which release chronically tense muscles. Lowen was creative in inventing such exercises. Attention is paid to respiration, frozen chests, locked pelvises, tensions in the throat, feeling sick (clients are often asked to vomit rather than suppress this feeling). Lowen paid particular attention to the legs which he saw as important in terms of balance and contact with the ground and introduced the concept of grounding. Unlike Reich who worked from the head down, Lowen believed in working from the feet up. Both stressed the central role of breathing.

Bioenergetics is best done as individual therapy, where the therapist can give the client individual attention. When it is practised in groups it usually follows one of the following formats or a mixture of each: the therapist works with one individual at a time, the rest of the group learn by observing; participants pair up and help each other with a bioenergetic exercise; each participant does an exercise on his or her own with the therapist doing rounds to make sure they are getting the most from the exercise.

Many people find bioenergetics bewildering at first because they are not used to the connections between bodily tensions and feelings.

You may be asked to remove much of your clothing. Clients are often asked to wear swimwear or leotards.

READING

Bioenergetics by Lowen, A. Penguin 1975 £4.95. Lowen developed his approach out of his work with Wilhelm Reich, and this book is his attempt to put his theories into a usable form for the interested lay reader. Bioenergetics is a study of the human personality through the energy processes of the body, and this book is a good place to start. You may also look for his book of exercises **Way to Vibrant Health** Harper & Row, 1977, £7.95. **Lifestreams; An Introduction to Biosynthesis** by Boadella, A. Routledge and Kegan Paul 1987, £6.50. Boadella, an English therapist, also worked with Reich and has developed a different approach to bodywork, bringing insights from Lowen and other Reichian influenced therapists, such as Stanley Keleman, whose books **Your Body Speaks Its Mind** and **Living Your Dying** both by Center Press are also worth reading.

CENTRES OFFERING BIOENERGETICS

Abshot Holistic Centre PO14, Bioenergetic Partnership, Bodyspace, British Association of Analytical Body Psychotherapists. BN2, Centre for Personal & Professional Development N17, Chiron Centre for Holistic Psychotherapy W5,

Healing Centre NW5, Human Potential Resource Group GU2, Open Centre EC1V, Spectrum N4.

TRAINING IN BIOENERGETICS
British Association of Analytical Body Psychotherapists. *Title of Training:* Body Oriented Psychotherapy in an Analytical Setting: Training for Practitioners. *Duration:* Five years; four training blocks of four days per annum plus seminars, group process workshops, supervision and individual therapy. *Entry requirements:* Previous experience in individual and group psychotherapy; current client load; references from therapist and/or supervisor. *Fees:* £1,000 per annum payable in instalments plus residential costs, individual therapy and individual supervision.

Biofeedback

Biofeedback training uses electronic gadgetry to feed back information about specific internal physiological states to the person using it. It is claimed that specific physiological states correspond to certain types of mental activity. For instance, a change in skin resistance from low to high and an increase in finger temperature corresponds to the person feeling more relaxed. These changes are signalled to the user by changes in sound tone or lights from the machine. Thus by using a small electronic box a person is able to monitor his or her particular level of relaxation. Further, from being able to monitor one's level of relaxation, it can be used to learn how to change one's own physiological responses and hence change how one feels.

Learning how to relax is one of the uses of biofeedback training, though it is not confined to this. It can be used to prevent and control stress related diseases, or to monitor changes in states of consciousness. After much research, Maxwell Cade, who pioneered biofeedback training in this country, was able to plot the significance of brainwave activity against states of consciousness. Alpha, beta and theta brainwave patterns correspond respectively to the state of consciousness one enters when meditating, to normal everyday consciousness and to the state of consciousness one enters when hypnotised.

The purpose of feedback training is to accelerate the process of learning how to relax, or how to meditate, or to know when one is in a hypnotic state. It is not intended that people should become hooked on the use of the machine to enter any particular mental state. The idea is that after training one becomes independent of the machine. It thus makes sense to take a course and use a machine rather than purchasing one for oneself, though it is possible to buy one. They range from under £100 for a relaxation meter to over £2500 for the 'Mind Mirror' (a brainwave monitor) developed by Maxwell Cade and Geoffrey Blundell.

READING

˜.ne Awakened Mind *by Cade, M. and Coxhead, N., Element 1987.* Subtitled *Biofeedback and the Development of Higher States of Awareness,* this book combines an outline of the principles of biofeedback regulation with the authors' exploration of its combination with meditation techniques to achieve a 'maximal mind-body awareness' leading to higher levels of consciousness. Another book worth seeking out is **Beyond Biofeedback** *by E and A. Green, Knoll 1989,* two of the originators of biofeedback techniques.

CENTRES OFFERING BIOFEEDBACK

Acumedic Centre NW1, Awakened Mind NW2, Belgravia Beauty SW1X, Biomonitors, Centre for Stress Management SE3, Pearl Healing Centre CR7, Women and Health NW1.

Client-centred therapy

This is sometimes called Rogerian counselling or therapy after its founder Carl Rogers. His theory, method, and research has had a profound effect on the world of counselling.

Client-centered therapy is both an attitude on the part of the therapist which affects the style of intervention, and a particular way of behaving with the client. The therapist is trained to listen in an empathetic way and respond to the client by reflecting back to the client his or her own thoughts and feelings.

Client-centered therapy is phenomenological in its orientation. This means that the way the client perceives the world is seen as valid. The therapist will not impose any interpretations on the client's behaviour or invalidate the way the client sees himself or herself.

Rogers states that if a therapist possesses three qualities then the client will benefit. Firstly if the therapist has the quality of empathy and the client perceives this then the client will find the therapy beneficial. Empathy is the ability to put oneself in the shoes of the client, to understand the way the client sees the world and to be able to see it through his or her eyes. It is not enough that the therapist is empathetic but this quality must be perceived by the client. An essential skill for an empathetic counsellor is listening.

Secondly the therapist must be real. He or she must be genuine. It is essential that the client does not receive 'double messages' such as the therapist saying 'Yes of course I don't mind you talking about homosexuality' whilst crossing legs and going red in the face. This requires that the therapist must have undergone therapy, as being real requires understanding oneself. It means an ability to listen and be open to oneself.

Thirdly if the therapist can show a non-possessive warmth towards the client, prizing the client in a non-threatening way, then the client will feel valued and supported.

Client-centered therapy is practised on a one to one basis and in groups. Most trainings in counselling study the Rogerian approach. See 'Counselling' section.

READING

The Carl Rogers Reader *by Rogers, C. Constable 1990, £8.95.* This is a recent title, a sort of 'portable Carl Rogers'. It covers all the main areas and ideas in his work. For a more in-depth view, read **Client Centred Therapy** £8.95 or his more popular **On Becoming a Person** £7.95 both published by *Constable.*. **Person Centred Counselling in Action** *Mearns, D. & Thorne, B. PBK 1988, £8.95.* Part of an excellent series, this book gives the background theory of Rogers' ideas and gives guidelines as to how these are used in therapy. The major themes, Empathy, Unconditional Positive Regard and others are explored in depth.

CENTRES OFFERING CLIENT-CENTRED THERAPY

Arts Psychology Consultants W14, Cabot Centre NW1, Centre for Personal & Professional Development N17, Clapham Common Clinic SW4, Eigenwelt London NW3, Equilibrium Therapy Centre SW18, Hayes Hypnotherapy Centre UB4, Healing Centre NW5, Heath Health Care NW3, Helios N1, Lifespace Associates SW3, London Focusing Centre SW4, London Lighthouse W11, Metanoia W5, New Cross Natural Therapy Centre, Psychosynthesis and Education Trust SE1, Psychotherapy Centre W1H, Refuah Shelaymah Natural Health Centre N16, Resonance MK14, Skills with People N5, Sunra SW12, Violet Hill Studios NW8, Whole Health Clinic NW3, Women Unlimited SW16.

Co-counselling

Co-counselling does not involve a professionally trained therapist. Two lay people meet to counsel each other for a set time. One assumes the role of client and talks to the other person, whose role is as a counsellor. When the allotted time is up they then switch roles and continue in a similar way.

This is a very simple idea, which was initially formulated by Harvey Jackins under the banner Re-evaluation Counselling. Courses were set up by him for people to receive guidance and training in these techniques. An emphasis was placed on learning how to practice the therapy without hurting or damaging one another.

The client is in charge and determines what he or she wants to talk about, for how long and how much he or she wants the counsellor to intervene. The counsellor's job is mainly to listen and pay attention to the client. Validation of the client's experience by the counsellor is seen as crucial, and this is imparted by the counsellor paying attention to the client and sticking with the material the client produces.

Repeating key phrases the client uses, and contradicting self-deprecatory statements are two of the few intervention techniques the counsellor uses.

Harvey Jackins set up the main organisation in America, and one of the main organisations in this country is Co-counselling International which is a breakaway from the former.

Intending co-counsellors participate in a 40 hour training course, and after the training join a network where they can meet prospective partners, and practise co-counselling. They usually meet once a week with the same partner for two hours, until they both decide to terminate the arrangement. They can then choose another partner.

This method has two advantages. Firstly it is cheap. After paying for the initial training course only a small fee is required to be on the network list. Secondly the two people remain on an equal level, and much of what seems mysterious in therapy intervention becomes obvious when playing the part of the counsellor.

There are many adult education classes in this subject. Refer to *Floodlight*.

READING

Fundamentals of Co-counselling Manual *by Jackins, H. National Island Publications1982, £4.50.* This is the basic 'textbook' of Re-evaluation Co-counselling as used in training workshops. It is an explicit guide to the method.
How To Change Yourself and Your World *by Evison, R. Co-counselling Phoenix1985, £4.95.* An English produced manual by people who broke away from the Jackins' Re-evaluation Counselling Network. Brings in many more (acknowledged) ideas from other therapies for use in the co-counselling situation.

CENTRES OFFERING CO-COUNSELLING

Alternative Medicine Clinic NW15, Cabot Centre NW1, Co-Counselling International NW3, Helios N1, Human Potential Resource Group GU2, London Co-counselling Community N4, London Co-counselling Community N4, National Association of Counsellors, Hypnotherapists and Psychotherapists CB1, Skills with People N5, Women and Health NW1.

TRAINING ON CO-COUNSELLING

London Co-counselling Community *Title of Training:* Co-counselling Training *Duration:* 40 hours (either once a week or over weekends) *Entry requirements:* **None** *Fees:* Refer to organisers *Comments:* Training courses are run periodically. Contact the centre for information. The course is run by Co-counselling International (London). They do a further skills course for those wishing to progress. Once trained on this course all two-way and group counselling sessions are free and you are free as a member to attend various workshops (day or residential) very cheaply. Must be able to give another person full attention without own distress disrupting the session.

Co-Counselling International *Title of Training:* Fundamentals of Co-counselling. *Duration:* 40 hours. *Entry requirements:* None. *Fees:* £Vary, but low to the unwaged and low waged. *Comments:* Some local authorities run courses. Once you have completed the course you can join Co-Counselling International and participate in groups very cheaply, or find partners to work together on personal growth.

Counselling

Counselling is not a particular form of therapy. We have included it in this section because of the many centres which offer counselling. The term covers a wide area of approaches, ranging from simple advice-giving to something which is indistinguishable from psychotherapy.

Counselling can be used to denote consultation and advice giving on a particular subject, as in Careers Guidance Counselling. Someone like a student counsellor may deal with practical problems like the late arrival of a grant cheque, or may give full blown psychotherapy. The Samaritans give telephone counselling to people who are in acute distress, and it is intended not so much to be an in depth exploration of someone's problems, but to provide whatever support, comfort and advice is needed to get someone through a crisis.

Counselling as a therapy is often associated with the client-centred therapy of Carl Rogers (see client-centred therapy section). The reflective technique evolved by Rogers, where the client's statements are not analysed but simply reflected back or rephrased, is often used by counsellors to help the client clarify issues. The focus of the counselling usually revolves around a specific issue or problem, such as sexual behaviour, financial situation or family crisis.

A few practitioners of alternative and complementary medicine also incorporate counselling into their approach. Many of the natural health centres offer counselling as well as body therapies. Because the term is so broad, it is as

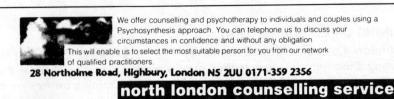

well to ask what kind of approach you will actually be getting, and what kind of training the counsellor has had.

The **British Association for Counselling** situated in Rugby is a large body which may help you with any questions about counselling and provide you with a practitioner in your area.

READING

The Counselling Handbook by Quilliam, S & Grove-Stephenson, I., Thorsons 1989 £5.95. A relatively recent book (Mar '90) aimed at clients and potential clients of counselling. It is a well researched, easy to read guide to most of the different styles/ approaches available and where to find them. One of its strengths is the discussions included with both therapists and clients, which may ease one's apprehensions before taking the plunge. **Handbook of Counselling in Great Britain** by Dryden, W. et al (Eds), Routledge 1989 £15. A large and expensive book produced in conjunction with the British Association for Counselling. Gives an outline of the major situations where counselling is used and the major themes that can be covered. Less expensive if you are considering being counselled is the pamphlet **Counselling and Psychotherapy... Is it for me?** by Hetty Einzig for the British Association for Counselling, a brief 30 page introduction to what to expect.

CENTRES OFFERING COUNSELLING

All Hallows House EC3R, Alternative Medicine Clinic NW15, Arts Psychology Consultants W14, Barnes Physiotherapy Clinic SW13, Bennett & Luck N1, Bodywise E2, Brackenbury Natural Health Centre W6, British Association for Counselling CV21, Cabot Centre NW1, Central School of Counselling and Therapy NW7, Centre for Counselling and Psychotherapy Education W11, Centre for Health and Healing W1V, Centre for Personal & Professional Development N17, Centre for Stress Management SE3, Changes NW3, Chelsea Complementary Natural Health Centre SW10, City Health Centre EC1Y, Clapham Common Clinic SW4, Clissold Park Natural Health Centre N16, College of Psychic Studies SW7, Dancing Dragon Massage N16, Dancing on the Path, Demigod SW10, Edgware Centre for Natural Health HA8, Eigenwelt London NW3, Equilibrium Therapy Centre SW18, Gestalt Centre London EC1Y, Gestalt Therapy in West London W3, Haelan Centre, Hampstead Healing Centre NW3, Hampton Holistic Centre for Homoeopath and Autogenic Training TW12, Hayes Hypnotherapy Centre UB4, Healing Centre NW5, Healing Fields Practice N7, Healing Workshops NW5, Health in Action E8, Heath Health Care NW3, Helios N1, Highbury Centre N5, Hillside Practice, Homoeopathic Centre W13, Homoeopathic Health Clinic HA3, Human Potential Resource Group GU2, Hypnotherapy/Psychotherapy Practice SW6, Identity Counselling Service NW1, Institute for Social Inventions NW2, Isis Counselling and Therapy Service SW17, Islington Green Centre of Alternative Medicine

N1, Kensington Consultation Centre SW8, Life Resources NW7, Life Works NW1, Living Centre SW20, Living Colour NW3, London Focusing Centre SW4, London Lighthouse W11, London Natural Health Clinic W8, Metanoia W5, Mill Hill Health Care NW7, Minster Centre NW2, Moving Line Counselling and Therapy, Natural Death Centre NW2, Natural Healing Centre HA4, Natural Medicine Centre BR2, Natureworks, Neal's Yard Therapy Rooms WC2H, New Cross Natural Therapy Centre , North London Counselling Practice NW11, North London Counselling Service N5, Pearl Healing Centre CR7, Primrose Healing Centre NW1, Psychosynthesis and Education Trust SE1, Ravenscroft Centre NW11, Refuah Shelaymah Natural Health Centre N16, Serpent Institute W12, Shirley Goldstein, Silver Birch Centre NW10, Skills with People N5, Sound Health SE8, South London Natural Health Centre SW4, Southfields Clinic SW18, Spiral W12, St James Centre for Health and Healing W1V, St. Marylebone Healing and Counselling Centre NW1, Sunra SW12, Violet Hill Studios NW8, Welbeck Counselling Service W1N, Westminster Natural Health Centre SW1V, Westminster Pastoral Foundation W8, Whole Health Clinic NW3, Women and Health NW1, Women Unlimited SW16, Wood Street Clinic EN5.

TRAINING IN COUNSELLING

CAER (Centre For Alternative Education And Research) *Title of Training:* Royal Society of Arts Counselling Skills In The Development of Learning *Duration:* 6 months part time. 3 day modules, residential over a month. *Entry requirements:* Some previous experience in working with people and personal counselling. *Fees:* Refer to organisers *Comments:* 'The residential aspect of this course provides for a depth of learning rarely encountered elsewhere'.

Centre for Counselling and Psychotherapy Education *Title of Training:* Diploma in Counselling and Psychotherapy. *Duration:* 4 years part time. *Entry requirements:* Prior therapy of one year, part time counselling training or equivalent. *Fees:* Refer to organisers *Comments:* Training in counselling and psychotherapy from a spiritual perspective. Training is accredited by the British Association for Counselling. Centre for Counselling and Psychotherapy Education is a member of the National Conference of Psychotherapy (UK).

Metanoia *Title of Training:* Diploma in: 1) TA Psychotherapy 2) Gestalt Psychotherapy 3) Integrative Psychotherapy 4) Person-centred Counselling *Duration:* 1-3)Four years. Ten weekends per year, plus clinical placement for 20 days. 4) Eight three day modules per year for two years, with one year of eight diploma preparation days (once a month) ending in an exam. *Entry requirements:* Degree in Psychology or related qualifcation. 2/3 day introductory courses required for 3) and 4) *Fees:* £1200 - £1600 per year *Comments:* Require personal psychotherapy for the duration of the training.

Westminster Pastoral Foundation *Title of Training:* 1) Certificate in Groupwork 2) Diploma in Group Psychotherapy 3) Certificate in Counselling Skills and Attitudes 4) Diploma in Advanced Psychodynamic Counselling *Duration:* 1) 2 years part time 2) 2 and a half years part time (minimum) 3) 2 years of 30 weeks, 3 hours per week 4) Range from 2 years full time to 4 years day release. *Entry requirements:* 1) Personal suitability 2) Completion of 1) or equivalent 3) Personal suitability 4) Basic training in counselling skills; experience of counselling; aged 25-60; personal suitability. *Fees:* Refer to organisers *Comments:* This broad ranging curriculum offers the prospective student, and experienced counsellor much to choose from. For full details contact the Training Department. Some courses are BAC accredited, and these trainings are recognised preparation for many other psychotherapy trainings. Also available are a variety of day and weekend seminars and workshops in counselling and specialist topics. Diploma in Supervision for experienced, trained psychodynamic counsellors or psychotherapists who are currently providing supervision.

School of Psychotherapy and Counselling *Title of Training:* Certificate in Fundamentals of Counselling. *Duration:* One year part time (3x10 week terms). *Entry requirements:* No formal qualifications necessary, but applicants will be expected to demonstrate a) high level motivation, b) given considerable of thought to counselling and issues relating to it, c) organisational ability and communicate ideas clearly, d) ability to study independently. *Fees:* Refer to organisers *Comments:* Course forms a sound basis for progress onto a more advanced level of counselling course. Provides a thorough grounding in fundamental skills of counselling, underpinned with a broad yet reasonably substantial foundation course in the various theoretical approaches to counselling. Students also have supervised practice sessions as well as the experience of a weekly personal development group.

Spectrum *Title of Training:* Foundation course in counselling skills. *Duration:* Foundation course is half a day per week for 1 year, plus 2 three-day groups. *Fees:* Refer to organisers

Equilibrium Therapy Centre *Title of Training:* Basic Counselling-Skills and Theory. *Duration:* Total 60 hours part-time over 5 months. *Entry requirements:* Open to anyone interested or who wishes to further present skills. No previous experience necessary. *Fees:* £500 each course (No VAT) *Comments:* Courses accredited by Associated Examining Board (A.E.B.) & can lead to a Diploma. The courses are run at their venue in Greenwich.

Healing Centre *Title of Training:* Training in Counselling.

Couple Therapy

Couple therapy is applicable to all couples, married or unmarried, homosexual or heterosexual, however long the partners have been together.

The couple are seen together so that both sides of any relationship conflict can be appreciated. However if it is impossible for both partners to be present, either because one partner does not want to be involved in therapy, or because the partner seeking therapy does not feel they can discuss their feelings with their partner at first, then one partner can go along independently. The therapist will then discuss with the client whether he or she wants to include the other partner at any stage.

Different areas will be covered in the course of therapy depending on what the problems are. Often conflict may be caused because the partners do not know how to communicate with each other, and misunderstandings may have escalated. The therapist can help the couple to develop ways of expressing their feelings without blaming each other. Sometimes there may be more specific problems, such as an unsatisfactory sex life, and in this case if the difficulties are not just due to a more general difficulty in communicating, these can be dealt with (see Sex Therapy section). Sometimes there may be a need for individual work if one or both partners have personal issues which need to be explored. Sometimes the issues may involve quite a practical solution, for instance if one partner needs to find a means of self-expression outside the relationship such as study or work, the therapy can be used to explore the possibilities.

In some cases it may be that the couple discover that they do not want to stay together. The therapist can then help them to negotiate a separation which is satisfactory in emotional terms. If there are children involved, the therapist may suggest that they become included in the sessions so that they can participate in this process. RELATE (formerly Marriage Guidance) gives free counselling to couples.

READING

Couples in Counselling by Gough, T. (Dartman, Longman & Todd 1989) £6.95. Most therapy approaches can be, and are used when working with couples. What is useful about this book is its down to earth appraisal of the issues that may be causing problems in a relationship, to either or both partners, and the techniques that may be applied to help resolve such difficulties.

CENTRES OFFERING COUPLE THERAPY

Alternative Medicine Clinic NW15, Association for Analystic and Bodymind Therapy and Training N10, Association for Marriage Enrichment W8, Association of Independant Psychotherapists N6, Astro-Psychotherapeutic Practice W3, Brackenbury Natural Health Centre W6, Cabot Centre NW1, Centre for Counselling and Psychotherapy Education W11, Centre for Personal & Professional Development N17, Chiron Centre for Holistic Psychotherapy W5, Clapham Common Clinic SW4, Ealing Psychotherapy Centre W3, Equilibrium

Therapy Centre SW18, Gestalt Therapy in West London W3, Hampstead Healing Centre NW3, Healing Centre NW5, Hillside Practice, Holistic Yoga Centre MK19, Identity Counselling Service NW1, Institute of Group Analysis NW3, Kensington Consultation Centre SW8, Living Colour NW3, London Institute for the Study of Human Sexuality SW5, London Lighthouse W11, Metanoia W5, Minster Centre NW2, North London Centre for Group Therapy N14, North London Counselling Practice NW11, Pearl Healing Centre CR7, Pellin Centre SW8, Ravenscroft Centre NW11, Skills with People N5, Sound Health SE8, Spectrum N4, Sunra SW12, Violet Hill Studios NW8, Women Unlimited SW16.

Dance Therapy

Dance therapy aims to release the natural flow of bodily expression which is unique to each individual. Movement is a way of communicating from direct physical experience which children use quite naturally. In growing up, we are often taught to restrict this joyful and expressive movement. Dance therapy concentrates on spontaneous, individual movements which proceed from the dancer's experience rather than on learning formal dance patterns.

Tribal societies have long used dance as a way of expressing feelings, of accomplishing the transition to other states of consciousness (for instance the trance state), and for connecting to their community and environment in a way which has meaning, often through the mythic significance of the dance. In Europe over the centuries since medieval times, dance has become more and more formalised, until the appearance of Isadora Duncan at the turn of the century with her free form, emotive dancing which shocked many of her straight-laced contemporaries.

Rudolph Laban, a German psychotherapist was the first to incorporate dance into his treatment of patients between the wars. Marian Chace, an American dance therapist, developed another form of dance therapy when she was asked to work with patients in a mental hospital, after psychiatrists there had been impressed by the improvements in patients who attended her dance classes privately.

Dance therapists differ widely in their approach. Usually therapy takes place in a group. First the participants are asked to do warming up exercises, and some material to be developed in the course of the class may emerge at this stage. Music may be played, but this is not necessarily the case. The therapist may reflect the dancer by mirroring his or her movements, drawing attention to particular gestures, or inviting the dancer to find words for the emerging feelings or connect more fully to them. Interaction between the group as a whole may also be encouraged. In some dance therapy classes the emphasis may be less on 'therapy' and more on 'creativity' where the dancers are encouraged to find their own style of dance to express their uniqueness.

Dance therapy can also be used in a Jungian framework. Here movement functions as a bridge to the unconscious mind. The movements, once developed and repeated, may come to embody symbols or mythological themes, which will then be discussed by therapist and client.

Dance therapy can be used in a wide variety of situations. It is useful for people who are unable to speak about their feelings, such as autistic children or psychotics. Those who suffer from physical symptoms related to stress or other emotional difficulties can also benefit, as well as those who are suffering from immobilising organic complaints such as Parkinson's disease or a stroke. It is also useful for people who tend to intellectualise too much.

READING

The Mastery of Movement *by Laban, R. Northcote House 1980, £8.95.* This is Laban's classic book on human movement, as we follow his methods of exploring the inner motivation of movement and its expression in emotion, intellect and values/meanings. Another book worth looking at is **Personality Assessment Through Movement** *by North, M. Northcote Press 1989.*

Centres offering Dance Therapy

Chantraine School of Dance NW6, Dancing on the Path SE22, Open Dance EC1V

Training in Dance Therapy

Laban Centre *Title of Training:* Postgraduate Studies in Dance Movement Therapy either as an MA or one year Diploma. *Duration:* 2 years full time or 3 years part time or 4 years part time + one additional term for each course for dissertation. *Entry requirements:* Minimum 25 years old (some exceptions to this). Honours degree in Dance or, degree in another area with experience in dance

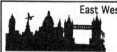

and/or Laban Centre Certificate in Special Education. Where English is not first language, the Cambridge Test of Proficiency in English. Refer to organisers for details of 'special entry' requirements. *Fees:* Refer to organisers *Comments:* Professional training develops the skills of observing, assessing significance of movement in self-expression and interaction. Students will undertake a research project in 2nd year, culminating in their dissertation. Laban's Summer School offers introductory courses in dance movement therapy. Other courses offered for practicing professionals in field of dance movement and psychology.

Hertfordshire College of Art and Design *Title of Training:* Postgraduate Diploma in Dance Movement Therapy (CNAA) *Duration:* 1 year full time modular course allowing for part time study over extended periods. *Entry requirements:* Relevant first degree, Dance, Movement Studies, etc. or equivalent professional qualification, Occupational Therapy, Psychotherapy, CQSW etc. Minimum 6 months full time prior relevant clinical experience. *Fees:* Refer to organisers *Comments:* One third of course Clinical Placements within hospitals, health centres, etc. Modular part time students in relevant clinical employment may be allowed to complete the placement module in their workplace. The College is a member of ECARTE an EC Arts Therapies Education Consortium giving them a European profile. The Course is part of an Arts Therapies Programme with shared modules with Postgraduate Diplomas and Masters in Art Therapy and in Dramatherapy.

Roehampton Institute of Higher Education *Title of Training:* Diploma in Dance Movement Therapy *Duration:* Two years part time *Entry requirements:* Programme open to graduates and others who can show evidence of a strong commitment to Dance Movement Therapy. *Fees:* Refer to organisers *Comments:* Programme aims to help students develop skills needed for the application of the principles and practice of dance movement therapy. Graduates of the Diploma programme should be able to facilitate DMT activities in clinical, educational and community settings. Also offer courses in Counselling in Formal and Informal settings; Diploma in Music Therapy and a Diploma in Counselling and Supervision.

Kando Studios *Title of Training:* Kando Technique Teacher Training. Duration: 36 modules of one and a half hours, plus homework. Can be done faster on a full time basis. *Entry requirements:* Available on enquiry *Fees:* £765 for training, £250 per annum license fee.

Open Dance *Title of Training:* Foundation course in Dance Therapy.

Encounter

Social convention dictates that we restrain ourselves. There are many times when we have to suppress certain feelings for social reasons, but we are also imprisoned by our own neurotic constraints. Whether the suppression is due to real external constraints or whether it is due to a neurotic withholding is something an encounter group tries to find out.

Will Schutz pioneered the 'open encounter', the version of the encounter group which was the most successful in this country, and which grew at a phenomenal rate in the late sixties and reached the height of its popularity in the early seventies.

Schutz would follow the energy in the group at any one moment. For instance if a member was tapping his foot he would ask him to exaggerate it and get in touch with what this impulse was about. If the person were to say he felt impatient with someone in the group and would like to kick him into action, Schutz would have him kick a cushion and get more in touch with this feeling and to express this pent up emotion. Where this would lead to would depend on many factors. It might be that many of the group also have this feeling towards the same person, but held back from saying so for one reason or another. It might be that the impulse was a frustration at his own feeling of getting nowhere, which would be further therapeutic grist for the mill. As more physical movement is required than in most other therapy groups, participants sit on cushions rather than on chairs so that they are not in any way obstructed.

Encounter groups give people permission to cut through social convention and politeness and openly encourage the expression of feeling and honesty. Rather than talking about feelings the encounter group encourages their physical expression. If you were to say you would like to hug a particular person in the group, you might be asked to go ahead and do it.

There are two other types of encounter groups, neither of which are as common as the 'open encounter'. Carl Rogers pioneered a form of encounter where he encouraged a more honest engagement between members and tried to induce an atmosphere of empathy, regard for the other members and genuineness in relating. It is called 'basic encounter'. Chuck Dederick pioneered the 'Synanon encounter' specifically for drug abusers. Members were asked to focus on one person and verbally attack him or her. Members would take it in turn to be target. The aim of this 'shock therapy' was to wake them up from an habitual lifestyle.

Encounter is practised in groups. Often the setting is residential. It may be a two, three or five day workshop. They have been known to go on for a month. If it is described as a 'marathon encounter', this means you are likely to get little sleep for the duration of the workshop. In this country the 'marathon encounter' usually lasts between twenty four and forty eight hours.

READING

Joy. . . 20 Years Later by Schutz, W. *Ten Speed Press, 1989, £7.95.* This is a revised edition of Schutz's original text on the principles and practice of his ideas. Although not so specific to the actual workings of an encounter group as his other book **Elements of Encounter** (long out of print, and never widely available in the UK), it nevertheless gives a good grounding in the encounter approach and what to expect. **Theories and Practise of Group Psychotherapy** by Yalom, I. Harper and Row, 1987, hardback £17.95. The chapters on Encounter and T-Groups (the origins of Encounter) in this book are excellent introductions to the method. The whole book is recommended to anyone who wants to look at the many and various 'human potential' approaches to group work.

CENTRES OFFERING ENCOUNTER

Centre for Personal & Professional Development N17, Healing Centre NW5, Human Potential Resource Group GU2, Open Centre EC1V, Resonance MK14, Spectrum N4.

Existential Psychotherapy

Existential psychotherapy can be considered more an approach than a therapy in the normal sense of the term, as it is against techniques and weak on a classification of intervention strategies on the part of the therapist. Indeed, the training of an existential therapist is quite different from that followed by trainees in many other psychotherapies. The trainee existential psychotherapist is expected to become steeped not only in psychological theory, but in the philosophy of existentialism. Most of all, she is encouraged in taking a particular attitude towards herself, towards others and towards life itself. To this end the trainee undergoes a form of apprenticeship with a supervisor who acts as a guide. The training therefore bears more resemblance to the guru/student relationship found in oriental religions than it does to western psychotherapy.

To understand existential psychotherapy it is necessary to know something about its philosophical underpinning. The work of the existentialists such as Heidegger, Boss, Sartre, Kierkegaard, Nietzsche and Husserl provided the philosophical movement upon which existential psychotherapy is based. Existentialism focuses on the 'givens of existence', such as being, death, alienation, authenticity, suffering, responsibility in choosing and meaning. These themes were also echoed by clients in psychotherapy and soon the the philosophy of existentialism filtered through into the psychotherapeutic arena. Existential psychotherapy grew to occupy a place of its own, with its own style of expression.

In this country, the psychiatrist Ronald Laing became famous in the 1960s for his existentialist approach in working with schizophrenics. He placed importance on understanding the subjective world of the client and attacked the swiftness of psychiatry in objectively labelling the so-called psychotic. He saw madness as an authentic experience which is in itself a healing process, through which one could journey and emerge on the other side. Laing set up the Philadelphia Association in London from which the break-away organisation, the Arbours Association was formed. This organisation turned private houses into therapeutic communities where the previously labelled schizophrenics were allowed to express their madness.

READING

Existential Counselling in Practice *by Van Deurzen-Smith, E., Sage 1988.* The first practical book written in the UK on this form of therapy. Quite readable for a book on a subject which many find intellectually difficult. She weaves the philosophy, and practice of the approach into an interesting framework. A heavier tome is *Yalom's Existential Psychotherapy, Harper and Rowe £17.95,* but for anyone interested in the flavour of the existential approach, try reading any of R.D. Laing's works, all published by Penguin.

CENTRES OFFERING EXISTENTIAL PSYCHOTHERAPY

Cabot Centre NW1, Clapham Common Clinic SW4, Eigenwelt London NW3, Heath Health Care NW3.

TRAININGS IN EXISTENTIAL ANALYSIS PSYCHOTHERAPY

Society for Existential Analysis *Fees:* Refer to organisers *Comments:* Plans for a one-year course in existential psychotherapy. Are also associated with a post qualifying diploma in existential psychotherapy (a two year training for those in this field). When phoning you will get through to Regent's College.

Family Therapy

There are a number of different schools of family therapy, but most follow a systems theory approach whilst drawing on different therapeutic models such as psychoanalytic psychotherapy, gestalt, transactional analysis, client-centred therapy, behavioural methods and psychodrama for some of their intervention tactics.

The focus is not on the individual family member. If any one individual suffers symptoms within the family, such as a child suffering from 'school phobia', this is considered a symptom of the family, and the family must be treated as a whole. It may be that the child will not go to school because of the distant relationship that has developed between the parents, and consequently the child feels a need to support the mother.

The aim is to discover how the behaviour of members within the family perpetuates the symptom, and to change the relationship between the members so that the symptom disappears. Emphasis is placed not on why the family is behaving the way it is, but on what present behaviour is causing the symptom.

Therapy may be carried out with one or two therapists working with the family. It is usually brief because of the difficulty often involved in bringing the whole family together at one time. Sessions are usually at least six in number.

Usually the family will go the therapist/s place of work, but sometimes the therapist/s will go to the family's home to undertake therapy or will make at least one attempt to go to the home of the family to see how they behave in their surroundings.

Family therapy is often suggested to families where one of the children has a problem, for instance an unruly teenager or a young child experiencing difficulties at school.

READING

Peoplemaking *by Satir, V. Science & Behaviour 1972, £6.95.* This was the first book to bring the benefits of the insights gained from family therapy to the general public. It's an easy read that brings many of the problems of family life into sharp focus, and has been generally hailed for its healing potential. Another similar title that is worth looking at is **Families and How to Survive Them** *by Cleese, J. & Skynner,* R., the latter being one of the principal developers of Family Therapy in the UK. **Family Therapy in Britain** *by Street, E & Dryden, W. Open University Press 1988, £12.50.* Another manual containing articles on the major approaches to Family Therapy in use in the UK, by many of the leading practitioners in their fields.

CENTRES OFFERING FAMILY THERAPY

Alternative Medicine Clinic NW15, British Association for Social Psychiatry, British Association of Psychotherapists NW2, Cabot Centre NW1, Centre for Personal & Professional Development N17, Clapham Common Clinic SW4, Healing Centre NW5, Heath Health Care NW3, Institute of Family Therapy W1M, Institute of Group Analysis NW3, Kensington Consultation Centre SW8, North London Centre for Group Therapy N14, Pearl Healing Centre CR7, Sunra SW12, Tavistock Clinic NW3, Violet Hill Studios NW8, Westminster Pastoral Foundation W8, Women and Health NW1.

TRAINING IN FAMILY THERAPY

Institute of Family Therapy *Title of Training:* 1) Introductory course in Family and Marital Therapy. 2) Part I, Training in Family Therapy 3) M. Sc in Family Therapy 4) Advanced Clinical Training in Family Therapy. 5) Introductory Course in Alcohol and Substance Abuse and the Family. *Duration:* 1) One year part-time 2) One year part-time 3) Two years part-time 4) Two years part-time 5) Twenty weeks part-time *Entry requirements:* See training prospectus available from the Training Dept at above address. *Fees:* Refer to organisers

Tavistock Clinic *Title of Training:* Programme of Training in Child and Family and Adolescent Psychiatry *Duration:* Four years full time. *Fees:* Refer to organisers *Comments:* Trainees are required to have personal psychotherapy at least three times a week at their own expense.

Maudsley Hospital Refer to organisers

Feminist Therapy

Feminist therapy is an attitudinal approach to the practice of therapy. It was founded by women who observed sexism and patriarchal values on the part of therapist and client which became reinforced within the therapy. Women found they were being undermined in their determination to grow when confronted with a sexist male therapist. They also found that some of the assumptions of traditional psychotherapy were based on social values which subtly affected the therapeutic encounter, whether the therapist was male or female.

Feminist therapy began at a grass roots level, and through consciousness raising groups, rape crisis work and work with battered women there has emerged a therapy with a clear philosophy.

Three common issues emerge in the therapy of women: anger, self-nurturance and autonomy or power. Women tend to turn their anger inwards rather than outwards. In feminist therapy the client is helped to be more expressive and to direct the anger to where it belongs. Women tend to have devoted themselves to others at the expense of themselves, and a consequence of this can be depression. In feminist therapy they are asked to take care of their own needs too. To gain autonomy women are asked to expand the options they allow themselves and are helped to confront the role restrictions society places on them, at home and at work.

Susie Orbach and Luise Eichenbaum founded the Women's Therapy Centre in London.

While feminist therapy is not exclusive to women, men have not opted for it. Virtually all the clients are women, and all of the therapists are. However, some male therapists have begun to explore the theme of men's socialisation and are reaching for new definitions of masculinity.

A feminist therapist may incorporate gestalt, client-centred therapy or T.A. into the therapy, but the essential ingredient is the emphasis that is placed on the individual worth of the client, and on her socialisation. Issues frequently dealt with are body image, eating problems, self-care and sexuality.

READING

What Do Women Want by *Eichenbaum, L. & Orbach, S. Fontana 1983, £3.50.* The authors are pioneers of the Feminist Therapy approach, and are co-founders of the Women's Therapy Centre. This book explores the many issues that women have to come to terms with to fulful their own emotional needs. A book for men as well. **Feminist Counselling in Action** by *Chaplin, J. Sage 1988,*

41

£8.95. Written for counsellors and therapists to understand a feminist approach, it is also useful for people who may be drawn to the approach. Further readings can be found in **In Our Experience; Workshops at the Women's Therapy Centre** *by Krzowski, S. & Land, P. (Eds) Womens Press £6.95.*

CENTRES OFFERING FEMINIST THERAPY

Astro-Psychotherapeutic Practice W3, Centre for Personal & Professional Development N17, Clapham Common Clinic SW4, Communication and Counselling Foundation SY25, Gestalt Studio NW5, Hayes Hypnotherapy Centre UB4, Hidden Strengths TW2, Human Potential Resource Group GU2, IBISS TW7, London Institute for the Study of Human Sexuality SW5, London Institute for the Study of Human Sexuality SW5, New Cross Natural Therapy Centre , Pellin Centre SW8, Psychotherapy Workshops for Women, Redwood Women's Training Association M24, Serpent Institute W12, Spectrum N4, Sunra SW12, Women Unlimited SW16, Women's Therapy Centre N7.

Gestalt Therapy

Fritz Perls was a Freudian trained psychoanalyst who became disenchanted with the practice of psychoanalysis. He was analysed by Reich for whom he expresses much affection and by whom gestalt thinking was heavily influenced. He set up the South African Institute of Psychoanalysis and then later went to America where, with his wife Laura Perls, he evolved gestalt therapy. In the sixties he introduced gestalt therapy to Esalen, California, the first growth centre. Rather than paying attention to why clients behaved the way they did as was common in psychoanalysis, he paid attention to what they did and how they behaved. He helped them become more aware of what their behaviour meant to them and what it signified to others. Thus gestalt therapy pays attention to the non-verbal more than the verbal. This does not mean that people talk less in gestalt groups, but that the focus of concern of the therapist is much more on the bodily messages than in more orthodox psychotherapies.

Another theme that Perls stressed was responsibility. He insisted clients take responsibility for themselves. If someone would say 'It feels good when you say that' he would ask them to rephrase it as 'I feel good when you say that', thus enabling them to become more in touch with their own feelings.

Talking to the 'empty chair' is the hallmark of gestalt therapy. If for instance you had not expressed your feelings to someone close to you, such as your mother, you may be asked to imagine her sitting in an empty chair, and to say the things you wished you had said to her. You may be then asked to switch chairs and to sit in the chair you imagined her sitting in, and pretend to be her responding to you. Thus a dialogue might ensue between yourself and what you imagine your mother would say to you. This unrehearsed dramatisation of how you see your relationship with your mother is likely to provide the group members and the therapist with a detailed and revealing story. The use of the 'empty chair' is not limited to being filled with persons. Parts of oneself can be placed there as well. For example, if you are the type of person who constantly criticises yourself, you may be asked to put the critical side of yourself in the empty chair and to have a dialogue with that side of yourself. Such a public display of the contents of one's own psyche engenders strong emotional bonds between the group members and can produce an intense emotional atmosphere.

People who could most benefit from this type of therapy are those who feel they have difficulty expressing their feelings, those who feel stuck, those who feel cut off from others and those who would like feedback on how people see them.

READING

Gestalt Therapy *by Perls, F, Goodman, P and Hefferline, R. Souvenir Press, 1974, £7.95.* The original work describing the theory of Gestalt therapy. Good to explore its basis thoroughly, but many people find it a difficult 'read'. Probably more accessible is his later book **The Gestalt Approach & Eye-Witness to Therapy** *(S & B, £8.95).* This was originally published as two books, the first being a last revision of his theoretical ideas, the second , transcripts of some of his films giving an insight into Perls 'live'. **The Red Book of Gestalt by** *Houston G. Rochester Foundation 1982 £3.50.* A delightful little book, self published and illustrated by line drawings, giving a simple, but not simplistic, introduction to how Gestalt Therapy works, both in group and individual settings.

CENTRES OFFERING GESTALT THERAPY

Alternative Medicine Clinic NW15, Arcadia Creative Therapy Centre SE6, Association for Analystic and Bodymind Therapy and Training N10, Centre for

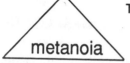

Personal & Professional Development N17, Chiron Centre for Holistic Psychotherapy W5, Gestalt Centre London EC1Y, Gestalt Consortium (The), Gestalt Studio NW5, Gestalt Therapy & Contribution Training SE13, Gestalt Therapy in West London W3, Hillside Practice, Isis Counselling and Therapy Service SW17, Jeyrani Health Centre E18, Lifespace Associates SW3, Metanoia W5, New Cross Natural Therapy Centre , Open Centre EC1V, Pellin Centre SW8, Pellin Training Courses SW8, Re-Vision NW2, Resonance MK14, Skills with People N5, Spectrum N4, Sunra SW12.

TRAININGS IN GESTALT THERAPY

Pellin Centre *Title of Training:* Pellin Integrative Counselling and Psychotherapy Training Course. *Duration:* 1-5 years part time training in London and residential training in Southern Italy. *Entry requirements:* Appropriate professional and life experience working with people. Nourishing personal characteristics. Discipline and integrity. Academic background in helping professions useful but not essential. *Fees:* Refer to organisers *Comments:* Pellin training is an integration os psychodynamic, behavioural and humanistic approaches to counselling and psychotherapy. Particular emphasis on Gestalt and unique element of Pellin theory and philosophy. Programmes are small with emphasis on personal attention, intensity and quality

Pellin Training Courses *Title of Training:* Gestalt Training Programme in Counselling and Psychotherapy. *Duration:* Three years part time. *Entry requirements:* Should be in the helping professions or wishing to find work with people. *Fees:* Refer to organisers

Gestalt Studio *Title of Training:* Gestalt Studio Training *Duration:* Three years plus two years supervision. *Fees:* Refer to organisers

Metanoia *Title of Training:* Gestalt Psychotherapy Diploma Training *Duration:* Three years. Modular basis of between one to eight five day workshops per year.

Entry requirements: Completion of introduction course on the fundementals of Gestalt (held three times a year) or its equivelent. Require degree in psychology and/or equivalent. *Fees:* £160 per workshop. *Comments:* Require personal psychotherapy for the duration of the training. Some burseries available.

Gestalt Centre London *Title of Training:* (1) Diploma in Counselling (2) Gestalt Centre Diploma (Psychotherapy) *Duration:* 1) Two years part-time. One evening weekly plus two weekends per term. 2) Five years part-time, as above. Each year can be taken as a separate module. *Entry requirements:* Experience of gestalt necessary. Degree/health care qualification or equivalent work and life experience. Must be able to demonstrate academic ability. *Fees:* Course fees are approx: 1) £960 per year; 2) £1500 per year; plus individual therapy fees *Comments:* The Psychotherapy training extends over five years to provide enough time for students to reach the level of emotional clarity and maturity required. Although the hours are part-time the course needs full-time committment.

Group-oriented Therapy

By group-oriented therapy we mean therapy where the group process is deemed to be important and worthy of analysis, and where the dynamics of the group compose part of the therapy, so that it becomes therapy *of* the group and *by* the group. Although no firm line can be drawn here, because many psychotherapies would argue that the dynamics of the group are important, the crucial thing is that the dynamics of the group take up a central role in the therapy and that historically the origins of the therapy evolved around group processes. In London the three major schools have different theoretical origins.

The 'group analytic' approach was developed by S.H. Foulkes. It was developed not only as a way of applying psychoanalytic knowledge to group practice, but takes into account factors specific to groups. In this type of group the therapist, or 'conductor' as they prefer to be called, may remain in the background much of the time, but can at times be much more active. The free floating group discussion is to group analytic therapy what free association is to psychoanalysis. Eight people (four men and four women) is seen as the optimum number for this type of group. Therapy is usually twice a week, one and half hours for each session.

The Tavistock approach to group work was developed by W. Bion. Bion (a Kleinian analyst) saw much of what went on in groups as issues over leadership. The therapist or 'consultant' usually stays in the background and offers interpretations about what is going on in the group. Groups can go on intensively for a week and are affectionately known as 'Tavi' groups.

The humanistic approach offers 'T-groups', sometimes referred to as sensitivity training groups. These groups meet residentially, often for a week. The focus is on the 'here and now' activity of the group and feedback and self-expression are a prime concern. The leader reflects, for instance, on how the group conducts itself, and the leader will focus not on 'what' decisions the group took but 'how' it went about deciding and which roles people took up in this decision making.

All of the above approaches are useful in learning both about how groups function and about your contribution to the group process. For those who feel they would like to know more about groups or for those who work in groups and need to understand more of group processes, all can be recommended, but remember that the style of each of the above schools are quite different from each other.

READING

Group Therapy in Britain by *Aveline, M. & Dryden, W. (Eds). Open University Press 1988, £12.50* . A manual, giving theoretical background and practical usage of the major approaches to group therapy. Another book worth looking at is by Yalom, reviewed in the 'Encounter' section. **Once Upon A Group** by *Kindred, M. Self published 1987, £3.00* A light-hearted look at what can be quite a heavy subject. The author draws out, in basic lay language, the themes and issues that can be dealt with in any of the group therapies practised today.

CENTRES OFFERING GROUP-ORIENTED PSYCHOTHERAPY

Association for Analystic and Bodymind Therapy and Training N10, Association for Group and Individual Psychotherapy N19, Centre for Personal & Professional Development N17, Gestalt Consortium (The), Group Relations Training Association TS14, Healing Centre NW5, Human Potential Resource Group GU2, Institute of Group Analysis NW3, London Association of Primal Psychotherapists NW5, London Lighthouse W11, Minster Centre NW2, New Cross Natural Therapy Centre, North London Centre for Group Therapy N14, Open Centre EC1V, Pearl Healing Centre CR7, Playspace NW1, Skills with People N5, Sound Health SE8, Tavistock Clinic NW3, Violet Hill Studios NW8, Will (Workshop Institute for Living Learning) .

TRAININGS IN GROUP-ORIENTED PSYCHOTHERAPY

Human Potential Resource Group *Title of Training:* Facilitator Styles Course *Duration:* Two years part-time. Approx 60 days in each year including regular meetings, one day per week & 3 weekend workshops each term, plus 2 x 5 day workshops per year. *Entry requirements:* For those in the teaching/training professions. The course is a balance of theoretical with experiential and practical work. *Fees:* Refer to organisers

Institute of Group Analysis *Title of Training:* 1) Introductory General Course 2) Qualifying Course in Group Analysis *Duration:* 1) Thursday afternoons 3

terms 2) One afternoon, one evening approximately 4 years. *Entry requirements:* 1) Open. 2) IGA approved Introductory General Course. *Fees:* Refer to organisers *Comments:* Courses held in London and Manchester. Also hold workshops, including The Art of Assessment, Empathy - the heart of the pscyhotherapeutic process, Introductory weekend in Group Analysis, Working with dreams. Special events conferences. One day seminars. Fees for these vary according to status, i.e., attendee of IGA Introductory Course.

Tavistock Clinic *Title of Training:* For training in group work apply to the institute. *Fees:* Refer to organisers

Group Oriented Therapy Westminster Pastoral Foundation *Fees:* Refer to organisers

Goldsmiths' College *Title of Training:* Diploma in Group Psychotherapy. *Duration:* Three years part-time (eves and some day attendance). *Entry requirements:* Degree or professional qualification. Fees: £1,100 p.a. part-time. *Comments:* The course emphasizes social context and cross cultural issues in group psychotherapy and public sector work. Graduates could gain employment in the NHS, GP practices, as staff consultants, as well as running groups in private practice.

Association for Group and Individual Psychotherapy *Title of Training:* Psychotherapy Training *Duration:* Three years part-time. Seminars and analytic groups twice weekly. Weekly evening and weekend day groups. Personal therapy, twice weekly required. *Entry requirements:* Applicants should have at least one year's personal psychotherapy with an approved psychotherapist before starting the course. *Fees:* Refer to organisers

Hypnotherapy

There are as many types of hypnotherapy as there are practitioners. They may have different aims, but they do share one characteristic. All begin with the therapist guiding the client into an hypnotic state. The client is simply required to respond positively to the direction of the therapist. Once in this state, what happens next will depend on the aims of the therapy and the background and training of the therapist.

Hypnotherapy tends to be symptom oriented. It offers help for tension, smoking, pain relief, obesity, psychosomatic ailments and phobias - the list is extensive. Some hypnotherapists claim to be able to uncover repressed material from the unconscious. Indeed, Freud gave hypnosis respectability when he got results from using it on his early clients, but later abandoned it when he found it induced idealisation of the analyst and when its effects proved to be transient. He replaced it with *free association* within psychoanalysis which would seem to have been the kiss of death to hypnosis as a treatment tool. Nevertheless the use of hypnosis it seems has grown unabated, but the type of therapy that it is offered within, as was mentioned earlier, varies a great deal from practitioner to practitioner. It may be the therapist will simply impose a counter suggestion upon the client such as 'when you leave here you will want to smoke less', or he or she may want to explore some of the client's unwanted feelings and will perhaps encourage the client to explore the physical manifestations of the feelings.

Usually a contract is agreed between therapist and client before hypnosis begins about what the aims of the therapy are and what suggestions will be given to the client. The therapist cannot make you do anything against your will in hypnosis, or make you do anything that is outside your normal code of ethics.

READING
Hypnosis by *Waxman, D. Unwin 1981, £3.95* . Subtitled 'A Guide for Patients', this is a thorough introduction to the history, development, and practice of classical hypnosis. One flaw however : the heavy bias against non-medical practitioners. Another introductory book is **Hypnotherapy, is it for you?** *by*

Sleet, R., Element 1989. **Hypnotherapy; A Modern Approach** *by Golden, W. et al. Pergamon 1988, £7.50.* Another book for practitioners, which can be of use to interested or potential clients. The authors use many of the 'newer' approaches to hypnosis, for example the non-directive approach developed from the work of Milton Erikson, who is now acknowledged as the greatest hypnotherapist of our time.

CENTRES OFFERING HYPNOTHERAPY

Acupuncture and Osteopathy Clinic SW1V, Alternative Medicine Clinic NW15, Alternative Therapies Centre N16, Association for Analystic and Bodymind Therapy and Training N10, Association of Natural Medicines CM8, Bexleyheath Natural Health Clinic DA7, Body Clinic NW11, Bodywise E2, Brackenbury Natural Health Centre W6, British Hypnosis Research DE22, British Society of Hypnotherapists SW6, Capital Hypnotherapy Centre W6, Care-Healing Centre W9, Centre for Stress Management SE3, Changes NW3, Chessington Hypnotherapy Clinic, Clapham Common Clinic SW4, Community Health Foundation EC1V, Edgware Centre for Natural Health HA8, Equilibrium Therapy Centre SW18, Hayes Hypnotherapy Centre UB4, Heath Health Care NW3, Helios N1, Homoeopathic Centre W13, Islington Green Centre of Alternative Medicine N1, Kingston Natural Healing Centre, Living Centre SW20, London Lighthouse W11, National Association of Counsellors, Hypnotherapists and Psychotherapists CB1, Natural Medicine Centre BR2, Natureworks, Neal's Yard Therapy Rooms WC2H, Pearl Healing Centre CR7, Psychotherapy Centre W1H, Sayer Clinic: Chelsea SW6, South London Natural Health Centre SW4, Sunra SW12, Violet Hill Studios NW8, Westminster Natural Health Centre SW1V, Wholeness E18.

TRAININGS IN HYPNOTHERAPY

National School of Hypnosis and Psychotherapy *Title of Training:* Diploma in Ericksonian Hypnosis, Psychotherapy and Neuro-Linguistic Programming *Duration:* 144 hours spread over 12/18 months, followed by one year's clinical supervision via the professional society. *Entry requirements:* Minimum 3 years in higher education and background in the caring professions; otherwise, mature candidates may be considered on demonstration of ability and commitment to undertake the courses. *Fees:* Refer to organisers *Comments:* No classes held at address, for enquiries only in writing or by telephone. Interviews by appointment.

National College of Hypnosis & Psychotherapy *Title of Training:* Diploma in Hypnotherapy & Psychotherapy *Duration:* 2 years, part time requiring 15 weekends class attendance and home study. *Entry requirements:* Graduate or good general education. Consideration given to experiential and professional qualifications. *Fees:* Refer to organisers *Comments:* Training is national, London, Cheshire and Glasgow. Recognised training faculty for the British Register of

Complementary Practitioners (Hypnotherapy) and founded on their initiative. Sole training faculty for National Register of Hypnotherapists & Psychotherapists. Also supplies external tutors to Institute of Advanced Nursing Education of the Royal College of Nursing and 'is the only organisation with training faculty and professional association in full membership of United Kingdom Standing Conference for Psychotherapy'.

Jungian Analysis

Analytical psychology is the more common name given to the psychotherapeutic approach founded by Carl Jung. Although Jung initially agreed with Freud's formulation of the unconscious he later came to view the unconscious in wider and more transpersonal terms. For Freud, the patient's history was detailed in the unconscious mind, and through the process of free association would yield up its secrets, secrets which had been buried during childhood, when natural desires and social demands came into conflict. Thus for Freud the unconscious was a chronicle of traumatic events and a repository of repressed infantile fantasies. Jung, however, came to a quite different view. He saw the content of the unconscious not just in Freud's terms, but also as something which reflected the history of the human species and the cosmic order. He called this particular unconscious the 'collective unconscious'.

The conscious and unconscious mind are seen as complementing and interacting with one another. The individual is seen as striving towards integration of these two aspects, and he called this process 'individuation'. Manifestations of the collective unconscious are to be found in dreams, symbolic language and fantasies. By exploring the meaning of these manifestations one can come to a deeper understanding of oneself. For instance, the 'archetypes' (such as the 'wise old man') which according to Jung, are part of the collective unconscious, could be known through understanding the symbols of one's dreams. Another central theme of Jung is the relationship between the 'masculine'

('animus') and 'feminine' ('anima') abilities within each of us. In this sense he was a pioneer of present day understanding of sexuality.

Jung advocated the 'eyeball to eyeball' encounter, where both analyst and client sit upright facing each other. Rather than focussing on the past he was more inclined to focus on the present and the future.

Two schools predominate in London. Firstly there is the classical school which has stuck closely to Jung's original writings. Then there is the Society of Analytical Psychology which while still working within a Jungian framework has assimilated the work of others on early childhood development.

READING

Memories, Dreams and Reflections by Jung, C. Fontana 1963, £6.99 . Jung's autobiography, full of insights into his life and the development of his ideas. A good place to start to explore Jungian analysis. **Practical Jung** by Wilmer, H. Chiron 1987, £9.95 . Subtitled 'The Nuts and Bolts of Jungian Psychotherapy', this is a fun, but seriously researched look at how Jungian Therapy works. Illustrated with cartoon-type line drawings. A more classical approach can be found in Fordhams, M. **Jungian Psychotherapy** (Wiley 1978, £9.95).

CENTRES OFFERING JUNGIAN ANALYSIS

Abraxas W2, Association of Independant Psychotherapists N6, Astro-Psychotherapeutic Practice W3, Biodynamic Psychotherapy and Teaching W3, British Association of Psychotherapists NW2, Centre for Personal & Professional Development N17, Graigian Community NW5, Heath Health Care NW3, Helios N1, Hillside Practice, Human Potential Resource Group GU2, Imprint SW19, Isis Counselling and Therapy Service SW17, Society of Analytical Psychology NW3.

TRAININGS IN JUNGIAN ANALYSIS

Association of Jungian Analysts Title of Training: Refer to organisers for details of training programme Fees: Refer to organisers

British Association of Psychotherapists Title of Training: 1) Individual Psychoanalytic and Analytical Psychotherapy with adults. 2) Training in Psychotherapy with children and adolesents Duration: Minimum of 4 years part-time (details available from trainings secretary). Entry requirements: 1) Degree in medicine, psychology or social science, or a relevant equivalent. Some experience of working with disturbed in a psychotherapeutic capacity. Fees: Varies each year from £1,030 in the first year to £500 in the fifth. Students must also pay for analysis and supervision. Comments: They are the oldest training organisation in the UK and have 450 members. The course is evening based so that students can continue to work while they study.

Society of Analytical Psychology Title of Training: Training in Adult Analysis.

Duration: Three years part-time. Two evenings per week and own analysis 4 times a week. *Entry requirements:* Candidates must have a degree or professional qualification (e.g. Social Work or Counselling). If the degree held has not included substantial study of psychology evidence of own study in this area required. Some clinical experience of patients also required. Candidates must be under 50 years of age. *Fees:* Refer to organisers

Kleinian Analysis

The work of Melanie Klein has had a major influence on the British Psychoanalytical school of thought. She lived and worked in London from 1926 onwards evolving theories of personality development which were to lead her to the creation of a variation of the style of treatment advocated by Freud. Though she accepted the common themes of psychoanalytic theory, such as the importance of the unconscious and the influence of early childhood upbringing on the later life of the individual, she also focused on some hithero unexplored areas of early development. She is most well known for her contributions towards understanding psychic development in the first two years of life and the emphasis she placed on aggression. Her focus was on the oral stage of development whereas Freud had devoted more attention to later stages of development.

She believed that the child in the first few months of life cannot make a clear distinction between himself as a separate entity and the world he inhabits. The child at this stage experiences the world in terms of what is pleasurable and what is unpleasurable. For instance he experiences the mothers breast, a warm cot, being picked up and held as good, and feeling hungry or cold as bad. The two prime emotions that the baby feels as a response to these good and bad experiences are warmth and anger respectively (Klein uses the terms love and hate). The infant may fluctuate between these two prime emotions rapidly as he does not have a developed sense of time or sequence of events. This rapidity of fluctuation can be observed when an infant in rage through hunger suddenly changes to feeling warmth and love towards the mother when fed. The mother is not only the object of these warm feelings but is also, in the child's mind, the object of rage when the child has unpleasurable experiences, and to the child she is then the bad mother. After a few months the child comes to realise that it is experiencing both rage and love towards his mother whom he can then see as a separate person from himself. The interplay between these two powerful emotions towards the same person sets up conflicts in the child which he has to deal with. Klein believed that the resolution of this conflict and the primitive way in which the child perceives the world lay the foundations for defences and for transference.

So how does the theory affect the practice of Kleinian analysis? Transference interpretations are likely early on in the therapy whereas in Freudian analysis they are usually allowed to develop before being interpreted. This transference tends to be focused on interpreting good or bad feelings that are directed towards the analyst to help the client realise that these feelings may be repetitions of earlier feelings towards the good and bad mother.

The couch is used. There may be a chair so that the client can have a choice of seating, though he may prefer not to sit facing as this may impede fantasy life.

The Kleinian approach would seem best suited to those who have a sympathy with the above ideas, who feel pent up with negative feelings, have difficulty making contact with others, who may feel anxious or who find it difficult to love others and be loved.

READING

Selected Melanie Klein *by Mitchell, J. (Ed). Penguin 1986, £5.99*. An excellent collection of Klein's work with analysis and comment by Juliet Mitchell. Shows the development of her ideas and how her therapy works. **My Kleinian Home** *by Herman, N. Free Association Books 1988, £9.95*. An account of the author's journey through four therapies, ending with a full Kleinian analysis. Moving and enlightening.

CENTRES OFFERING KLEINIAN ANALYSIS

Tavistock Clinic NW3.

Men's Therapy

Historically, men only therapy groups evolved initially as a response to the Women's Movement in the early 1970s. Groups such as *Achilles' Heel* and *Red Therapy* attempted to link left wing and feminist politics with therapy.

The rationale behind men's therapy is that men may find it easier to talk about issues such as misogeny or sexuality honestly in an all men group. Exponents of these groups see men as relying largely on women for their emotional support. In a men's therapy group they may be able to become less competitive with other men, and develop deeper friendships with them. Through this process they may become less dependent on women for emotional support, and more able to give them emotional support when necessary. The aim is to develop less polarisation in relationships into 'opposite sex' roles and characteristics. This is seen as not only benefitting the men involved by releasing them from a narrow 'masculine' role, but also their relationships with partners, children and others.

Men leading men's groups may employ a variety of methods and approaches. Some may explicitly explore the theme of masculinity. In some groups, the political or social effects of men's therapy may be seen as the most important effects of the work, while in others are more focused on individual, psychological change, though these two aspects are seen as inseparable in practice.

CENTRES OFFERING MEN'S THERAPY

Association of Independant Psychotherapists N6, Astro-Psychotherapeutic Practice W3, Bodywise E2, Brothers SE14, Centre for Personal & Professional Development N17, Hayes Hypnotherapy Centre UB4, Healing Centre NW5, Helios N1, Islington Green Centre of Alternative Medicine N1, Man To Man NW3, Skills with People N5, Sunra SW12, Wild Dance W2, Working With Men SE5.

Trainings in MENS THERAPY

Spectrum Refer to organisers

Working With Men *Title of Training:* 1) Sexuality course for Men 2) Working with perpetrators of sexual abuse 3) Working with adult survivors of Child Sexual Abuse. *Duration:* 1) 10 weeks part time, 1 hour weekly + home work daily Other courses range from one day to four days. *Entry requirements:* 1) interview with facilitator Others, application form. *Fees:* Refer to organisers *Comments:* One of few centres working with both perpetrators and survivors. Also offer individual counselling/therapy and other therapy groups for men. Refer to organisers for details.

Music Therapy and Voice Therapy

Music has been used for healing purposes for many centuries. Culturally it is used to unify groups, for relaxation, stimulation or to evoke a particular mood or response. It evokes feelings, and is also a powerful means of expressing feelings and communicating non-verbally. It can promote a feeling of bonding and closeness in a one to one therapeutic relationship or within a group. Music can provide a safe context through which feelings which otherwise might seem unacceptable can be expressed, acknowledged and subsequently understood. Like the other creative arts, it can provide an objective framework through which the individual can bring to light perhaps hitherto hidden aspects of his or her experience, and reflect on them objectively within this framework.

Though the use of music in a therapeutic way is usually expressive - it involves playing an instrument or singing (voice therapy), it may also involve listening to music.

Music therapy has wide applications. It can be used to help those with mental or physical handicaps develop skills and satisfying means of expression. It is also useful in developing self-confidence and concentration, releasing feelings and increasing vitality.

CENTRES OFFERING MUSIC THERAPY

Centre for Health and Healing W1V, Healing Voice TW10, Institute For Arts In Therapy & Education N16, London Lighthouse W11, Mu Sum Ba - Living Rhythm BN27, Nordoff-Robbins Music Therapy Centre NW5, Pearl Healing Centre CR7, Refuah Shelaymah Natural Health Centre N16.

CENTRES OFFERING VOICE THERAPY

Augenblick Centre, Healing Voice TW10, Helios N1, Highbury Centre N5, IBISS TW7, Neal's Yard Therapy Rooms WC2H, Playspace NW1, Primrose Healing Centre NW1, Silver Birch Centre NW10, Skills with People N5, Sound Health SE8, Sound Moves SE20.

TRAINING IN MUSIC THERAPY

Nordoff-Robbins Music Therapy Centre *Title of Training:* City University Post-Graduate Diploma in Nordoff-Robbins Music Therapy *Duration:* 1 year full time September-July *Entry requirements:* Preferably a degree/diploma in music. Piano perfoming standard to grade 8 minimum. Entry to course is based on an audition which takes into account life experience, attitude etc. as well as musical considerations. Personal therapy is not a requirement. Auditions held throughout the year. *Fees:* Course fees at present £2750, overseas £4650. *Comments:* This training offers the only Nordoff-Robbins Music Therapy training in Great Britain, there are only two other courses in Germany and the USA.

Neuro-linguistic Programming

In the early seventies Neuro-Linguistic Programming (NLP) was developed by Richard Bandler, John Grinder, Leslie Cameron-Bandler, Judith DeLozier and Robert Dilts. In 1975 and 1976 Richard Bandler and John Grinder were the co-

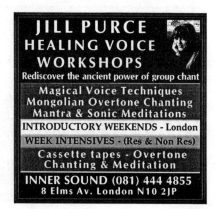

authors of *The Structure of Magic I* and *The Structure of Magic II*, which are still considered to be the definitive books on NLP. They claimed to have isolated important factors which underlie the work of well-known therapists. These factors were seen to be common to the three therapists they studied. The three therapists were Fritz Perls, Virginia Satir and Milton Erikson.

Rather than pay attention to the therapists' notion of how therapeutic change occurred Grinder and Bandler noted patterns in the communication in these different therapist/client relationships and from these drew the conclusion that these patterns were the 'magic' ingredient that elevated these practitioners above the rest. In this sense a parallel can be drawn with Carl Rogers' thesis that it is not so much the particular technique or theory the therapist uses that brings about psychotherapeutic change, but the underlying attitudes of the therapist, even if he or she is unaware of having these attitudes.

They believed that each client should be approached differently. Therefore, they gave microscopic attention to how the client acted and looked, and from these signs could identify mechanisms of perceptions for each person. For example they were able to deduce whether or not a person was using visual recall rather than auditory recall from noting shifts in pupil size, breathing, direction of gaze and head movements. The therapist can then communicate to the other person in the appropriate mode, thus inducing rapport.

NLP is a technique based therapy used mainly in a group setting. As a client you will not only be the recipient of these techniques but will, by participation, learn some of these skills for yourself. Some of the techniques are mirroring and matching, and reframing, pacing, V/K disassociation and anchoring. An emphasis is on 'accessing' an 'anchor', that is, recalling good experiences and using them as resources for the future. This is done by superimposing good feelings from a past event onto a situation that has unpleasant feelings, so that the unpleasant feelings become less potent.

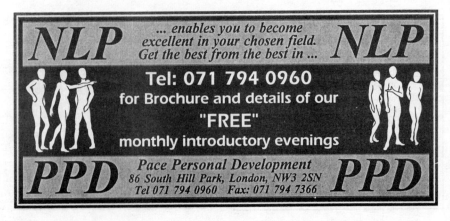

READING

Frogs into Princes by *Bandler, R. & Grinder, J. Real People Press 1978, £6.95.* This was one of the first books on NLP and in a burgeoning literature, it stands as probably the nearest one can come to 'experiencing' NLP in a book. It contains edited transcripts of weekend workshops and covers all the basics of the subject with live interaction between the authors (as workshop leaders) and the participants. **What is NLP?** *Eric Robbie, Self-Published 1989, £2.95.* A small pamphlet, actually an extended version of the author's article in *Innovative Therapies in Britain* (Eds. Dryden & Rowan, Open Univ. Press), which gives a concise history of NLP, a good exposition of its theoretical background, and examples of how it works in practice. It is also written in 'English', rather than 'American'. Available from specialist bookshops.

CENTRES OFFERING NEURO-LINGUISTIC PROGRAMMING

Alternative Medicine Clinic NW15, Association for Neuro-Linguistic Programming N16, British Hypnosis Research DE22, Care-Healing Centre W9, Changes NW3, City Health Centre EC1Y, Community Health Foundation EC1V, Equilibrium Therapy Centre SW18, Human Potential Resource Group GU2, Islington Green Centre of Alternative Medicine N1, Pace Personal Development NW3, Raphael Clinic NW6, Ravenscroft Centre NW11, Skills with People N5, Wholeness E18.

TRAININGS IN NEURO-LINGUISTIC PROGRAMMING

British Hypnosis Research *Title of Training:* Diploma in Ericksonian Hypnosis, Psychotherapy and NLP. *Duration:* One year, part time. Two level training: practitioner level and advanced level. Each level involves 6 weekends, 12 supervision days and 20 evenings. *Entry requirements:* 1) Professional qualificiation in one of the caring professions. 2) A first degree as evidence of academic achievement. 3) Experience or employment in an area related to the subject matter of the course. *Fees:* Refer to organisers *Comments:* Skill based training held at St Ann's Hospital, London. Emphasis is placed on supervising each students whilst they work with actual patients. (Volunteer patients are supplied by BHR).

John Seymour Associates *Title of Training:* Neuro-Linguistic Programming Diploma. *Duration:* Part time - 24 days in total. *Entry requirements:* Completion of Introduction to NLP weekend. *Fees:* Refer to organisers *Comments:* Full money back guarantee on any individual seminar. Fully recognised by Association Neuro-Linguistic Programming. Free brochure and quarterly newsletter to all on the mailing list.

Pace Personal Development *Title of Training:* (1) NLP Foundation Skills. (2) NLP Practitioner. (3) NLP Master Practitioner. (4) NLP Advanced Master Practitioner. (5) Other special courses and seminars. *Duration:* (1) 9 days. (2) 15 days. (3) 24 days. (4) 48 days. (5) Other courses from 1 day to 10 days; evening seminars. *Entry requirements:* (1) Open to all. (2) Practitioner entry requirement is Foundation Skills. (3) Master Practitioner entry requirement is Practitioner Certificate. (4) Advanced Master entry requirement is Master Practitioner. Fees: (1) £750 + VAT. (2) £1,070 + VAT. (3) £1,700 + VAT. (4) £350 + VAT or £550 + VAT. *Comments:* Courses start at various times throughout the year. Pace Personal Development is endorsed by John Grinder (originator of NLP). We use some of the world's finest NLP trainers.

Personal Construct Therapy

George Kelly proposed this theory of personality and a method of treatment in 1955. Though it has gained a major foothold in academic circles and now ranks as a major theory of personality, it has not been widely used as a form of treatment.

According to Kelly we all have a personal construct system. 'Construct' because we construe people, events and situations. 'Personal' because we construe in a highly personal way, and 'system' because the constructs are related to each other in a particular order or system.

Whilst PCT draws on a number of other therapies for techniques it also claims a number of techniques of its own, namely enactment, self-characterisation, fixed role therapy and repertory grid analysis.

Enactment is used on a one-to-one basis, and is an informal role-play technique. A situation is elaborated and the therapist and client act out the situation. The aim of this is to allow the client a fresh and detached view of a familiar situation.

The client may be asked to write a biography of him or herself as if written by a good friend. This is analysed by the therapist and is used as an evaluation technique in establishing the client's self image. This technique is known as self-characterisation.

The fixed-role technique is rather novel. Once the therapist has a picture of how the client sees him or herself and the world, a fictional character is created by the therapist. This fictional character views the world in a way which is quite different, though not opposite, from the way the client does. The client is then presented with a description of this fictional character and is asked to pretend to be this person for at least a week. The aim of this is for the client to note how others react to the new character, and from this the client will review his or her own construct system.

The repertory grid technique may involve filling out a questionnaire that asks for ways the client pictures his or her world. It is then used for further analysis.

Personal Construct Therapy can also be practised in a group. George Kelly saw a group as a vehicle for its members to elaborate their construct system. By being a member of a group one has the opportunity of seeing how others see you and one can gain a new perspective on how people relate to each other.

Fay Fransella has pioneered work in PCT with stutterers at the Royal Free Hospital.

READING

Theory of Personality by Kelly, G. Norton 1955 (63), £5.95. This book consists of the first three chapters of Kelly's major work **The Psychology of Personal Constructs,** and gives the basic background and theory to Personal Construct Psychology. Another book to look for is **Inquiring Man** by Bannister, D. & Fransella, F. (Croom-Helm 1986).

CENTRES OFFERING PERSONAL CONTRUCT THERAPY

Clapham Common Clinic SW4, Heath Health Care NW3.

Postural Integration

Similar to Rolfing (see the section on 'Body Approaches') from which it is derived, but rather than just physical manipulation of the body, as in Rolfing, postural integration delves into the emotional issues connected with body tensions. It takes the form of a manipulation of deep tissue combined with Reichian analysis and awareness of the body through movement.

The format of the session is similar to Rolfing, ten sessions of up to two hours. The client is encouraged to focus on breathing and feelings whilst the practitioner works on the body. New physical movements are encouraged with a focus on their meaning to the client.

CENTRES OFFERING POSTURAL INTEGRATION

Centre for Release and Integration TW10, New Cross Natural Therapy Centre , Open Centre EC1V, Sound Health SE8.

TRAINING IN POSTURAL INTEGRATION

Centre for Release and Integration *Title of Training:* Training in Postural Integration *Duration:* 3 years part time *Entry requirements:* Experience in bodywork or body-oriented psychotherapy. *Fees:* Refer to organisers *Comments:* First year, 'Foundation in Bodywork' can be taken as a self-contained unit, with a 'Certificate in bodywork' being awarded with successful completion.

Open Centre *Title of Training:* Postural Integration. *Duration:* Two years. *Comments:* For details contact Silke Ziehl on (081) 549 9583

Primal Integration

Primal Integration is a term coined by Bill Swartley to describe the very free-form type of primal work he developed (independently of Arthur Janov - see 'Primal Therapy' below) within a growth model.

Primal Integration works with very early preverbal experiences from the womb, birth and infancy, as well as with later experiences, in an eclectic way. The emphasis is on self-direction and self-regulation and allowing spontaneous growth processes to unfold rather than employing a highly structured or directed programme. The work is frequently undertaken in groups with a minimal leader-determined structure but with appropriate ground rules for safe working. Thus primal material is allowed to emerge under its own dynamic but is not directly aimed for.

There is not usually an individual intensive when commencing the work as is the case with Primal Therapy. Intensives are usually on a group basis and undertaken at a later stage in the work.

Primal material is worked with through bodywork, through transference (see Psychoanalysis for a definition of 'transference'), through face to face work and a variety of other ways.

CENTRES OFFERING PRIMAL INTEGRATION

International Primal Association, Open Centre EC1V, Primal Integration Programme N8.

Primal Therapy

Arthur Janov, the founder of primal therapy, holds that the seat of neurosis lies in the past and that the maltreatment of children, some of society's child-rearing practices, pain and lack of love in upbringing all contribute to this. Neurosis consists of pain that is warded off, and which lies deep within the person, profoundly affecting feelings towards self and others. By re-experiencing this pain and hurt and expressing it, neurosis will dissolve.

The process of therapy is sequential. First the client is asked to submit an autobiography and history. There then follow two interviews. If the client is accepted for treatment a three week intensive process begins. During the three weeks the client is seen daily for up to three hours. After the three weeks the client enters individual or group therapy for up to a year.

The therapy usually takes place in a room that is sound protected, with cushions and mattresses. The lighting is usually dim.

During the therapy the focus is on the client's hurt. Time is spent going over incidents of neglect or abuse. Freedom is given to physical expression of these feelings, whether it is curling up into a foetal position, screaming abuse, or sobbing with pain, while the therapist acts supportively to enable this healing of past pain.

READING

The Primal Scream *by Janov, A. Shere 1973, £4.99*. Some people find the claims made by Janov in this book somewhat extravagant, but it makes compulsive reading and there can be no denying that Primal regressive therapy can be a powerful therapeutic tool. The Primal Issue Revisited *by S&S (Eds) in Self & Society 1987, £1.50*. A special issue of the *Journal of Humanistic Psychology* devoted to developments in primal type work. Worth seeking out to look at the wide range of practitioners working and their different approaches.

CENTRES OFFERING PRIMAL THERAPY

Association for Analystic and Bodymind Therapy and Training N10, Healing Centre NW5, Hillside Practice, London Association of Primal Psychotherapists NW5.

TRAININGS IN PRIMAL THERAPY

London Association of Primal Psychotherapists *Title of Training:* Primal Psychotherapy Training *Duration:* Three years part-time, two to three evenings per week. *Entry requirements:* Must have been in primal therapy at least one year and have a good academic degree. *Fees:* £750 per annum payable in three instalments, plus cost of personal therapy.

Psychoanalysis

Classical full scale Freudian psychoanalysis requires the client, referred to as patient or analysand, to attend a fifty minute session with an analyst four or five times a week, for at least three years. It thus means a huge investment in time and money which is one of the reasons it is not as widely practised as psychoanalytic psychotherapy (see below).

The reasons for such prolonged and regular contact are to be found in the theory initially formulated by Freud. Two cornerstones of the theory are transference and resistance. Such prolonged contact revives feelings and impulses one originally had towards significant figures from the past (usually one's parents) which become directed towards the analyst. This is transference. Time is needed for resistances to emerge too. Resistance is the withholding from oneself and the analyst of one's psychic interior. By helping the patient to become more aware of the workings of the unconscious in transference and resistance, he or she can become free of neurotic symptoms.

The basic rule is that the analysand 'free associates', in other words says whatever comes to mind. The analyst pays attention to the emergence of transference and resistance and tries to tease them out further.

The analyst may intervene in various ways, but usually by confrontation or interpretation, for example 'you're really angry at me and you express this by being continually late', or 'you seem to feel you have been mistreated by fate and dealt an unfair hand'.

Classically, the analysand lies on the couch with the analyst sitting behind, out of sight. Usually the analysand does most of the talking.

Analysts often work early in the morning or early evening, to accommodate their clients' employment schedules.

READING

What Freud Really Said by *Stafford-Clark, D. Peng 1967, £4.50*. As its title suggests, this book explains in down to earth terms the major ideas of the father of psychoanalysis. He also examines the context in which Freud developed those ideas.

CENTRES OFFERING PSYCHOANALYSIS

Arcadia Creative Therapy Centre SE6, British Psycho-Analytical Society and The Institute of Psycho-analysis, Hayes Hypnotherapy Centre UB4, Heath Health Care NW3.

TRAININGS IN PSYCHOANALYSIS

British Psycho-Analytical Society and The Institute of Psycho-analysis *Title of Training:* Training in the Psycho-analysis of Adults *Duration:* Minimum of four years *Entry requirements:* (1) Medically qualified or undergoing medical training or (2) good university degree or its equivelent. *Fees:* Refer to organisers *Comments:* Trainees must undergo personal psychoanalysis (five sessions per week). Seminars and supervision are provided. If the trainee does not have sufficient experience of working with psychiatric patients he/she may be required to get more experience. Loans may be provided if the student does not have sufficient funds.

Psychoanalytic Psychotherapy

Psychoanalytic psychotherapy takes its lead from psychoanalysis. It upholds the basic psychoanalytic theory but takes into account some the realities of commitment of time and money. Unlike psychoanalysis, sessions are usually only once or twice, though sometimes three times a week with a fifty minute hour.

Also, unlike psychoanalysis, patient and analyst sit upright facing each other, and the engulfing intensity of the relationship which distinguishes psychoanalysis is tempered as the patient's everyday life becomes more the currency of the transactions.

PSYCHOANALYTIC PSYCHOTHERAPY

Psychoanalytic psychotherapy is a name that covers a wide range of psychotherapies that either hold to the basic Freudian theory or to one of the neo-Freudian theories. When one thinks of visiting a psychotherapist this is what most people expect to get.

READING
Introduction to Psychotherapy by *Brown, D. & Pedder, J. RKP 1979, £8.95.*
Although not only on the psychoanalytic approach, this book provides a good background introduction to how psychotherapy is practised.

CENTRES OFFERING PSYCHOANALYTIC PSYCHOTHERAPY
Arbours Consultation Service, Association for Group and Individual Psychotherapy N19, Association of Independent Psychotherapists N6, British Association of Psychotherapists NW2, British Psycho-Analytical Society and The Institute of Psycho-analysis, Centre for Psychoanalytical Psychotherapy NW4, Centre of Integral Psychoanalysis W11, CHI Centre SW6, Clapham Common Clinic SW4, Ealing Psychotherapy Centre W3, Gerda Boyesen Centre W3, Hayes Hypnotherapy Centre UB4, Heath Health Care NW3, INTAPSY W8, Isis Counselling and Therapy Service SW17, Lavender Hill Homoeopathic Centre SW11, London Centre for Psychotherapy NW3, Natureworks, Philadelphia Association NW3, Psychotherapy Centre W1H, Re-Vision NW2, Sound Health SE8, Tavistock Clinic NW3, Women's Therapy Centre N7.

TRAININGS IN PSYCHOANALYTIC PSYCHOTHERAPY
Arbours Association *Title of Training:* Training Programme In Psychotherapy. *Duration:* Three years. *Entry requirements:* Personal maturity and academic competance. *Fees:* Refer to organisers *Comments:* Trainees are required to be in individual psychoanalytic psychotherapy at least three times a week for the duration of the training. Training is individual psychotherapy. Trainees are expected to complete a six month placement in one of the Arbours therapeutic communitites. All prospective students must complete at least two terms on the Associates programme before beginning the full training.

Philadelphia Association *Title of Training:* Psychoanalytic Psychotherapy and Phenomenology *Duration:* Min four years, open ended, (one night per week and seminars plus therapy plus supervision). *Entry requirements:* Must have completed 1 year Introductory course, must have been in own therapy for at least a year and have relevant experience of working with disturbed/distressed people. *Fees:* £600 p.a. course fees. Therapy and supervision privately arranged, no VAT. *Comments:* Within the practice of psychotherapy and community therapy the P.A. is concerned with the phenomenological approach and critique. There is no set curriculum as the training programme is tailor made to each group.

Women's Therapy Centre *Title of Training:* Working with women - a psychodynamic approach. *Duration:* One year, Three hours per week. *Entry requirements:* Students must be currently working with women and have a counselling element in their work. They must already have some training and skills in the general area of counselling or groupwork. Also some baic knowledge and interest in psychoanalytic theory. *Fees:* £700 p.a. payable termly. *Comments:* The focus is on women's psychological development. Selection is by application form and individual interview.

London Centre for Psychotherapy *Title of Training:* (1) One year introductory course in Analytical Psychotherapy (2) Three year qualifying course in Analytical Psychotherapy. *Duration:* (1) One year part-time. (2) Three years part-time. *Entry requirements:* (1) Applicants should be graduates or professional in the health field. *Fees:* Refer to organisers

Association for Group and Individual Psychotherapy *Title of Training:* Psychotherapy Training *Duration:* Three years part-time. Seminars and analytic groups twice weekly. Weekly evening and weekend day groups. Personal therapy, twice weekly required. *Entry requirements:* Applicants should have at least one year's personal psychotherapy with an approved psychotherapist before starting the course. *Fees:* Refer to organisers

Outreach Counselling *Title of Training:* Introductory Diploma Course in Counselling and Community Skills. *Duration:* One to three years. *Fees:* Refer to organisers

Centre for Psychoanalytical Psychotherapy *Title of Training:* (1) Introductory Course (2) Clinical course Duration: (1) One year. (2) Three years. *Entry requirements:* Professional qualification in psychology, medicine or social work or appropriate experience in caring capacity. *Fees:* Refer to organisers *Comments:* Consultation and supervision, individual or group.

Tavistock Clinic *Title of Training:* An Interdisciplinary Programme of Training in Adult Psychotherapy for Experienced Professional Workers in the Health and Social Services. *Duration:* Four years full time. *Entry requirements:* Must be a clinical psychologist. *Fees:* Refer to organisers *Comments:* Trainees are required to have personal psychotherapy at least three times a week at their own expense.

Association of Independent Psychotherapists *Title of Training:* Analytical Psychotherapy. *Duration:* 3-4 years part-time. Wednesday evening seminars and lectures. 2 years of individual and group supervision. *Entry requirements:* 1) Aged 30 - 60. 2) Experience of working with people in emotional distress (paid or voluntary). 3) Completion of a foundation course or counselling skills course. 4) 200 hours of psychotherapy. Fees: £950 p.a. plus cost of psychotherapy and supervision. *Comments:* Personal therapy required, minimum of twice a week. Course starts October - early application recommended.

Psychotherapy Centre *Title of Training:* Psychotherapy *Duration:* Four years, part-time or full-time, days or evenings, minimum 5 hours per week at the Centre plus own time elsewhere. *Entry requirements:* Having therapy oneself from a practitioner at the Centre is the first and most important element of the training. *Fees:* £500 per year plus therapy costs (£25 or more per appointment.) *Comments:* 'The training has evolved in the light of decades of experience and research, and is motivated by concern for the welfare of the patients, without theory or drugs.'

INTAPSY *Title of Training:* Diploma Course in Psychodynamic Psychotherapy. *Duration:* Four years. *Comments:* The course leads to professional practice and membership of an international association of professional practitioners.

Psychodrama

Jacob Moreno created psychodrama. He began experimenting with the use of role playing with children as early as 1908 and evolved his method in the intervening years before his death in 1974.

Moreno felt that 'all the world's a stage'. He believed that we adopt rigid roles and act them out and so focused his work on freeing spontaneous expression through make-believe situations.

Psychodrama is psychotherapy married to the theatre. The therapist is called the director, and the client the protagonist. The client produces a scene from his or her life that is loaded with feeling - it may be getting a salary rise at work, leaving home, or whatever, and this becomes the drama that the protagonist and the other members of the group enact. The director tries to recreate the scene in all its vividness with a here and now quality.

As in the theatre the director encourages members to visualise what the surroundings are, and may point out where the imaginary door or window is and ask members to keep these in mind when dramatising the incident. The director may also use props as in theatre improvisation.

The group members do not learn lines for the characters they are playing, but feed on the descriptions given by the protagonist of how they are likely to respond in certain situations. Thus they slowly build up a picture of their assumed character, and modify it by a process of improvisation and rehearsal. The protagonist may switch roles to gain insight into another character's position. Such insight is often a revelation to the client.

If a group member does not appear to be acting out the character as the protagonist remembers him or her, the director may ask another group member to play the character.

If the group members feel the protagonist is not saying what he or she really feels in the situation, they are allowed to go up behind that person and say what they think he or she really feels. The protagonist has the option of rejecting or adopting this new thought.

Eventually a climax is reached and catharsis occurs. The cast then sit down and assimilate what transpired. Members may relate how they felt playing their particular character.

Another client may then choose to relate another incident, and so the process goes on.

READING

The Essential Moreno by Fox, J. (Ed) Springer 1987, £14.95 . Moreno was, of course, the father of Psychodrama and the editor here has made an excellent selection from his work, showing the development of his ideas and how they work in practice. **Acting In** by Blatner, H. Springer 1976, £15.95 . Blatner worked with Moreno towards the end of his life and this book has long been thought of as *the* basic textbook of psychodramatic methods. **Psychodrama: Inspiration and Technique** by Holmes, P. & Karp, M. (Routledge £14.99), a collection of articles by twelve psychodramatists who have developed beyond the ideas of Moreno.

CENTRES OFFERING PSYCHODRAMA

Bodyspace, Cabot Centre NW1, Eigenwelt London NW3, Healing Centre NW5, Holwell Centre for Psychodrama and Sociodrama EX31, Open Centre EC1V, Playspace NW1, Spectrum N4.

TRAINING IN PSYCHODRAMA

London Centre for Psychodrama and Group Psychotherapy *Title of Training:* Psychodrama and Group Analytic Psychotherapy Training *Duration:* Three and a half years, part time. *Entry requirements:* Minimum age 23. Training or experience in Mental Health Field. Attended Psychodrama workshops or registered practitioner. Provide professional and personal references. *Fees:* Refer to organisers *Comments:* 'Involves training in both psychodrama and group analysis and is unique in this respect'.

Psychosynthesis

Psychosynthesis is sometimes called a 'transpersonal' psychology. It is one of the psychologies which emphasise the importance of the spiritual dimension, and of developing higher levels of consciousness and self actualisation.

Its founder, Roberto Assagioli, was trained in psychoanalysis but became dissatisfied with Freud's preoccupation with the 'basement' of the psyche, and with the existing concepts of repressed feelings and neurosis. While acknowledging the importance of bringing to light these feelings for psychological health, Assagioli felt that there was also a 'higher' unconscious as well as the 'lower' unconscious. The 'higher' unconscious is the source of inspiration, imagination and 'peak' experiences - experiences of unity or joy which transcend the individual's sense of existing as a separate, isolated unit. Assagioli studied Indian philosophy and religion and sought to marry western psychology which emphasises the importance of the individual and the personality, with eastern mysticism's concern with higher levels of consciousness.

In psychosynthesis the psyche is seen as being made up of many different parts : our body, feelings and mind; the different roles we play in life which are all part of our overall personality but which may seem in conflict; and our experience of the depths and heights of the psyche. The process of psychosynthesis is to synthesise these often seemingly different and even contradictory parts. What unites all these elements is the self, a conscious experience of ourselves which is not identified with any one part, but which can observe and direct awareness of them.

Assagioli also emphasised the importance of what he called the 'will'. By this he did not mean will in the sense of will power, but the ability to make choices and to mould our selves and lives which is based on a deep experience of our own individuality.

Psychosynthesis therapists may use a variety of techniques. They may ask you to engage in an inner dialogue with particular parts of yourself, or lead you through a guided fantasy to clarify your feelings about a particular issue. They may encourage you to draw or paint from material which arises in the course of therapy. Therapists also draw on techniques used in other therapies such as gestalt and psychodrama. While the basic theory has been applied as a kind of psychotherapy, it also has applications in education, medicine and religion.

READING
Psychosynthesis; A Collection of Basic Writings *by Assagioli, R, Thorsons 1976.* In this book, Assagioli outlines his theory, and its difference to the other psychotherapies. He then describes the techniques that are used. A very full explanation but some people find it quite a difficult read. **What We May Be** *by*

Ferruci, P., Thorsons 1982. Ferruci was originally a student of Assagioli, and later his collaborator. This book is a manual of self help exercises in psychosynthesis. Well laid out and easy to read and use.

CENTRES OFFERING PSYCHOSYNTHESIS

Art from Within N5, Bodywise E2, Brothers SE14, Communication and Counselling Foundation SY25, Cortijo Romero UK LS7, Healing Fields Practice N7, Helios N1, Institute of Psychosynthesis NW4, Isis Counselling and Therapy Service SW17, Islington Green Centre of Alternative Medicine N1, London Focusing Centre SW4, Moving Line Counselling and Therapy, North London Counselling Service N5, Psychosynthesis and Education Trust SE1, Re-Vision NW2.

TRAININGS IN PSYCHOSYNTHESIS

Communication and Counselling Foundation *Title of Training:* 1) Professional

Psychosynthesis & Education Trust

COUNSELLING SERVICE

❑ Professional and experienced counsellors
❑ Individual assessment and placement
❑ Sessions available at London Bridge and throughout Greater London

For a copy of our brochure and more information ring us on the Counselling Service.
Tel. No:
0171 403 7814
or write to us at 92/94 Tooley Street, London Bridge, London SE1 2TH

The Psychosynthesis & Education Trust offers diploma courses in counselling & therapy as well as personal growth and professional development programmed.
For more details contact the trust on 0171 403 2100 or write to the above address.

ISIS

Counselling & Therapy Service

Isis Counselling and Therapy Service is a network of qualified and experienced counsellors and psychotherapists in London.

We have therapists trained in various therapeutic approaches including psychosynthesis, psychoanalytic psychotherapy, psychodynamic counselling, gestalt, stress management, integrative psychotherapy, existential therapy and Jungian psychology.

All our members abide by the British Association for Counselling Code of Ethics.

If you are interested in finding a counsellor or would like to know more about the Service, please telephone us on

0181 769 0675 or 0181 656 9209.

Training in Psychosynthesis and Counselling Skills and Attitudes/Diploma programme. *Duration:* 3 years, part time. *Entry requirements:* By application and interview plus Foundation Course of one week. *Fees:* Refer to organisers *Comments:* Training programme offers a theoretical model including the height and depth of the psyche, utilising ideas from Alice Miller and John Bowlby regarding abuse, deprivation, the image of the inner child; an integrated counselling skills and attitudes model including principles of person-centred and psychodynamic counselling within broader principle of healing. Training encourages the trainees' own synthesis of self.

Institute of Psychosynthesis *Title of Training:* Diploma in Psychosynthesis Psychotherapy. *Duration:* 4 years part-time. 9 weekends, 1 week residential, plus some evenings, plus personal therapy, per annum. *Entry requirements:* Completion of prerequisite course Fundamentals of Psychosynthesis. *Fees:* Refer to organisers

Psychosynthesis and Education Trust *Title of Training:* Professional Training Programme in Psychosynthesis Counselling and Psychotherapy. Three Diplomas offered. *Duration:* The professional counselling training is designed to be completed within three years on a part-time basis and is offered in different formats for people living within the greater London area and for others who are living further afield. An optional fourth year of training (Advanced Diploma Course)is offered for people seeking to practice psychotherapy professionally. *Entry requirements:* Prospective students must: 1) enroll in an introductory course 'The Essentials of Psychosynthesis'. 2) Make a written application 3) Undertake an assessment interview. Apply to organisers for more specific criteria. *Fees:* Fees for the three year course are paid in 36 monthly instalments by standing order, except for personal therapy fees which are paid direct to the therapist. Apply to organisers for more details. *Comments:* Over the three years students must have a minimum of 72 individual sessions with an approved therapist. Intake interviews are in January for the first term beginning in April of each year. Applications must be received by 20th January.

Re-Vision *Title of Training:* 1) Professional training in Counselling and Therapy within a transpersonal and integrative perspective. 2) Post-Diploma Psychotherapy Training *Duration:* Part time over 3/4 years 1) First 2 years 1 wknd per month plus 1 week summer residential, 3rd year 2 days per week over 3 ten week terms. 2) One additional year part time 1 day per week.(i.e. total four years) *Entry requirements:* Six day intensive basic course 'The Way of Psychosynthesis" Selection Criteria are:- professional qualifications; previous therapy; experience in helping professions; capacity for independent study; intended application of training; maturity. *Fees:* Fees per year 1) £1450.00 2) £1970.00 3) £2200.00 4)£1900.00 (approx) Individual therapy extra. *Comments:* Weekly personal therapy over the period in training required. Training groups are kept small (12-16 persons). Small tutorial groups for educational and pastoral support. Student association. The course integrates practical methods of working with the relationship derived from psychoanalysis, with active Humanistic methods within a transpersonal perspective that honours the journey of the soul. Use of video feedback for counselling practicals.

Rebirthing

Rebirthing is the process of reliving one's own birth and of coming to terms with the original experience. It is therefore a regression technique. Frederick Le Boyer, a leading exponent of natural birth, has suggested that birth can be painful for the baby and that this might affect the baby's outlook on the world. If it was harsh then the person might grow up to view the world in a negative way. Rebirthers argue that if one can regress to the initial birth and live it through, one can change negative thoughts and attitudes.

There are two different types of rebirthing in this country. One was founded by Leonard Orr on the West Coast of America in the 1970s and the other was developed by Frank Lake.

Orr rebirthing involves using a breathing exercise. The therapist and client occupy a quiet room and pillow and blankets may be used to cover the client if necessary. The client is asked to lie down and breathe in and out in a regular way without pausing. A contract is made beforehand about how long this will continue. Usually it is for an hour or until the client experiences a breathing release, which is the eventual aim of rebirthing.

An Orr rebirther also employs 'affirmations'. These are sentences which are repeated by the client such as 'Every breath I take, increases my aliveness' or 'I feel much love for people'. They affirm how the client would like to feel or be, and are intended to counteract negative attitudes.

Sometimes clients are asked to be reborn in water, as this is closer to the original experience of birth. A bath is usually used for this, and so that the client can remain submerged. He or she may be asked to use a snorkel.

The other type of rebirthing is usually done in a group. One member chooses to be reborn. The other members physically assemble themselves into a simulated womb around the member who lies on the floor in a foetal position. Cushions are liberally employed and are used as buffers between the group 'womb' and the 'foetus'. Gradually the members apply increasing pressure (usually by sitting on or pressing against the 'foetus') which simulates the growth of the foetus in the contained environment. The 'foetus' decides (usually when overcome with claustrophobia) to get out from the enclosing walls and makes its way out of an opening. This is a physically demanding exercise.

Both of these techniques are quite different so make sure you know which one you have signed up for.

READING

Rebirthing: The Science of Enjoying All of Your Life, Laut, P., Trinity 1983. An excellent manual of rebirthing techniques as originated by Leonard Orr. It shows how it works, how sessions may proceed and gives affirmations to further the growth process. Clinical Theology by Lake, F., (Dartman, Longman & Todd). 1980. This is Lake's major work on his approach, a fusion of theological, analytical/psychodynamic, and existential ideas. It doesn't give a clear outline of how his approach is used. His ideas are usually defined as being 'Primal Integration'. There have been two special issues of Self & Society which cover this approach, 'Birth and Rebirth' and 'Voices from the Past', both of which may be available from specialist shops or direct from Self & Society.

CENTRES OFFERING REBIRTHING

Helios N1, Metanoia W5, Primrose Healing Centre NW1, Rebirthing Centre SW18, Sunra SW12, Violet Hill Studios NW8, Women and Health NW1.

TRAINING IN REBIRTHING

Loving Relationships Refer to organisers

Relaxation Training

Relaxation training is a method of inducing in the client the relaxation response. The relaxation response was identified by Wallace and Benson as a decrease in blood pressure, respiratory and heart rate and an increase in alpha and theta brainwaves and skin resistance. These physiological changes correspond to a state of calm and well being. There are a variety of approaches which bring about the relaxation response, such as biofeedback, autogenic training, hypnosis, tai chi, yoga and some forms of meditation, all of which are covered elsewhere in this book. There is another method, however, which is to systematically tense and let go of various muscles in the body to achieve a state of reduced tension, which is the main focus here. This method of progressive relaxation was developed by Jacobson.

Relaxation training takes place in quiet surroundings with the client in a rested position. The client is asked to focus on relaxing the muscles one by one, usually starting from the feet. First the client is asked to tense a foot and then relax it, and to notice the difference between the foot when it is tense and when it is relaxed. This tensing and relaxing is done systematically throughout the muscles of the body. At times the client will be directed to focus on parts that have been tensed and relaxed, such as the right hand side of the body and asked how this compares with the left hand side of the body which has not yet undergone the process. By comparing differences the client is helped to gain awareness of muscular tension and how to relax all of the muscles throughout the body. The client may be asked to practise at home and supplied with an instruction led audio tape as an aid.

Relaxation training was incorporated into behaviour therapy when Joseph Wolpe adopted it to help hypertense people relax. It has also been used for helping people suffering from anxiety. On its own, the relaxation response will help reduce anxiety, but will not effectively help in situations which provoke anxiety unless it is used within a programme of desensitisation or another psychotherapy.

Relaxation training is something that can be learned quite quickly so that one can practise it on one's own. It is possible to learn from audio tapes alone and there are an abundance of such tapes on the market.

As mentioned above, there are many techniques for inducing the relaxation response, relaxation training being only one of them. It does not suit everyone and there are a significant number of people who find, for one reason or another, that they cannot learn the relaxation response. Some people even have an aversion to it, and are therefore advised to try a different approach entirely.

Courses offering relaxation may provide one of the approaches listed above or the one focused on here, or a combination of these.

READING

The Relaxation Response by Benson, H., Fontana 1977 £2.95. A description of relaxation response discovered by the author, and an outline of techniques and exercises to develop it for oneself. You Must Relax by Jacobson, E., Unwin 1975, £3.95. A popular introduction to his work, outlining the dangers of tension and its effects on oneself and society, followed by a 'manual' of techniques in Progressive Relaxation.

CENTRES OFFERING RELAXATION TRAINING

Alternative Medicine Clinic NW15, Alternative Therapies Centre N16, Belgravia Beauty SW1X, Biomonitors, Centre for Personal & Professional Development N17, Changes NW3, Clapham Common Clinic SW4, College of Healing WR14, Equilibrium Therapy Centre SW18, Green Wood College W6, Hampstead Healing Centre NW3, Hayes Hypnotherapy Centre UB4, Heath Health Care NW3, Kando Studios NW6, Life Resources NW7, London Focusing Centre SW4, London Lighthouse W11, Neal's Yard Therapy Rooms WC2H, Pearl Healing Centre CR7, Ravenscroft Centre NW11, Satyananda Yoga Centre, Skills with People N5, South London Natural Health Centre SW4, St James Centre for Health and Healing W1V, Sunra SW12, Violet Hill Studios NW8, Women and Health NW1.

TRAINING IN RELAXATION

Alternative Medicine Clinic Title of Training: Training for Carers and Professionals. Duration: Part time and full time. Fees: Vary.

Sex Therapy

This is a short term therapy designed to help couples who are suffering from a range of sexual difficulties including premature ejaculation, impotency, vaginismus (an involuntary spasm of the vaginal muscles which makes penetration impossible), non-ejaculation and orgasmic problems. As it is a therapy for couples it could be considered part of family or couple therapy with a specific issue in focus, though due to the work of Masters and Johnson it has grown into a therapy in its own right.

Usually, though not always, a male and female therapist work with the couple. The couple are asked to give their medical history so that any organic reasons for the sexual problem can be eliminated. After some discussion about the nature of the problem the couple are asked to follow homework assignments. The first stage is often an exercise called 'sensate focus' where the couple are asked to touch each other and to communicate to each other how it feels and what is, or is not, pleasurable. They are asked to abstain from sexual intercourse and genital and breast touching is usually forbidden. In the second stage breast and genital touching is allowed but intercourse and orgasm are not. The path of the third stage depends on the presenting problem. For instance, if the couple is a heterosexual one and impotence is the problem, the woman is taught how to manipulate the penis in specific ways and she is instructed to insert the penis into the vagina, thus relieving the man of the responsibility. However, many sex therapists nowadays do not adhere any more to such a 'performance orientated' programme, and find it more important to help couples relieve the pressures that are caused by the performance orientation in their sex lives.

It is not necessary to go along with a partner at first to receive sex therapy. Some people prefer to go on their own to build up confidence before they talk with their partner.

For sex therapy to be effective the couple should still be able to communicate with each other and it works best if there is a specific behavioural problem with sex, such as one of those listed above. In fact there can be a great deal of overlap between sex, couple and family therapy. There may be other attitudes, problems or conflicts at the root of the difficulties and in this case couple or family therapy might be more suitable. If there is still love between the couple and a mutual desire to work on the problem then sex therapy has a good success rate.

READING

Sex Therapy in Britain by *Cole M. and Dryden, W. (Eds)* . Another textbook giving articles by leading practitioners on various approaches to, and themes in, sex therapy. Quite a heavy read. Before taking the plunge into therapy, you may want to look at the many self-help books on the market, for instance, **Treat Youself to Sex** by *Brown and Faulder, Penguin 1977* or **Sex Problems; Questions and Answers** by *Cole and Dryden, Optima 1989.*

CENTRES OFFERING SEX THERAPY

Alternative Therapies Centre N16, Centre for Personal & Professional Development N17, Chinese Clinic W1V, Clapham Common Clinic SW4, Equilibrium Therapy Centre SW18, Healing Centre NW5, Identity Counselling Service NW1, London Institute for the Study of Human Sexuality SW5, London Institute for the Study of Human Sexuality SW5, Neal's Yard Therapy Rooms WC2H, North London Counselling Practice NW11, Pearl Healing Centre CR7, Redwood Women's Training Association M24, South London Natural Health Centre SW4, Spectrum N4, Welbeck Counselling Service W1N, Women and Health NW1.

TRAININGS IN SEX THERAPY

London Institute for the Study of Human Sexuality *Title of Training:* Training to Certificate and Diploma Level. Course takes the form of 5 modules: (1) Basic counselling skills (2) Human sexuality (3) AIDS counselling (4) Sex education (5) Sex therapy. Certificate is awarded on satisfactory completion of (1) *Fees:* Refer to organisers

Stress Management

Two researchers, Rosenman and Friedman, found that people could be divided into two categories which they called 'A' and 'B'. 'Type A' people tend to suffer from hurry-up sickness; they are aggressive, have difficulty relaxing, have few friends and tend to be workaholics. 'Type B' have opposite characteristics. 'Type A' people have a tendency to develop hypertension, heart problems, stomach aches, ulcers, diabetes and alcoholism. It is the 'Type A' person who may want to consider participating in a stress management programme.

The treatment programme is holistic and many techniques such as hypnosis, biofeedback, behaviour therapy and massage are combined with information on diet and exercise. It also employs 'cognitive restructuring' which is a means of teaching clients new ways of interpreting what they themselves and others do or say. These individual and often habitual interpretations are an important aspect of the 'stress response' in that they determine a person's stress related behaviour.

Practitioners vary in the emphasis they place on the above treatments. Some put physical exercise above all else and some see cognitive restructuring as more important, so it is worth seeing details of the programme before opting for this type of therapy to see if it suits your needs.

Many stress management consultants teach clients to hypnotise themselves. Some practitioners use relaxation audio tapes and will sell these to you. If biofeedback is taught then technical equipment to monitor physiological activity may to be used to help clients relax more (see Biofeedback).

Stress management is practised in group settings. Programmes tend to be short and deliver a package of treatments for managing stress. For those who wish to delve more deeply into their own psyche and their relationships with others, some of the other therapies mentioned in this book might be preferable.

READING

Stress Management by *Charlesworth, E., Cogi 1989.* Of the many stress books available, this is one of the most comprehensive. The authors look at what stress is physiologically and gives exercises using most relaxation techniques, including progressive relaxation, imagery and visualisation, autogenics and diet. **Guide to Stress Reduction** by *Mason, L.J., Cel. Arts 1985.* A nicely presented collection of stress reduction techniques. Less comprehensive than the above but probably easier to use.

CENTRES OFFERING STRESS MANAGEMENT

Acumedic Centre NW1, All Hallows House EC3R, Alternative Medicine Clinic NW15, Alternative Therapies Centre N16, Awakened Mind NW2, Brackenbury Natural Health Centre W6, Brunel Management Programme UB8, C.H.I Clinic SW6, Centre for Personal & Professional Development N17,

Centre for Stress Management SE3, Changes NW3, Clapham Common Clinic SW4, College of Healing WR14, Equilibrium Therapy Centre SW18, Falcons SW11, Green Wood College W6, Hayes Hypnotherapy Centre UB4, Health Management IG10, Heath Health Care NW3, Helios N1, Homoeopathic Centre W13, Homoeopathic Health Clinic HA3, Human Potential Resource Group GU2, IBISS TW7, Isis Counselling and Therapy Service SW17, Jeyrani Health Centre E18, Kingston Natural Healing Centre, Life Directions W1X, Life Resources NW7, London Focusing Centre SW4, McCarthy Westwood Consultants SW11, Natureworks, Neal's Yard Therapy Rooms WC2H, Pearl Healing Centre CR7, Primrose Healing Centre NW1, Ravenscroft Centre NW11, Sayer Clinic: Chelsea SW6, Silver Birch Centre NW10, Skills with People N5, Sound Health SE8, Spiral W12, St James Centre for Health and Healing W1V, Universitas Associates SM2, Violet Hill Studios NW8, Welbeck Counselling Service W1N, Wholeness E18, Women Unlimited SW16.

TRAINING IN STRESS MANAGEMENT

Centre for Stress Management Refer to organisers

Transactional Analysis

Eric Berne, a Canadian psychoanalyst was the founder of transactional analysis or T.A. as it is also known. As its name indicates, transactional analysis concerns itself with the analysis of transactions, a transaction being a unit of communication. In 1964 Berne wrote the bestseller *Games People Play*, which describes particular ways in which people relate to each other, which he calls 'games'. These are habitual and often destructive with titles like 'Kick Me', 'Wooden Leg' and 'Yes - But'. In his follow-on book, *What Do You Say After You Say Hello?* he develops his original ideas and posits that we live our lives in terms of a 'script'. A script is a life plan which we live out from decisions made in childhood, decisions which we still act upon although we have forgotten about them.

Through learning about the theory of games and scripts it then becomes possible to use these as a map to understand one's own history and one's present way of relating to others.

Part of the initial sessions of most T.A. groups is educational. Clients are taught the language and theory, which is subsequently put to use when analysing a member's behaviour in a group. For example a client may be provoking others in the group to become angry, whilst denying any responsibility for this. The therapist may interpret this behaviour as a game of 'Kick Me', a masochistic game of manipulating others into a persecutory role, so that the 'victim' can cry 'why does it always happen to me'. Further analysis might follow as to why certain people chose to take on the persecutory role.

T.A. provides a set of theories with which clients can see life and relational patterns more clearly. Once understood, the original decisions upon which these patterns are based can be changed, and as a result of this, the client's behaviour can then become more appropriate.

T.A. provides a palatable and often amusing jargon. Unlike most therapies which keep the theoretical jargon out of the consulting room, T.A. employs it as part of the process of understanding.

READING

What Do You Say After You Say Hello? by Berne, E., Corgi 1975. Probably a better place to start looking at Berne's ideas than **Games People Play.** It oulines the principles of TA and covers many of the developments of his ideas including the 'script theory'. **TA Today** by Stewart, I. and Joines, V., Lifespace 1986. Subtitled A New Introduction to T.A., this is a comprehensive textbook of the theory and practice of T.A. Widely recommended to clients by most TA practitioners and the obvious work to refer to understand how T.A. could work for you.

CENTRES OFFERING TRANSACTIONAL ANALYSIS

Heron Training Workshops, Lifespace Associates SW7, Lilly Stuart Resource Development Consultants SE7, Metanoia, Minster Centre NW2, Open Centre EC1.

TRAININGS IN TRANSACTIONAL ANALYSIS

Metanoia W.

Transpersonal Psychotherapy

The term 'transpersonal psychotherapy' covers a wide area, and can be used to describe Jung's analytical psychology and psychosynthesis (qv). It emphasises the spiritual aspect of people's experience, and the search for meaning. It has its roots in both eastern and western religious traditions on the one hand, and in Abraham Maslow's work on peak experience and the psychology of what he called 'self actualising' people on the other.

A key concept in transpersonal psychology is the belief that the central organising principle of the individual's life is the 'self'. The 'self' goes beyond the personal sense of I or ego, and is seen to include this personal sense with an awareness of the collective and universal. This self is also sometimes called 'soul' in transpersonal therapy. The self is seen to unit the different parts of the personality in an experience of wholeness.

Myth and archetypes are used to connect the individual with the collective and historical search of the human race for meaning. Crises are not seen as 'illness' or even 'problems' but rather as part of the process of the individual becoming more aware. Dreamwork, symbols, guided imagery, fantasy and meditation are used in sessions, as well as more extroverted methods of gestalt dialoguing with empty chairs, dialogue between the client and a part of themselves. The therapist may also make use of the 'Chakras' model. The chakras are the eight energy centres of the body according to Indian philosophy, which are situated at various points from the base of the spine to the top of the head. Work here may include for instance visualising an energy blockage at a particular chakra, and exploring what it means in terms of the client's life. Astrology may also be used to clarify the life events of the client.

CENTRES OFFERING TRANSPERSONAL PSYCHOLOGY

Association of Independant Psychotherapists N6, Centre for Counselling and Psychotherapy Education W11, Centre for Personal & Professional Development N17, Centre for Transpersonal Psychology W2, Dancing on the Path, Hampstead Healing Centre NW3, London Focusing Centre SW4, Studio E NW6, Violet Hill Studios NW8.

TRAINING IN TRANSPERSONAL PSYCHOLOGY
Centre for Transpersonal Psychology *Title of Training:* Refer to organisers for details. *Fees:* Refer to organisers

OTHER PSYCHOTHERAPIES

Adlerian
Adlerian Society for Individual Psychology SE7, Centre for Personal & Professional Development N17.

Anti-smoking Therapy
Alternative Medicine Clinic NW15, Alternative Therapies Centre N16, Cabot Centre NW1, Capital Hypnotherapy Centre W6, Changes NW3, Clapham Common Clinic SW4, Edgware Centre for Natural Health HA8, Equilibrium Therapy Centre SW18, Hayes Hypnotherapy Centre UB4, Heath Health Care NW3, Hong Tao Acupuncture and Natural Health Clinic HA5, Islington Green Centre of Alternative Medicine N1, Neal's Yard Therapy Rooms WC2H, Psychotherapy Centre W1H, South London Natural Health Centre SW4, Violet Hill Studios NW8, Women and Health NW1.

Bereavement Counselling
Alternative Therapies Centre N16, Bereavement and Loss Workshops N15, Bodywise E2, British Association for Social Psychiatry, Centre for Personal & Professional Development N17, Changes NW3, Clapham Common Clinic SW4, College of Psychic Studies SW7, Equilibrium Therapy Centre SW18, Hampstead Healing Centre NW3, Hayes Hypnotherapy Centre UB4, Healing Centre NW5, Heath Health Care NW3, London Lighthouse W11, Natural Death Centre NW2, Neal's Yard Therapy Rooms WC2H, North London Counselling Practice NW11, Pearl Healing Centre CR7, Refuah Shelaymah Natural Health Centre N16, Skills with People N5, Sound Health SE8, South London Natural Health Centre SW4, Trinity Hospice SW4, Violet Hill Studios NW8, Westminster Pastoral Foundation W8, Women and Health NW1, Women Unlimited SW16.

Biosynthesis
Open Centre EC1V.

Child psychotherapy
Anna Freud Centre NW3, British Association of Psychotherapists NW2, Centre for Personal & Professional Development N17, Children's Hours Trust N7, Healing Centre NW5, Heath Health Care NW3, Homoeopathic Health Clinic HA3, Institute of Group Analysis NW3, Women and Health NW1.

Creativity

Arts Psychology Consultants W14, Changes NW3, Circle of Creative Arts Therapy N8, Cortijo Romero UK LS7, Human Potential Resource Group GU2, IBISS TW7, Institute for Social Inventions NW2, Kando Studios NW6, London Focusing Centre SW4, Open Gate, Ravenscroft Centre NW11, Technologies for Creating N5, Tobias School of Art RH19, Universitas Associates SM2, Violet Hill Studios NW8.

Drama Therapy

Cabot Centre NW1, London Lighthouse W11, Women and Health NW1.

Dream Therapy

Abraxas W2, Art of Dream Fulfilment N16, Astro-Psychotherapeutic Practice W3, Cabot Centre NW1, Centre for Personal & Professional Development N17, Hampstead Healing Centre NW3, Healing Voice TW10, Imprint SW19, London Focusing Centre SW4, Pearl Healing Centre CR7, Playspace NW1.

Eating Problems

Alternative Medicine Clinic NW15, Alternative Therapies Centre N16, British Association of Psychotherapists NW2, Cabot Centre NW1, Centre for Personal & Professional Development N17, Changes NW3, Clapham Common Clinic SW4, College of Psychic Studies SW7, Edgware Centre for Natural Health HA8, Equilibrium Therapy Centre SW18, Gestalt Centre London EC1Y, Hayes Hypnotherapy Centre UB4, Heath Health Care NW3, Homoeopathic Health Clinic HA3, Neal's Yard Therapy Rooms WC2H, Pearl Healing Centre CR7, South London Natural Health Centre SW4, Violet Hill Studios NW8, Women and Health NW1, Women's Therapy Centre N7.

Enlightenment Intensive

Healing Centre NW5, Helios N1, Holistic Yoga Centre MK19.

Integrative Psychotherapy

Astro-Psychotherapeutic Practice W3, Cabot Centre NW1, Centre for Personal & Professional Development N17, Clapham Common Clinic SW4, Health Connection SW17, Heath Health Care NW3, Inner Track Learning GL7, Insight W2, Isis Counselling and Therapy Service SW17, London Focusing Centre SW4, Maskarray E3, Metanoia W5, Minster Centre NW2, Nafsiyat Inter-Cultural Therapy Centre N4, Open Centre EC1V, Pan Academy SW19, Photo-Language Workshop, Playworld, Re-Vision NW2, Social Effectiveness Training NW4, Sound Health SE8, Swedenborg Movement BR6, Universal Training RH2, Violet Hill Studios NW8, Workshops with a Difference TW2.

Management

Brunel Management Programme UB8, Human Potential Resource Group GU2, Life Directions W1X.

Music therapy

Centre for Health and Healing W1V, Healing Voice TW10, Institute For Arts In Therapy & Education N16, London Lighthouse W11, Mu Sum Ba - Living Rhythm BN27, Nordoff-Robbins Music Therapy Centre NW5, Pearl Healing Centre CR7, Refuah Shelaymah Natural Health Centre N16.

Regression

Alternative Medicine Clinic NW15, Alternative Therapies Centre N16, Bexleyheath Natural Health Clinic DA7, Centre for Past Life Healing NW1, Centre for Personal & Professional Development N17, Equilibrium Therapy Centre SW18, Hayes Hypnotherapy Centre UB4, Helios N1, Pearl Healing Centre CR7, South London Natural Health Centre SW4.

Reichian Therapy

Centre for Personal & Professional Development N17, Healing Centre NW5, Open Centre EC1V.

Resonance Therapy

Abshot Holistic Centre PO14, Healing Voice TW10, Open Gate .

OTHER TRAININGS

Drama Therapy

Hertfordshire College of Art and Design Refer to organisers

Roehampton Institute of Higher Education *Title of Training:* Certificate in Dramatherapy. *Duration:* 20 weeks part time. *Entry requirements:* Appropriate professional qualifications or experience and/or appropriate first degree. *Fees:* Refer to organisers *Comments:* This programme, run in conjunction with the Institute of Dramatherapy introduces students to the theory and practice of dramatherapy and play therapy.

Integrative Psychotherapy

Association for Analystic and Bodymind Therapy and Training *Title of Training:* Diploma in Psychotherapy *Duration:* 2 years: one evening per week, weekend larger group training, six-day intensive training, residential in Cornwall. *Entry requirements:* Must have completed 2-year (minimum) therapy to satisfaction of both therapist and client, or be in ongoing therpy, or be willing to run therapy concurrently with course. Degree an advantage, but not essential. *Fees:* Refer to organisers *Comments:* Training groups is kept small and intimate (maximum 10). Includes interpretation of group dynamic, gestalt therapy, hypnotherapy, relaxation techniques, therapeutic holding, regression therapy etc.

Chiron Centre for Holistic Psychotherapy *Title of Training:* Chiron Holistic Psychotherapy (Body Psychotherapy) 1) Basic Training 2) Diploma Phase *Duration:* 1) 3 years part time 2) 2 years part time *Entry requirements:* Detailed application form and assessment interview. Previous therapeutic experiences, i.e., individual/group theray), life experience, emotional maturity, intellectual capacity, experience working with people. *Fees:* Refer to organisers *Comments:* Teaching predominantly based on experiential learning. Main theoretical orientation is a combination of body concepts (Neo Reichian) and Gestalt philosophy. Chiron is a member of the United Kingdom Standing Conference for Psychotherapy (UKSCP).

Creative Arts and Therapy Consultants *Title of Training:* Diploma in Integrative Arts Psychotherapy *Duration:* 3 years part time. 1 day a week, 6 weekends a year. *Entry requirements:* Graduate status and/or qualification in and work experience in helping profession. Active interest in the arts. The Institutes certificate in Art Therapy or similar. Must have completed at least one year in personal therapy and agree to undergo therapy and supervision throughout the training. *Fees:* Refer to organisers *Comments:* The course is divided into 3 levels. Entry may be gained at any level, according to qualifications and clinical experience as a therapist. Ideally suited to those already working in counselling, social work, nursing, teaching, youth work, theatre and similar fields. Course content is 80% practical and 20% theoretical incorporating in-depth study into Psychology of Art.

Living Art Training *Title of Training:* The Living Art Training *Duration:* One year part-time of twelve weekends and a week in the country. *Entry requirements:* Application can only be made after taking a living art seminar weekend, and having a private interview. *Fees:* Refer to organisers *Comments:* No art experience necessary.

Minster Centre *Title of Training:* Diplomas in Integrative Psychotherapy and Counselling. *Duration:* Four to five years part-time. 7-9 hours per week. *Entry requirements:* First degree in any subject; non-degree training (eg. in social work or health care); suitable and equivalent life experience. *Fees:* Approx. £2000 per annum. *Comments:* Personal therapy required. Intake every September. Diplomas are BAC recognised. The training focuses on integration and helping students to develop a personal style.

Serpent Institute *Title of Training:* (1) Diploma course in counselling (2) Diploma course in psychotherapy. *Duration:* (1) Two years (2) Three years. *Entry requirements:* Acceptance for the course is based on the applicant's readiness and own self development as well as ability and commitment. *Fees:* Refer to organisers

Comments: Theoretical framework is Goddess spirituality - the valuing of the feminine principle within everyone. Training is for both sexes, with some single sex opportunities within it.

Spectrum *Title of Training:* 2) 1st and 2nd year psychotherapy course. *Duration:* 2) Two residentials, one day per fortnight plus 3 weekends over a year. *Entry requirements:* Individual. *Fees:* Refer to organisers

Monkton Wyld Court *Title of Training:* Art of Loving *Duration:* One year. One weekend per month plus 5 day residential. Entry requirements: Completion of a questionnaire. *Fees:* £900.00. *Comments:* Relationship skills exploration, held in a community based centre in Dorset. Possible to commute from London to this retreat in the country.

Centre of Integral Psychoanalysis *Title of Training:* ABC of Analytical Triology - Integral Psychoanalysis. *Duration:* 10 weeks with 2 classes per week of hone hour each. Some weekends. *Entry requirements:* None. Open to general public and specialised professionals such as nurses, teachers and therapists. *Fees:* Refer to organisers *Comments:* Although it is a short course, content is enriching and can immediately be applied with practical and effective results. 'Integral Psychoanalysis is recognised internationally as the 21st century therapy'.

CAER (Centre For Alternative Education And Research) *Title of Training:* Institute for the Development of human Potential (IDHP) Diploma in Human Development and Facilitation Skills *Duration:* Two years part time with an introductory 6 month Foundation Course. *Entry requirements:* Post graduate or significant personal development experience, or professional experience. *Fees:* Refer to organisers *Comments:* The IDHP Diploma is the only residential one currently offered. It has a significant transpersonal element and draws on the benefits of the environment. The Diploma course runs annually and was the first course in Humanistic Psychology in Europe.

Metanoia *Title of Training:* Integrative Psychotherapy Training. *Duration:* Three year part-time. Ten weekends approx once a month. Commences September every year. *Entry requirements:* Individually assessed. *Fees:* £850 p.a. approx. *Comments:* Psychoanalytic, humanistic and cognitive behavioural components.

Centre for Personal & Professional Development *Title of Training:* PG Diploma and MSc in Psychotherapy or Psychosexual Therapy. *Duration:* 2 years part-time, 1 day per week, two semesters per year. Approx 90 hrs contact per semester + 150 hrs study. *Entry requirements:* 1) First degree or professional qualification AND 2) 120 hours counselling or psychotherapy training. *Fees:* Approx. £2000 p.a. and supervision. *Comments:* Intake annually each Autumn. Next intake September-December '94. It combines a wide range of Humanistic Psychotherapy (e.g Gestalt, Bioenergetics, Systemic etc) with Sexuality and Gender Studies. Training in Forensic Psychotherapy. The training may include work in Psychosexual Clinic.

Pan Academy *Title of Training:* PanLife Training *Comments:* A course for social and global pioneers. The PanLife training is designed to help you develop yourself and your project to the maximum potential.

Mind Clearing

Holistic Yoga Centre *Title of Training:* Mind Clearing Training Training to run Enlightenment Intensives *Duration:* Mind Clearing Training is part time over a period of four months. Enlightenment Training is a ten day residential course. *Entry requirements:* To join the mind clearing training courses, must have received at least 40 hours clearing. For the Enlightenment Masters course, must have completed a three day intensive course. *Fees:* £600 for Mind Clearing, £400 for Enlightenment training. *Comments:* Apply for details as the couses are run infrequently. The courses are based on the work of Charles Berner.

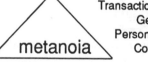

INTRODUCTION TO BODY THERAPIES

It could be said that in the twentieth century western world we have a curious and often paradoxical relationship with our bodies. While many are no longer dependent on hard manual labour to earn their living, most of us spend our working lives sitting in offices using only our heads or performing repetitive manual tasks which impose a strain on the body, while the rest of our way of life also offers little in the way of creative physical expression. Cars and public transport, while greatly convenient have obviated the need to walk anywhere. In the big cities, especially London, we usually live crammed together and have little more than the prospect of a Sunday afternoon walk in the park with the hundreds of other people looking for a dose of nature in the urban jungle.

Though a modern city lifestyle seems to offer little opportunity for us to express natural physical energy, paradoxically our culture also seems to be very concerned with the body in some ways. We are surrounded with images of fitness and beauty on billboards, TV and in films giving impressions of how our bodies ought to look. The 99% of us whose bodies don't measure up to this fantasy ideal may end up feeling self-conscious or dissatisfied with our physique. This pressure to focus on how the body looks from the outside can also leave us out of touch with how it feels from inside and from an immediate experience of our physical self expressing itself in its own unique way.

Western philosophy has tended to see mind and body as separate and science too has played its part in fostering the idea that our bodies are somehow different from our real selves. Modern medicine tends to treat the body in this way and on the whole deals with it as a machine, replacing defective parts if they malfunction, or readjusting the body with drugs and other chemicals, sometimes without much sense that the physical level might be connected with other levels of experience - emotional, mental or spiritual.

We have a long life expectancy now in the modern west, due largely to improved sanitation and nutrition. But we still fear the spectre of disease as much as ever. Perhaps more because most people living in this secular, semi-atheistic culture have little belief in the prospect of an after-life. So with little prospect of a hereafter, most people are even more anxious to conserve the life they have in the here now. Modern medicine has made advances particularly in the areas of surgery, vaccination and medicines. However, we are becoming increasingly dependant on modern medicine and drugs to cure quite common or relatively minor complaints. Modern drug therapy can be like using a hammer to crack a nut. By continual increasing reliance on this powerful method of disease control, we are in danger of upsetting the natural powers which the body has to cure itself. The more we rely on intervention from outside, the more we are in danger of losing our own innate power to heal ourselves, and others.

Alternative and Complementary Medicine

Not all the therapies and practices dealt with in the 'Body' section of this book come under the banner of 'Alternative Medicine'. For instance, the Alexander

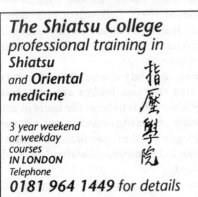

technique is an educational method which seeks to teach people to use their bodies in a more natural way, and to regain a freedom of movement which may have been lost. Similarly tai chi, which is a system of physical movements, is very much part of a wider philosophical and spiritual system and outlook. The title 'Body' is intended as very broad, and we have used it to include all approaches - therapeutic, educational and inspirational - which encompass the whole person through the medium of the body.

In the ever-growing field of holistic health there is still a lot of debate about what these much used words such as 'holistic', 'alternative medicine', 'complementary medicine' and 'natural therapies' mean, and different people define them in different ways. Most practitioners feel that their therapy is not 'alternative' to conventional medicine in the sense that it is a case of 'either/or' - either you go for traditional treatment or you go to a homoeopath - but rather that it broadens the patient's choice about how to get treatment.

The term 'complementary' is now being used more to stress that these natural therapies can be used alongside conventional medicine. 'Complementary'

can also be used in the sense that different natural therapies may be needed to treat one patient and therefore complement each other. Sometimes these complementary therapies are referred to as 'natural' therapies because on the whole they aim to work by co-operating with natural processes, rather than trying to override them as conventional medicine often does.

'Holistic' too seems to be a word which has as many meanings as there are different people using it. One possible definition is that it is an approach which takes into account the whole person, and the whole range of their experience; physical, mental, emotional and spiritual within their whole environment; physical, social and personal.

The Holistic Approach

The holistic approach to health does not just treat symptoms in order to 'get rid' of them. It tries to treat the underlying causes of the symptoms, which may be found in considering the patient's history, lifestyle, relationships, temperament and his or her whole outlook on life. Within the holistic framework, disease is not seen as a matter of chance, or as an affliction which comes purely from outside the body, but more as the whole organism's attempt to reach once again a state of harmony and equilibrium with itself and its environment. An illness, especially a chronic one, can be the body's way of drawing attention to the fact that something needs to change in the sufferer's lifestyle, that he or she may need something they are not getting, that some part of him or her self which was previously unacknowledged is seeking recognition, or it can even be part of an overall point of spiritual crisis or growth, part of a reorientation of life purpose.

An experienced holistic practitioner will look at particular symptoms in any of these contexts as appropriate. The holistic approach stresses the responsibility the individual has for his or her own health and well-being. This may mean taking active steps to change the things which cause illness where possible. This is not to say that the patient is in some way to blame for his or her malaise, but that we have the power to cure ourselves, or at least to change our attitude to

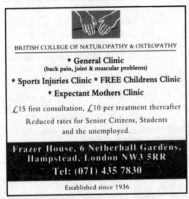

our disease. Alternative medicine offers the opportunity to co-operate with the processes by which the body heals itself.

The core of the holistic approach is that it sees all aspects of the human being as connected and interrelated: body, mind, emotions and spirit.

Diagnosis

Most people turn to complementary medicine when conventional medicine has failed to cure them, or offers no treatment. It is often stubborn, chronic conditions such as backache, migraines, asthma, menstrual problems, insomnia, arthritis or chronic indigestion with which the practitioner is presented.

Alternative therapies have their own methods of diagnosis - an acupuncturist will take your pulses, an osteopath will examine your spine, and a shiatsu practitioner will feel your abdomen. There are also specific forms of alternative diagnosis which you may want to try if you want more information. Iridology examines the eyes for signs of physical weakness and Kirlian photography shows the electrical field round the body and in this way detects early signs of illness. These alternative diagnostic methods can be most useful in helping people to develop a more positive and balanced attitude towards their bodies, thus preventing illnesses.

Most forms of diagnosis in complementary therapies are non-invasive; they do not probe into the body but are carried out by observing the signs given by the body.

Choosing a Particular Therapy

So how to choose the approach which will be most effective for you? It is easy to feel bemused by all the therapies on offer. Most people choose either by having a particular therapy recommended to them by a friend, or by reading something about a therapy and feeling attracted to that particular approach. With the descriptions of the therapies in this book, we offer some guidelines about the kinds of ailment they may deal with best. However, it is by no means obvious that if you have a bad back you should visit an osteopath, although this may be a good start. The pain in your back could also be due to other physical or psychological problems.

Reading about the different therapies can give you a good lead. Then, follow your instincts. If you feel interested in a particular therapy or don't like the sound of another you probably do have a real sense of what might or might not be helpful for you. It must also be stressed that if you have not already done so, you should always consult your doctor if you have any troublesome symptoms, just to be sure that your complaint is not one which would be better treated by modern medicine. You may also think of discussing any alternative treatment with your doctor, who is hopefully understanding and not totally dismissive of alternative medicine. There are some contra-indications for particular natural therapies. For instance, shiatsu is not recommended for people with cancer, because the stimulation of the metabolism can spread the cancer cells throughout the body. In pregnancy care should be taken with some of the therapies listed here. Once again, your doctor can give advice, and the complementary therapy practitioner needs to be informed of the full details of your condition.

Some of the centres listed in this book which offer more than one therapy give advice on which one would be most effective. Practitioners should tell you if they think that their form of therapy is not appropriate for your symptoms, or may even suggest another form. However, it must be stressed that what works for one person will not necessarily work for another, even if they have the same complaint. Some are now offering consultations specifically to help people choose.

Finding the Right Practitioner

At present there is no law in the U.K. which stipulates that a practitioner of alternative therapies must have reached an agreed standard and must be registered. Complete quackery is not so much the problem - there are probably

 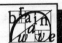

few people with no qualifications who set themselves up to treat people. However, although a practitioner may seem to be qualified, there is little way of knowing whether their qualification has demanded that they undertake the necessary study and experience to make them effective. In this sense, letters after the name are no guarantee of good service!

For osteopaths, medical herbalists and chiropractors there are registers compiled by governing bodies, and you can write off for registers of members to be sure of getting a well-qualified practitioner. If in doubt about practitioners of other therapies it may be as well to ask about their training - how long it was, how intensive, how much experience they had and also if they are insured, so that if anything does go wrong, at least you have the chance of a successful comeback.

There is of course also the question of rapport. It is important that you trust the practitioner and feel able to talk to him or her. If you feel uncomfortable with a therapist and this fails to change, it might be best to try another one who you feel more able to get on with. You might also like to consider whether the sex of the practitioner matters to you. Some people find it easier to talk about their health problems with someone of the same sex, and some with members of the opposite sex. Again, follow your gut feeling in this, and don't be afraid to ask for the practitioner you want.

Length and cost of treatment

There is no way of saying how long you may have to persevere with any particular treatment. This all depends on the kind of illness you have, the seriousness of the condition, how long you have had it, whether and how well you may be able to change any of the conditions which may be contributing to it and many other factors. If you are worried about how long it make take (and consequently how much you may have to pay) ask the practitioner after the initial session if they can give you any idea of how many sessions you will need.

Few practitioners are so hard up for patients that they will string out a treatment longer than necessary. Similarly, if at any time you feel you are getting nowhere and want to try another therapy, talk with the practitioner about it. They may also be able to throw some light on a new approach, or be able to explain why the treatment does not seem to be having the desired effect.

Cost too is variable, depending on the experience of the practitioner, and sometimes where he or she practises. Initial consultations usually cost more and last longer for homoeopathy, acupuncture and osteopathy because the practitioner will have to take some time to make the diagnosis. A few practitioners will give discounts for the unwaged. Some training institutes of body therapies such as massage and Alexander technique offer sessions given by trainees at a cheap rate. Homoeopathy is available on the National Health Service at the Royal Homoeopathic Hospital, and there are some homoeopathic GPs, though many of these work in the private sector and therefore charge for treatment. While finding the money for the cost of these treatments may be quite a problem for the low waged, we include details of centres which do offer lower rates for cases of hardship.

What the Centres are Like

Centres vary enormously. Some are really people's homes where perhaps a couple of people practice. Others may be rented rooms, and some are large, permanent buildings which may include restaurants and bookshops. Appointments are always necessary, although some centres run an emergency service or acute clinic. Even if they do, it is advisable to ring beforehand. Some centres have secretaries or receptionists who are always by the telephone to take your call, others make do with an answerphone.

Finding Practitioners Outside the Centres

If for any reason you want to find a practitioner who does not work in a centre there are several ways in which this can be done. Some training institutes or governing bodies provide registers of qualified practitioners. We list these after each therapy with 'register' after their name, rather than a postcode. In this way you can at least be sure that the therapist is qualified. You can telephone the training institute in question and ask them about the length and thoroughness of their training before you ask for the register. Some practitioners are listed in the local Yellow Pages. Local health food shops, community centres, specialist bookshops or wholefood restaurants sometimes have practitioners' cards on noticeboards, though you may have to check their qualifications for yourself in this case. There are also some directories available which list practitioners who advertise in them.

Another way of finding a practitioner is to apply to the Institute of Complementary Medicine, who run a referral service for the general public and the British Register of Complementary Practitioners, which is now recognised by the government. They can give you the names of practitioners of a particular therapy in your area. However they are not allowed to recommend a particular therapy for a particular complaint.

TRAINING IN BODY THERAPIES

Why Train?

Alternative and Complementary Medicine is a growing concern. The number of people who are consulting practitioners of the natural therapies is increasing every year. At the moment, there are hardly enough practitioners to meet this demand, and most good practitioners are extremely busy. Healing people in this way can of course be tremendously satisfying, and it is also a great responsibility. The training can be long and expensive, but most people who really feel motivated to undertake a course find the time and money in some way.

Before you start training, it is helpful to decide what level of skill you want in your chosen therapy. There are three different levels of expertise.

(1) Awareness of the principles, and to a certain extent the practice of a particular therapy, to a level where one can practice it on oneself. The degree to which one can do this depends very much on the therapy in question. For instance, Bach flower remedies can be self-applied very successfully, but osteopathy is not suitable for self-treatment.

(2) Application of the principles and practice to friends and relatives. This requires more skill and training, and though it may give a great deal of satisfaction, will probably not involve any financial reward.

(3) Treatment of members of the public. To do this, a practitioner needs insurance and preferably the protection of a governing body, if there is one for their particular therapy.

It is a good idea to ask yourself what level of training you really want. You may decide that (1) is a good place to start, and to that end you may then choose a less intensive, introductory course. If you want to train to treat the general public, then this is a much more serious undertaking. It is certainly makes sense to find out as much as you possibly can about the therapy you are thinking of training in. It is not unknown for people to discover at the end of a three year course that they do not want to practice that therapy.

Finding the Right Course

There are many different courses around, and they vary a great deal in terms of time commitment, teaching methods and cost. What constitutes a satisfactory course varies enormously from therapy to therapy. Before enrolling for any course, it is advisable to shop around and this will give you an idea of what the norm is for training in your chosen therapy. A shorter, cheaper course may seem more attractive in some ways than a lengthy intensive course, but it may not provide you with the skills and experience you need to practice successfully and well. Though it is difficult to make hard and fast rules because different therapies require different levels of knowledge and experience, there are some guidelines when looking at trainings.

(1) How long has the training institute been established? What kind of experience do the teachers have?

(2) On completion of training, will you be eligible for membership of a professional association which has its own register, code of ethics and disciplinary procedures? Homoeopathy, acupuncture, chiropractic, osteopathy, naturopathy, medical herbalism, reflexology, Alexander technique, polarity therapy and aromatherapy all have professional bodies to which qualified practitioners may belong. With other therapies this is not the case however, and so this criterion cannot be applied.

(3) How much home study is required? How much clinical training will you get? Will you receive thorough tuition in the philosophy and theory of the discipline? There should be a good deal of all of these elements.

(4) What kind of teaching facilities does the training institute have?

(5) Is the personal development of the trainee taken into account? To be able to help other people some measure of self knowledge and stability is necessary.

(6) For courses in homoeopathy, chiropractic, acupuncture and medical herbalism there should be a great deal of time devoted to the study of anatomy and physiology.

(7) Look carefully at the amount of tuition time given. It may seem that the course is long and takes place over a year or two, but if it is taught over weekends at six monthly intervals the actual time you are going to get being taught may be very little.

The Institute of Complementary Medicine offers a list of courses which they think provide a satisfactory training to those thinking of studying a particular therapy. Of course, if you simply want to learn about a therapy out of interest, or to practise on your family and friends in a modest way, the correspondence course or low time commitment course may be just what you want. However, if you are intending to treat the public the above are important considerations.

Entry Requirements

Once again, entry requirements vary enormously from college to college and therapy to therapy. For some courses, notably some of those in homoeopathy and acupuncture, training in orthodox medicine is required. Some require that applicants are medical doctors, or at least that they have been trained in nursing, or in one of the paramedical professions. For courses in reflexology, aromatherapy, massage and Alexander technique there are often no formal educational requirements, and the personal qualities and suitability of the applicant will form the basis for selection.

In general to become an effective practitioner in a natural therapy, you will need a genuine desire to help people, a certain amount of sensitivity and a lot of stamina to cope with the physical and emotional demands of healing.

Getting Clients
Some professional bodies place the same restrictions on advertising as those which govern medical doctors. However, to offset this these bodies will usually have a register of qualified practitioners which is sent out to enquirers. Many people starting out choose to work at a centre through which they can get clients more easily. However, practitioners of natural therapies are in great demand, especially those where the training is long and intensive.

Future Legislation Governing Practitioners - 1996
In Britain at the moment, there is little legislation governing practitioners of alternative and complementary medicine. Due to this we have been able to benefit from the proliferation of these therapies. However, this is not the case in Europe, as each country currently has different laws governing the industry. The increasing power of the European Union is likely to lead to calls for standardisation throughout Europe. This will need complex legislation, including watchdogs, training bodies and associations to represent practitioners. However, the constant growth of the EU is likely to delay the process of legislation for some time to come, as countries continuing to apply for membership of the EU will have yet more views on the industry.

The biggest fear of practitioners, and those wishing to train in a particular therapy, is that they will be excluded from any 'legal' list of practitioners drawn up by the government because they have trained with the wrong organisation, or they belong to the wrong professional body. It is worth remembering when choosing a training course that the more obscure courses may not be included if and when legislation comes.

On the positive side, the next ten years may see more standardisation in

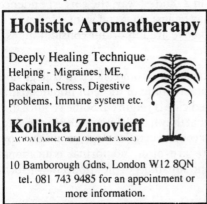
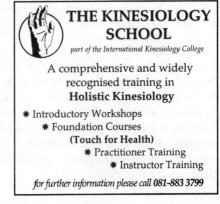

training courses, and a system of accreditation developing. As yet there is some doubt about who is going to be doing the accreditation; whether it will be a government body or a body formed of those within the Alternative and Complementary medical professions. The latter would of course be more acceptable to practitioners.

If you have any doubts about the validity of training courses, or if you would like an update on the legislation, contact the organisations below.

Useful Contacts

Institute for Complementary Medicine, *PO Box 194, London SE16 1QZ. (0171) 237 5165.* Referral service for the public to complementary practitioners, and network of public information points around the country. They run the British Register of Complementary Practitioners, advise on trainings to those thinking of training and publish the Journal of Complementary medicine. The ICM also works in research in several areas of complementary and alternative medicine and is associated with training courses overseas.

British Holistic Medical Association, *Trust House, Royal Shrewsbury Hospital South, Shrewsbury, Shropshire, SY3 8XF. (0743) 261155.* Membership/networking organisation for those interested in promoting holistic approaches to health care. Produce quarterly newsletter and professional journal, organise conferences and workshops. Produce self-help books and tapes and general information about holistic medicine, available mail order. Send SAE for full details. Members receive the qrtly 36-page newsletter *Holistic Health,* get discounts on self-help tapes, books and events and details of regional group activities. Membership for different categories: health care professional, health care student, and open membership for the public. Sliding scale from £15-£45 depending on income.

Council for Complementary and Alternative Medicine *179 Gloucester Place, London NW1 6DX 9 (0171) 724 9103* Set up to provide a forum for communication between professional associations and complementary practitioners.

THE BODY APPROACHES

Acupuncture

Acupuncture is the ancient Chinese healing art which, at least until recently, was the standard form of medical treatment in China. How the system was discovered is unknown, but one theory is that as far back as the stone age healers noticed that small areas of the skin at certain points on the body became sensitive when a particular organ was affected by illness. These areas indicate the acupuncture points of which there are about 800. The points are linked together by their association with a particular organ or function and form pathways or meridians as they are called, through which the life energy or ch'i flows.

The ch'i energy is made up of two forces, *Yang* and *Yin* energy. Yang corresponds to the masculine, positive, active principle and Yin to the feminine, negative, receptive principle. Good health is maintained while these two forces are balanced, and while the energy is flowing freely through the meridians.

The art of the acupuncturist is to restore any imbalances in energy and to unblock the pathways by stimulating the points along them where there may be a blockage. This is done in one of three ways. Usually very fine needles made of silver or stainless steel are inserted a little way into the skin. The needles may be just left there to have their effect, or they may be stimulated by the acupuncturist who may twirl them or push them gently in and out of the point. Sometimes moxa (dried mugwort, a pleasantly aromatic plant) may be burnt over the point, and this is a popular form of self-treatment practised in some countries. Thirdly the points may be massaged or gently scratched with the fingers.

When you visit an acupuncturist for a treatment, he or she will first take a case history of your complaint and will try to build up a picture of any imbalances in energy by asking you about such things as your food preferences, your reactions to heat and cold, and your emotional reactions in certain circumstances. Then they will take your pulses. Although these are taken at the wrist as they are by any ordinary doctor, the acupuncture pulses are a more complex and subtle aid to diagnosis than the one recognised by western medicine. There are six pulses on each wrist, and these are felt with three fingers by the acupuncturist, who will note the quality and relative strength of each one. Having made the diagnosis in this way, the needles will be inserted.

The idea of having needles stuck into your skin may be very alarming, especially if it brings back memories of injections and innoculations! But there is usually no pain involved in the treatment because the needles are very fine and inserted very lightly, usually only a little way into the skin. The needles are

ACUPUNCTURE

sterilised, but since the advent of AIDS many acupuncturists are making extra sure of hygiene by using disposable needles.

The treatment may last from 20 minutes to an hour. After a treatment some people feel relaxed, some elated or as if they are walking on air. Occasionally you may feel worse before you feel better. You will probably need to go for treatment once or twice a week for chronic ailments, and more often for an acute illness. Acupuncture is also very effective if used preventatively. Traditionally, a treatment at the turn of the season will keep your energy balanced and maintain good health.

The effectiveness of acupuncture in relieving pain has been shown rather dramatically by stories of major operations carried out in China using only skilfully applied needles for anaesthesia. These are rather special cases, but acupuncture can be used effectively for relief of less acute pain. While acupuncture can theoretically cure any reversible disease it is best when there is no actual damage to organs or tissues, and especially for chronic conditions which conventional medicine cannot deal with. Complaints such as headaches, toothache and inflamed gums, colds and asthma, digestive disorders, menstrual disorders, obesity, rheumatism and 'nervous' problems can all benefit from treatment.

READING

Alternative Health - Acupuncture by Dr Michael Nightingale, MacDonald £3.95. This consumer's guide to acupuncture concentrates on the actual treatment itself seen from the patient's viewpoint. It answers practical questions about acupuncture as well as providing background information about this popular therapy. The author tries to dispel the concerns of first time patients. **Traditional Acupuncture - the Law of the Five Elements** by Diane Connelly, Centre for Traditional Acupuncture £9.99. Diane Connelly is a qualified acupuncturist and author. This book is primarily intended for students of the discipline. It is also useful for the interested lay person. This book has been popular for the depth and seriousness with which it approaches its subject.

CENTRES OFFERING ACUPUNCTURE

Academy of Systematic Kinesiology KT5, Acumedic Centre NW1, Acupuncture and Osteopathy Clinic SW1V, Acupuncture Clinic of North London, All Hallows House EC3R, Alternative Medicine Clinic NW15, Alternative Therapies Centre N16, Association of Natural Medicines CM8, Bennett & Luck N1, Bexleyheath Natural Health Clinic DA7, Body Clinic NW11, Bodywise E2, Brackenbury Natural Health Centre W6, British Acupuncture Association and Register M33, British College of Acupuncture WC1N, British School of Oriental Therapy and Movement SE21, Bumblebees Natural Remedies N7, Camden Osteopathic and Natural Health Practice NW5, Chelsea Complementary Natural Health Centre SW10, Chinese Clinic W1V, Chung San Acupuncture School W2, City Health Centre EC1Y, Clapham Common Clinic SW4, Clinic of Alternative Therapies E18, Clissold Park Natural Health Centre N16, College of Homoeopathy Clinic SE13, Edgware Centre for Natural Health HA8, Edmonton Acupuncture Clinic N9, Equilibrium Therapy Centre SW18, Faculty of Traditional Chinese Medicine of the UK, Fook Sang Acupuncture and Chinese Herbal Practitioners Training College UK NW11, Forty Hill Natural Therapy Centre, Gerda Boysen Clinic W3, Haelan Centre, Haelen Centre, Hale Clinic W1N, Heath Health Care NW3, Helios N1, Hong Tao Acupuncture and Natural Health Clinic HA5, Insight Care N1, Islington Green Centre of Alternative Medicine N1, Jeyrani Health Centre E18, Kingston Natural Healing Centre, Lever Clinic EN1, Life Works NW1, Living Centre SW20, London Lighthouse W11, London Natural Health Clinic W8, London School of Acupuncture and Traditional Chinese Medicine (Clinic) EC1Y, London School of Acupuncture and Traditional Chinese Medicine EC1Y, Lotus Healing Centre NW8, Natural Healing Centre HA4, Natural Medicine Centre BR2, Nature Cure Clinic W1M, Natureworks, Neal's Yard Therapy Rooms WC2H, New Cross Natural Therapy Centre , Nine Needles Health Care Centre TW9,

Northwood Hills Acupuncture Clinic HA6, Notting Hill Traditional Acupuncture Clinic W11, Portobello Green Fitness Centre W10, Primrose Healing Centre NW1, Private Health Centre E7, Putney Natural Therapy Clinic, Raphael Clinic NW6, Sayer Clinic: Chelsea SW6, Sayer Clinic: Croydon CR0, Silver Birch Centre NW10, South London Natural Health Centre SW4, Southfields Clinic SW18, St James Centre for Health and Healing W1V, Sunra SW12, Traditional Acupuncture Centre SE1, Traditional Chinese Medicine Clinic UB5, Violet Hill Studios NW8, Westminster Natural Health Centre SW1V, Wimbledon Clinic of Natural Medicine SW19, Women and Health NW1, Wood Street Clinic EN5.

TRAINING IN ACUPUNCTURE

British College of Acupuncture *Title of Training:* Postgraduate Training in Acupuncture *Duration:* Three years *Entry requirements:* Applicants should be registered members of one of a number of professions, e.g. doctor, osteopath, naturopath, chiropractor, dental surgeon, vetinary surgeon, physiotherapist, nurse. *Fees:* Refer to organisers

Chung San Acupuncture School *Title of Training:* (1) Training in acupuncture (2) Training in Chinese herbal medicine. *Duration:* (1) Three years part time, weekends. (2) 2 years part time *Entry requirements:* (1) Must have 'A' levels in science subjects. (2) Must have chinese medical background (e.g. qualification in Acupuncture. *Fees:* Refer to organisers

College of Traditional Chinese Acupuncture *Title of Training:* Licentiate in Acupuncture. *Duration*: Three years part time. *Entry requirements:* Minimum 5 GCE 'O' levels/GCSE's and 2 GCE 'A' levels, or equivalent level of general education. Professional qualifications and work experience will be taken into account in considering applications from those not holding the above. *Fees:* Refer to organisers *Comments:* The College specialises in the 5 Element System of Acupuncture. The emphasis of the training is on the development of the practitioner in terms of clinical and personal growth. 4 intakes per year, March and September with a choice of attendance days. 8 year credit system of advanced training for graduates.

Faculty of Traditional Chinese Medicine of the UK Refer to Organisers.

Fook Sang Acupuncture and Chinese Herbal Practitioners Training College UK *Title of Training:* Combined course in Traditional Chinese Medicine, including Genuine Chinese Acupuncture, Chinese Herbal Medicine, Diagnosis. *Duration:* Three years part time, weekend attendance. *Entry requirements:* Minimum 'O' and 'A' levels, or equivalent. Higher Degree being preferable. Ability to work hard is an important quality to be taken into consideration. *Fees:* Refer to organisers *Comments:* Director of Studies and founder of the College, Dr B L K Lee (Canton, China), is internationally experienced Practitioner and Consultant Lecturer on Chinese acupuncture and herbal medicine.

International College of Oriental Medicine *Title of Training:* Acupuncture and Masseur Course. *Duration:* Three years full-time, fourth year part-time. *Entry requirements:* Minimum of 2 'A' levels preferred, but will consider serious applicants individually. *Fees:* Refer to organisers *Comments:* Because this is a full time course it attracts local authority grants.

London School of Acupuncture and Traditional Chinese Medicine (Clinic) *Title of Training:* (1) Full-time course in acupuncture and Traditional Chinese herbal medicine. (2) Full-time course in acupuncture and moxibustion. (3) Postgraduate course in Chinese herbal medicine. *Duration:* (1) Four years (2) Three years (3) Two years *Fees:* Refer to organisers

London College of Chinese and Oriental Medicine *Title of Training:* Training in Chinese Herbal Medicine and Acupuncture. *Duration:* Four years. 48 days per year. 9.30-5pm. *Entry requirements:* The main criteria is an intention to help others. *Fees:* Refer to organisers

Traditional Chinese Medicine Clinic *Title of Training:* Acupuncture and Chinese Herbal Medicine *Duration:* One to two years. *Entry requirements:* Graduate or equivalent in medical or biological science. *Fees:* Refer to organisers

Acupuncture Nine Needles Health Care Centre *Title of Training:* 3 year course in Oriental Medicine including acupuncture, shiatsu, moxibustion, etc. *Duration:* Evenings part-time, three days a week. *Fees:* Refer to organisers

London School of Acupuncture and Traditional Chinese Medicine *Title of Training:* Diploma in Acupuncture. *Duration:* Three years full-time (approx 20 hours per week, 30 weeks per year.) Entry requirements: 5 'O' levels, 2 'A' levels, 21 years of age, mature entrants considered on work experience if no exam results. *Fees:* £3,600 p.a. inclusive *Comments:* One intake per year, first week of October. All applicants are interviewed. They want students who have an awareness of the job of becoming a therapist and commitment to becoming a professional acupuncturist. Their uniqueness is emphasis of clinical training throughout the course.

Aikido

Aikido is a Japanese martial art developed by Morihei Uyeshiba who popularised the art after the Second World War. He felt that the object of a martial art should not be to win, but to promote harmony and co-operation, a message which was as sorely needed in the post war world as it is today.

The word comes from 'ai' which means 'union', 'ki' which is 'life force' and 'do' which means road or way. The object of aikido is to achieve harmony and union with the life energy which is in and around all of us. Power is not a matter of physical strength, but comes from strengthening and deepening the connection with this life force. As with tai chi chuan, the expert does not exert his or her strength over the opponent, but uses the attacker's own force for defence. The student must learn that winning itself is not important, and a contest between two practitioners is not so much a fight to the death as a dance in which there is a high degree of co-operation.

Although aikido can be an effective method of self-defence, responsibility is taken for not inflicting unnecessary harm on the attacker. The method should have given the practitioner sufficient skill and awareness to make it unnecessary for them to use the same kind of brute tactics as the aggressor. Strength comes from concentration and awareness, and for this reason aikido is a spiritual discipline as well as a form of self defence. In becoming more in tune with the 'ki' or life energy, one also becomes more centred or rooted in the 'hara'. The 'hara' is the physical centre of gravity in the body and is located about two inches below the navel. It is also the symbolic centre of the top and bottom halves of the body, a point where the physical and mental spheres meet.

Aikido is usually taught in classes of about 20 people. Tuition is given in the 'dojo' or practice hall, a word which also means the hall where Zen monks practise meditation. Teachers have their own approach to discipline in the dojo; some are stricter than others and require a certain etiquette to be maintained inside. Keeping a formal etiquette is in itself a kind of discipline which is seen to reinforce the discipline involved in learning a martial art. A class usually lasts about an hour, and there is a uniform of jacket, belt and baggy trousers. As with most martial arts beginners move up through a series of 'gradings' or examinations to attain higher levels of proficiency. Because the emphasis is on developing inner strength, there is no need to be physically strong to practice Aikido.

READING

Aikido: The Way of Harmony by *John Stevens, Shambhala £12.95.* This definitive, profusely illustrated book covers the essential elements of the philosophy and practice of Aikido, the Japanese martial art that has been embraced by modern psychology and many western bodywork therapies. Useful to beginners and experienced practitioners, with descriptions and photographs of the main Aikido techniques and interesting insights into the history of Aikido and the life of its founder, Uyeshiba Morihei. Written by one of the main western Aikido teachers in Japan, under the direction of one of the founder's ealiest students.

CENTRES OFFERING AIKIDO

British Ki Aikido Association NW1, Cabot Centre NW1, Natureworks, Women and Health NW1.

Alexander Technique

Named after the creator, Australian F. Matthias Alexander, the Alexander technique is the application of a subtle guidance by a practitioner in the movement of the client. Alexander practitioners call themselves 'teachers' and their clients 'students'. They aim to re-educate the students by enabling them to 'unlearn' their habitual poor habits of movement.

Observing a teacher and student at work, it looks as if very little is happening. Imagine a typical scene: the teacher seems to spend much time holding the back of the student's head with one hand and jaw of the student with another, and guiding the student gently out of a chair, little by little, then sitting him or her down again. What is happening is that the student is learning by being taken slowly through a simple movement, in this case standing up. When the student is about to fall into a poor use of the body, the teacher will stop them and make them aware of what they are doing. The teacher will lead the student through these movements time and time again until the student learns a new way of moving and the misuse disappears.

The student may be asked to take up other positions such as as 'the monkey' (standing like a monkey), or asked to lie down on a table whereupon the teacher may lift and gently rotate the arms and move the legs.

At about the seventh session many people experience a feeling of walking on air. As the sessions continue they may report more energy and an ease in physical mobility.

Many of the students are actors or musicians. Musicians practise it because they are prone to bad posture huddled over their instruments and actors because they need to claim more versatility in their movements.

Some people notice alterations in the structure of their body, such as the disappearance of stoops and the hollow back. Some people claim to notice little difference.

The usual arrangement for lessons is three times a week for the first two weeks, twice a week for the next five weeks and once a week thereafter until about thirty visits have occurred. There are enormous variations upon the figures just quoted, mainly depending on the progress of the student. Students are asked to dress in loose clothing.

Each lesson lasts for half an hour. Many teachers practise outside of normal working hours. Alexander technique is also sometimes taught in week long intensives.

READING

Body Learning by *Michael Gelb Aurum Press £5.95.* The approach to learning and the techniques outlined herein can transform your life if you read and practise the methods outlined in this extremely well illustrated introduction to the Alexander Technique. **Art of Changing** by *Glen Park, Ashgrove Book £9.50 Cassette £6.95.* This book takes a deeper look at the Alexander technique introducing the basic exercises to aid personal growth and transformation, and to deal with physical and mental stress. Glen Park then develops this study to encompass the way in which the emotional and spiritual dimensions may be furthered with reference to Alexander's system of working. The cassette is a useful adjunct to the book, helping the student to work through the exercises and combine them with awareness of the chakra centres.

CENTRES OFFERING ALEXANDER TECHNIQUE

Acupuncture and Osteopathy Clinic SW1V, Alexander Teaching Centre EC1V, Augenblick Centre, Bloomsbury Alexander Centre WC1B, Bodywise E2, Brackenbury Natural Health Centre W6, Bumblebees Natural Remedies N7, City Health Centre EC1Y, Clapham Common Clinic SW4, Clissold Park Natural Health Centre N16, College of Homoeopathy Clinic SE13, Constructive Teaching Centre, Edgware Centre for Natural Health HA8, Gestalt Centre London EC1Y, Hale Clinic W1N, Highbury Centre N5, IBISS TW7, Kingston Natural Healing Centre, Living Centre SW20, Natural Medicine Centre BR2, Natureworks, Neal's Yard Therapy Rooms WC2H, New Cross Natural Therapy Centre , Notting Hill Traditional Acupuncture Clinic W11, Primrose Healing Centre NW1, South London Natural Health Centre SW4, Sunra SW12, Violet Hill Studios NW8, Westminster Natural Health Centre SW1V, Wimbledon Clinic of Natural Medicine SW19, Women and Health NW1, Wood Street Clinic EN5.

TRAININGS IN ALEXANDER TECHNIQUE

Constructive Teaching Centre *Title of Training:* Training Course for Teachers of the F Matthias Alexander Technique. *Duration:* Full-time course over three years. *Entry requirements:* Students should be aged between 18 and 35, and must go through introductory and probationary periods. *Fees:* £1,175 per term. *Comments:* The training course is approved by the Society of Teacher of the Alexander Technique.

North London Teacher Training Centre *Title of Training:* Alexander Technique *Duration:* 3 years full time, 16 hours per week. *Entry requirements:* Some experience in Alexander technique, introductory lessons at the school. *Fees:* Refer to organisers *Comments:* Train teachers of Alexander technique.

Allergy Therapy

It has been accepted for a long time now that pollen can cause an allergic reaction called hayfever which can spoil the sufferer's enjoyment of summer. It was not until recently however that research carried out by a London hospital convinced the medical profession that common foods could also cause a wide range of physical and mental symptoms in some people. Formerly such symptoms might have gone unrecognised and been treated by painkillers or tranquillisers.

An allergic reaction takes place when the body reacts to a substance which has been eaten, inhaled or in contact with the body in some other way, as if it were harmful, even though the substance is not in any way a threat to the organism. The immune system rejects the substance, and in its attempts to do so causes allergic symptoms. White flour, dairy products and food additives are often the culprits in food allergy.

Allergy can be involved in ill health in different ways. Sometimes the patient's symptoms, which can range from headaches, digestive problems, depression, palpitations and arthritic pains, are due to the allergy alone, and by not eating the food which causes the allergic reaction the symptoms are cured. Sometimes allergy is implicated in a particular illness, and helps to aggravate the symptoms. This is more controversial, and research has not been at all conclusive. An example of this was the claim that schizophrenia could be precipitated by food allergy. While this is debatable, it is certainly true that if the immune system is weakened by allergy, it may be less able to contend with any other disturbance which is present in the body.

The increase in environmental pollutants such a car fumes, industrial waste and pesticides has also had its part to play in causing ill health. These substances can be harmful, and the body's reaction may represent a response to a genuine threat, rather than being a strictly allergic reaction. Dr Peter Mansfield and Dr Jean Monro have investigated the effects of chemicals in the environment on chemically sensitive children. Although it is a moot point whether reactions to these substances are allergic or simply intolerant, allergy therapy can still be used here to identify the possible source of the patient's symptoms.

There are various methods used to diagnose an allergy. The patient may be put on a very restricted diet of foods which are usually non-allergenic. Then other foods will be reintroduced into the diet one by one, and the reactions of the patient to each food are charted. Another method is the 'scratch test' where the surface of the skin is lightly scratched and different substances are applied to it. Any irritation or inflammation may be an indication of an allergic reaction. A variant of this test is the introduction of the substances by injection into the skin and noting any skin reactions. The cytotoxic blood test uses a sample of blood to which the suspected allergens are introduced, and the effects monitored. Analysis of hair will show the long term effects of allergy, although it will not show recent developments. Applied kinesiology can be used to test muscle strength in the presence of a potential allergen.

Once the cause has been found, the foods or substances which cause the allergy can be eliminated from the diet or environment. One form of treatment offered by some therapists is the 'neutralising dose'. If the allergen is greatly diluted to the level of a homoeopathic potency and injected, the body will build up a resistance to the substance and be able to tolerate it again. However, to many people it may seem easier just to stop eating what the body rejects.

For information about allergy, contact Action Against Allergy.

READING
Food Allergy and Intolerance *by Jonathan Brostoff and Linda Gamlin, Bloomsbury Publishing £4.99.* This explains comprehensively and simply how certain foods can cause problems for some people and how by identifying and eliminating the culprits they can improve their health. Includes chapters on chemical sensitivity, the mind and body connection and problems in childhood. Also links common ailments with food allergies and details elimination diets to be followed. **Arthritis - The Allergy Connection** *by John Mansfield, Thorsons £4.99.* Dr. Mansfield explores a revolutionary new approach to alleviating one of the most crippling diseases known. He describes effective ways of dealing with the way in which food allergy may affect the development of arthritis including desensitisation and avoidance of stimulants. His ideas are reinforced by the results of clinical trials and scientific evidence.

CENTRES OFFERING ALLERGY THERAPY
Action Against Allergy, All Hallows House EC3R, Alternative Medicine Clinic NW15, Association of Natural Medicines CM8, Bayswater Clinic W2, Brackenbury Natural Health Centre W6, Breakspear Hospital WD5, Clapham Common Clinic SW4, Colon Health W9, Food and Chemical Allergy Clinic CR0, Heath Health Care NW3, Homoeopathic Health Clinic HA3, Hong Tao Acupuncture and Natural Health Clinic HA5, Life Resources NW7, Natural Healing Centre HA4, Natural Health Clinic HA3, Neal's Yard Therapy Rooms WC2H, Pearl Healing Centre CR7, Psychotherapy Centre W1H, South London Natural Health Centre SW4, Wimbledon Clinic of Natural Medicine SW19, Women and Health NW1.

Applied Kinesiology / Touch for Health

Applied Kinesiology is a manipulative therapy. It involves testing muscles with the hands for any signs of weakness, which if present may show a disturbance in the fuctioning of an organ. In this way, it is useful as a diagnostic technique. Kinesiologists are particularly interested in this weakness if it occurs in a set of muscles on only one side of the body, for this indicates an imbalance which, they believe, can be the first stage in the development of a particular health problem.

The technique was first developed by Dr George Goodheart, an American chiropractor. He linked his discoveries about muscular weakness with oriental medical ideas of energy flow through the body in 'meridians' (see 'Acupuncture'). Through the meridians, the muscles are linked to particular organs. Whatever underlying problem is revealed by the muscle tests, it is usually treated by working on the reflexes to strengthen the muscles, massaging meridians and in some cases by diet.

Applied kinesiology is often used to diagnose food allergies. Muscles are tested before and after the ingestion of foods suspected of causing allergy. If the muscles are weaker a few seconds after the patient has chewed the suspected food, this indicates the presence of an allergy.

The difference between Applied Kinesiology and Touch for Health is that the former is used by professionals for diagnosis and treatment of patients, while Touch for Health is taught to the general public as a self-help technique for preventative health care.

CENTRES OFFERING APPLIED KINESIOLOGY

Academy of Systematic Kinesiology KT5, Alternative Medicine Clinic NW15, Clapham Common Clinic SW4, Edgware Centre for Natural Health HA8, Islington Green Centre of Alternative Medicine N1, Kinesiology School N10, Neal's Yard Therapy Rooms WC2H, South London Natural Health Centre SW4, Violet Hill Studios NW8.

Aromatherapy

Aromatherapy is a treatment method which uses essential oils extracted from flowers, plants, trees or spices. These are massaged into the body, inhaled, sprinkled in baths or in some cases ingested.

Aromatic substances were used in healing throughout the ancient world, notably by the Egyptians who buried jars of frankinsense and myrrh alongside their pharohs in their tombs, and who used the same perfumes for both medical and cosmetic effect. Proponents of aromatherapy have to this day developed the art for purposes as diverse as the healing of wounds, treating skin cancer and banishing wrinkles.

The essential oils used in aromatherapy are highly concentrated and have to be extracted from large quantities of the mother plant. They are expensive to buy and need to be stored carefully in the right conditions and temperature, and these factors place some limitation on the popular use of aromatherapy. The oils

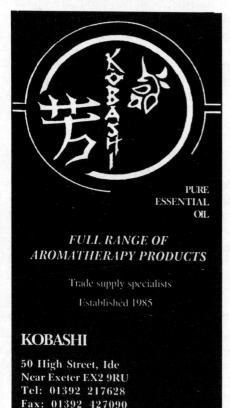

are absorbed into the body through the skin. Although it is not known how aromatherapy works, since research has shown that if a drug is administered in this way its effects may be different from those it produces if it is taken orally, it may be that it is the method of application used in aromatherapy which enables the therapeutic effect of the oils.

The practitioner will decide on the essential oils which will be most efficacious for the client. Sometimes diagnosis is made using radiesthesia. This technique uses a pendulum - a small object such as a ring or a bead used as a weight and attached to a length of string or thread about a foot long. The therapist then asks questions, either about the health of the patient, or about what particular remedy is indicated and the pendulum responds with a 'yes' or 'no' answer.

Having selected the appropriate oil the aromatherapist will probably want to spend some time preparing the skin because diet, pollution and make-up have dulled the receptivity of the modern skin. Inhalation is used for the treatment of head and lung complaints. About six to ten treatments may be required, although beneficial effects may be felt earlier.

As might be expected, aromatherapy is most effective used in the treatment of the skin, in healing wounds and burns, and treating shingles, acne and stress related conditions. The massage with which the oils are applied adds to the therapeutic effect of the treatment.

READING

Practical Aromatherapy *by Shirley Price, Thorsons £3.50.* A simple explanation of all aspects of aromatherapy and how it can be used to good effect as a self-help therapy. Included is an illustrated section on aromatherapy massage techniques and also how to blend pure essential oils for different purposes. Suitable for the lay person and practitioner alike. **Aromatherapy, An A-Z** *by Patricia Davies, C.W. Daniel £9.95.* A book which provides the answers to such questions as: 'can I combine aromatherapy with other therapies or even conventional medicine? Which oil could help my skin? How are essential oils obtained from plants?' A popular and suitable reference work for students and practitioners of aromatherapy.

CENTRES OFFERING AROMATHERAPY

Acupuncture and Osteopathy Clinic SW1V, All Hallows House EC3R, Alternative Medicine Clinic NW15, Alternative Therapies Centre N16, Aromatherapy Associates SW6, Belgravia Beauty SW1X, Bennett & Luck N1, Bexleyheath Natural Health Clinic DA7, Bluestone Clinic W1N, Body Clinic NW11, Bodywise E2, Brackenbury Natural Health Centre W6, Bretforton Hall Clinic WR11, Centre for Health and Healing W1V, Changes NW3, Chelsea Complementary Natural Health Centre SW10, Chessington Hypnotherapy Clinic, Clapham Common Clinic SW4, Clissold Park Natural Health Centre N16, College of Homoeopathy Clinic SE13, Equilibrium Therapy Centre

SW18, Falcons SW11, Gerda Boyesen Centre W3, Gerda Boysen Clinic W3, Green Wood College W6, Helios N1, Holistic Aromatherapy Practice W12, IBISS TW7, Institute of Clinical Aromatherapy SE6, Institute of Traditional Herbal Medicine and Aromatherapy N8, Islington Green Centre of Alternative Medicine N1, Jeyrani Health Centre E18, Kingston Natural Healing Centre, London College of Massage W1P, London Lighthouse W11, London Natural Health Clinic W8, Lotus Healing Centre NW8, McCarthy Westwood Consultants SW11, Micheline Arcier Aromatherapy SW1X, Muswell Healing Arts N10, Natural Medicine Centre BR2, Naturecare SW16, Natureworks, Neal's Yard Therapy Rooms WC2H, New Cross Natural Therapy Centre, Portobello Green Fitness Centre W10, Primrose Healing Centre NW1, Putney Natural Therapy Clinic, Raphael Clinic NW6, Register of Qualified Aromatherapists NW1, Sayer Clinic: Croydon CR0, Shirley Goldstein, Silver Birch Centre NW10, South London Natural Health Centre SW4, Sunra SW12, Therapy Made Unique E18, Tisserand Institute BN3, Violet Hill Studios NW8, West London School of Therapeutic Massage W11, Westminster Natural Health Centre SW1V, Whole Health Clinic NW3, Wholistic Health and Life Extension LA5, Women and Health NW1, Wood Street Clinic EN5, Yoga Dham HA2.

TRAINING IN AROMATHERAPY

Aromatherapy Associates *Title of Training:* (1) Diploma Course (2) Foundation Diploma Course *Duration:* (1)Twelve days full time (2) 1 year part time Entry requirements: (1) Knowledge of massage and anatomy and physiology. (2) No prerequisites *Fees:* On application.

Institute of Clinical Aromatherapy *Title of Training:* 1) Aromatherapy for Beauty Therapists (Certificate) 2) Clinical Aromatherapy (Diploma) *Duration:* 1) 3 days (9.00 till 7.00) 2) 8 days (9.00 till 7.00) *Entry requirements:* 1) Practising Beauty Therapists only 2) Massage, Anatomy & Physiology *Fees:* Refer to organisers *Comments:* 'We are the longest established aromatherapy school in the UK. Eve Taylor, our principal, teaches all over the world.' The Clinical Aromatherapy Diploma is recognised by the International Federation of Aromatherapists. Accommodation is available on the premises. Large free car park. All food during the day is included in the fee, there are NO extras apart from accommodation, if required.

London School of Herbology and Aromatherapy *Title of Training:* Aromatherapy Massage Course. *Duration:* 9 months part-time (100 hours). *Entry requirements:* None: students are trained in all aspects of required knowledge. *Fees:* Refer to organisers *Comments:* Training in both Chinese traditional approach, and western medical approach. Both courses include clinical practice.

Micheline Arcier Aromatherapy *Title of Training:* Aromatherapy Diploma Course. *Duration:* 8 days over two long weekends. *Entry requirements:* Qualified in anatomy, physiology, face and body massage with 2 years practical experience. *Fees:* Refer to organisers

Shirley Price Aromatherapy Ltd. *Title of Training:* Aromatherapy training courses including diploma standard with reflexology techniques. Basic massage course, anatomy and physiology correspondence course, diploma course, 4 post-diploma courses. *Duration:* Diploma course in two parts, 3-9 months depending on qualifications already held in Anatomy and physiology and basic massage. *Entry requirements:* For diploma course, students must have a recognised qualification in basic massage and anatomy and physiology. *Fees:* Refer to organisers *Comments:* Accredited school of the International Federation of Aromatherapists. Courses held at venues throughout the UK including London.

Tisserand Institute *Title of Training:* Holistic Aromatherapy *Duration:* Nine months full time. Part time is two years. *Entry requirements:* GCSE biology or equivalent. *Fees:* Refer to organisers *Comments:* Incorporates massage and reflexology, touch for health. Training courses are held in London at Royal Masonic Hospital, Hammersmith, London W6.

Institute of Traditional Herbal Medicine and Aromatherapy *Title of Training:* Aromatherapy Bodywork Diploma Course. *Duration:* One year part-time, 200 hours, over 16 weekends. *Entry requirements:* None specified, interview requested. *Fees:* £1,595 inclusive, with reductions for Massage/Amatomy and psychology examptions. *Comments:* Graduates may join a leading professional association - The Register of Qualified Aromatherapists. The Institute teaches traditional Chinese medicine as an energetic and physical basis for aromatherapy diagnosis and treatment.

Jeyrani Health Centre *Title of Training:* Creative Healing - to be used with aromatherapy. *Duration:* 2 weekends. *Entry requirements:* Course open to healers, massage therapists, aromatherapists, nurses and doctors. *Fees:* Refer to organisers *Comments:* Excellent results with specific techniques for each condition. Special treatments are used in cases such as: asthma and chronic bronchitis, cardiac toner, female treatments.

Raworth Centre *Title of Training:* 1) Diploma in Holistic Aromatherapy 2) Individual Modules for Practising Therapists & Medical Personnel *Duration:* 1)6 months 2 days per week OR accelerated learning programme 3 months - 4 days per week OR weekend study 8 months of alternative weekends. *Entry requirements:* 1) None stated. *Fees:* Refer to organisers *Comments:* 'First in UK to offer Holistic Aromatherapy, has since developed into a veritable polytechnic of natural medicine'. Own premises, 16 staff, in-house clinic. Accredited by 11 national and international professional bodies. Unique to the Centre - Natural Health Practitioner's Diploma, 1 year part time.

Essentials for Health *Title of Training:* Diploma in Aromatherapy *Duration:* 150 hours part-time over 10 weekends *Fees:* £970 inclusive

IBISS *Title of Training:* Practitioners courses in Anatony & Physiology, Aromatherapy, Reflexology, Massage, Practical Body Work. Tools for Change. Living, Dying and Dancing. (LDD) *Duration:* LDD course for one year. Others are one year part-time for 4 modules, alternate weekends. *Entry requirements:* At the discrection of the facilitator, but Anatomy & Physiology and Body Work are essential before attempting other modules. *Fees:* Approx £320 per module. LDD £800 per year.

Violet Hill Studios *Title of Training:* Wholistic Aromatherapy *Duration:* Nine months part-time 210 hours in total, 7 hours per week. *Entry requirements:* None *Fees:* Three modules. Complete course £970. Mod 1) £350 Mod 2) £490 Mod 3) £280. *Comments:* Course is recognised by the A.O.C. It is a whole approach to aromatherapy, a student will gain knowledge in breathing techniques self-care, healing and back care. Contact Mother Earth Aromatherapy School (0181) 450 2470 for more details.

Ayurvedic Medicine

Ayurveda (which means 'science of life') is the traditional medicine of India which has been practised for over two and a half thousand years. It is based on texts which, among other things, describe operative techniques, how infection can be transmitted during surgery and even describes the body as being composed of cells long before Western medicine had made such important discoveries.

According to this system of medicine there are five elements (doshas) - earth, air, fire, water and ether. There are also three basic qualities of energy - rajas (active), ramas (passive) and sattva (unifying, wise). It is the correct balance of these, constantly changing with environmental conditions, which constitutes health.

Diagnosis involves observing the quality of 32 pulses, taking a personal history, considering astrological information and observing the condition of the body. Treatment can be with herbs, exercises, diet, breathing techniques, massage, urine treatment, yogic cleansing techniques or surgery.

Ayurvedic medicine is the main form of medicine available to people living in India. The training is long and thorough, and involves some knowledge of western medicine.

Unani medicine is an offshoot of Ayurveda, and includes ideas based on Greek and Arab sources. Siddha medicine is another form which has incorporated the use of minerals for treatment.

CENTRES OFFERING AYURVEDIC MEDICINE
Alternative Medicine Clinic NW15.

Bates Eyesight Training

This is a natural method of eyesight improvement through eye exercises. It was devised by Dr William H Bates, an eye specialist who gave up orthodox methods in order to find a more satisfactory way of treating bad eyesight. He published his bestseller, *Better Eyesight Without Glasses*, detailing these exercises in 1919. Various exercises are recommended. 'Palming' involves covering the eyes with the palms of the hands for 10 minutes at a time, two or three times a day. This excludes all light and relaxes the eyes. 'Shifting and swinging' involve deliberately imitating the natural minute and constant shifting movements of the eyes around an object, or objects. 'Splashing' involves splashing the eyes with hot and cold water repeatedly morning and night. Bates believed blinking reguarly - once or twice every ten seconds - was also of great importance. He also recommended remembering colours or beautiful scenes while 'palming', because he found this improved vision in actuality. A practitioner of the Bates eyesight training will give these and other exercises to be practised every day.

Aldous Huxley, who as a young man could hardly see to read, is perhaps the most famous of those who have been helped by this method, as he explains in his book, *The Art of Seeing*.

CENTRES OFFERING BATES EYESIGHT TRAINING
Bates Association of Great Britain BN43, Pearl Healing Centre CR7.

TRAINING IN BATES METHOD
Bates Association of Great Britain *Title of Training:* The Bates College: Professional Teacher Training in the Bates Method. *Duration:* Two years, part time (20 weekends). *Entry requirements:* Flexible. *Fees:* £1,200 per annum approximately. No VAT. *Comments:* Bates College offer 'the only fully structured course under Bates regulations in the UK'. Introductory workshops are available in most areas.

Biodynamic Massage and Psychology

Biodynamic massage and biodynamic psychology were formulated by Gerda Boyesen, a Norweigan psychologist, physiotherapist and Reichian analyst. As in Reich's psychology, Biodynamics works on the premise that the mind and body function together in any emotional process, and that shocks, traumas and continually repressed feelings can build up chronic physical and psychological blocks. This is especially true if during childhood the growing child did not feel in a safe enough environment to be able to express its feelings. The modern world too tends to exacerbate these feelings of insecurity and stress, and the body may be holding itself in a permanent state of alert and tension.

Boyesen, through her work as a physiotherapist, found that blocked energy builds up in the form of fluids trapped between muscles and nerves. Her unique contribution to Reichian therapy was that she found that in massaging the patient to disperse this build up of fluids, the intestine was activated in a spontaneous peristaltic movement. This movement was not to eliminate foods, but rather a kind of psychic clearing process which occurs when emotion is allowed to follow its natural process of expression. This she likened to the concept in Chinese medicine that every organ has two functions. One function is physical, and one is esoteric or 'meaningful'. According to Boyesen, the meaningful function of the intestine is to digest stress.

The cornerstone of the theory and practice of biodynamic massage is that the healthy organism has the power to express and resolve, to digest all emotional traumas and shocks once the body has ceased to armour itself in patterns of chronic tension and blocks.

The therapist works using a stethoscope to listen to the noises inside the abdomen. There are many different sounds made by the intestines and the therapist is guided by these which are not just the sound of food being digested, but responses to the massage. The sounds mean that the therapist has been able to set free the emotional energy that has become trapped in a particular part of the body. The therapist may massage any part of the body. If enough energy is being released in a 'biodynamic updrift' the therapist may stop the massage, and instead encourage the client to tune in to his or her own 'stimuli from within'. These may take the form of memories, emotions, physical movements or expansive breathing.

Biodynamic massage is helpful in the treatment of migraines, high blood pressure, digestive problems and muscular pain as well as stress, anxiety and depression. It helps to maintain good health and brings about a greater sense of aliveness.

CENTRES OFFERING BIODYNAMIC MASSAGE

All Hallows House EC3R, Association of Biodynamic Psychotherapists NW6, Biodynamic Psychotherapy and Teaching W3, Brackenbury Natural Health Centre W6, Cabot Centre NW1, Centre for Personal & Professional Development N17, Chiron Centre for Holistic Psychotherapy W5, Clapham Common Clinic SW4, Gerda Boyesen Centre W3, Healing Fields Practice N7, Hidden Strengths TW2, Highbury Centre N5, Hillside Practice, Neal's Yard Therapy Rooms WC2H, Psychotherapy Workshops for Women, Sound Health SE8, Violet Hill Studios NW8.

CENTRES OFFERING BIODYNAMIC PSYCHOLOGY

Augenblick Centre, Cabot Centre NW1, Centre for Personal & Professional Development N17, Gerda Boyesen Centre W3, Gerda Boysen Clinic W3, Healing Fields Practice N7, Kingston Natural Healing Centre, Raphael Clinic

NW6, Sound Health SE8, Violet Hill Studios NW8.

TRAININGS IN BIODYNAMIC MASSAGE AND PSYCHOLOGY

Gerda Boyesen Centre *Title of Training:* (1) Three Year Certificate Course in Biodynamic Psychology. (2) Two Year Advanced Training Course in Biodynamic Psychology and Psychotherapy. *Duration:* (1) Three years (2) Two years. *Entry requirements:* Prefer graduates, but life experience can be substituted for a university degree. The biggest demand is for emotional maturity and sensitivity. *Fees:* £1,500 per annum plus personal therapy fees, plus ITEC course in first year. Individual sessions at £15. *Comments:* Personal therapy is required whilst in training, a total of 30 hours per year. The cost is £20 per hour. Much of the training is given by Gerda Boyesen personally.

Chiron Centre for Holistic Psychotherapy *Title of Training:* Basic Biodynamic Massage. *Duration:* 1 year part time comprising 4 terms of 12 weeks each (144 hours). *Entry requirements:* Detailed application form and assessment interview. *Fees:* Refer to organisers *Comments:* Chiron is a member of the National Consultative Council for Alternative and Complementary Medicine (NCC). 'Our emphasis is less concerned with techniques but with presence, relationship and process'. Emphasis is placed on the whole person and integration of the physical, mental, emotional and spiritual aspects. Certificate holders are invited annually for revision days and offered to join a massage association to guarantee professional standards.

TRAININGS IN BIODYNAMIC PSYCHOLOGY

School of Holistic Systems Therapy *Title of Training:* Modular training in Psychodynamic Bodywork and Counselling (4 certificated modules). *Duration:* Mod 1) One term - ten weeks, one evening per week, four long weekends (Fri eve Sat and Sun), two Saturdays. Mod 2) Two terms, one day per week, five long weekends. Mod 3) Three terms (one year), one day per week, five long weekends, one five-day intensive group therapy, three hours per week clinical supervision. Mod 4) as 3) plus an additional year of clinical practice with supervision. *Entry requirements:* 1) Five G.C.S.E.'s or equivalent or life experience. Each year is then taken on completion of previous. Minimum age 21 years. *Fees:* Mod 1) £650 payable in advance, plus exam fee, books and professional uniform. 2) 3) and 4) £650 per term plus approximately £25 per week for personal psychotherapy minimum ten per term. *Comments:* Requires personal psychotherapy for the duration of the training from module 2) onwards. Intake module 1) January, April, September. The profesionally certificated modules allow each person to find their own level of professional practice according to their current capacity and economic situation.

Chiropractic

Chiropractic is a method which uses manipulation of the joints and especially the spine by the hands to restore and maintain health.

The system was devised by Dr Daniel David Palmer at the turn of the century when he cured his janitor of deafness by manipulating his spine. Although there are obvious similarities between chiropractic and osteopathy, the main differences lie in the slightly different styles of manipulation used, and that chiropractors are more likely to use X-rays and orthodox physiological tests such as blood samples and neurological examination for diagnosis. Like osteopathy it is based on the idea that displacement of the vertebrae causes disease, but while traditional chiropractic theory states that these impair the functioning of the nervous system, osteopaths maintain that the resultant disease is caused by impaired circulation.

The chiropractor will take a detailed medical history and make a physical examination, possibly using the tests outlined above. He or she will also feel the spine and joints with their hands to locate tissue changes and assess the range of mobility present. Then the appropriate manipulation is carried out. This takes the form of twists and pulls with the chiropractor and patient in a number of different positions.

A chiropractor should have undergone an intensive 4 year training at a recognised college. Conditions which respond well to chiropractic are not surprisingly low back pain, slipped discs, sciatica, headaches, migraines, digestive disorders and even asthma. Some cases of arthritis may be suitable and respond to treatment.

CENTRES OFFERING CHIROPRACTIC

Bumblebees Natural Remedies N7, Chiropractic Clinic NW11, Edgware Centre for Natural Health HA8, Hale Clinic W1N, Heath Health Care NW3, Institute of Pure Chiropractic ONX, Natureworks, Neal's Yard Therapy Rooms WC2H, New Cross Natural Therapy Centre , Sayer Clinic W8, Sayer Clinic: Chelsea SW6, Sayer Clinic: City EC2M, Sayer Clinic: Covent Garden, Sayer Clinic: Croydon CR0, Sayer Clinic: Marble Arch W1H, South London Natural Health Centre SW4, Wood Street Clinic EN5.

TRAINING IN CHIROPRACTIC

Anglo-European College of Chiropractic *Title of Training:* BSc. Chiropractic (CNAA). *Duration:* Four year full-time (Five year programme from 1993) Both full-time programmes incorporate one year's clinical training. *Entry requirements:* As per University: 3 'A' levels or equivalent. Some chemistry is required. Mature candidates (that is, over 23) are considered on an individual basis. *Fees:* Refer to organisers *Comments:* We are the only Institution offering graduate status in Chiropratic in the Continent of Europe. There are reciprocal arrangements with many other countries world-wide who accept the BSc Chiropractic for the purposes of their local State Licensing arrangements. All Chiropractors in Europe, upon completion of their full-time course, have to complete a further one year pre-registration period in Clinical Practice before they may practice independently.

Colonic Irrigation

Sometimes also called colonic hydrotherapy, colonic irrigation is the cleansing of the large intestine (or bowel) by passing water through and out of it via the rectum.

The function of the colon is to extract minerals, nutrients and excess water from food after is has passed, partly digested, out of the stomach and small intestine. Food is moved through the intestine by means of regular muscular contractions (called 'peristalsis') towards the rectum from which it is excreted. However, bad diet, stress, emotional trauma or the side-effects of medicines and drugs can interfere both with this movement, and with the colon's ability to absorb and it can become blocked with toxic waste matter. This not only further interferes with digestion, but is also believed to fester and release poisonous substances into the blood stream. These eventually reach and affect the vital organs, and this, according to the theory of colonics, is the cause of bad health. The aim of colonic irrigation is to unblock the colon and flush out the toxins so that it is restored to healthy functioning.

A series of four to eight colonic irrigations is usually suggested for new clients. A sterile speculum is placed in the rectum, and then a small tube through which water flows into the colon. The water is extracted through a separate tube, and the contents on the colon can be watched through a transparent window as they come out.

The process itself is not unpleasant. The recipient's lower half is kept covered

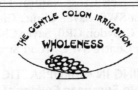

throughout so that they do not feel undignified or embarrassed. The temperature and pressure of water is monitored by the practitioner, and hot and cold water may be alternated to stimulate the bowel. It should take about half and hour.

Immediately afterwards, recipients may need to open their bowels. Bacteria which normally lives in the gut and which is important to the digestion of food is replaced with an implant.

With the initial course of treatment, the practitioner may recommend a change of diet, or the taking of a particular dietary supplement to maintain the healthy functioning of the colon. Treatments are often taken two to four times a year.

While in trained hands, colonic irrigation is safe, in the hands of untrained people it can be dangerous and should *never* be attempted at home. The Colonic International Association has a list of trained practitioners.

READING

Tissue Cleansing through Bowel Management *by Bernard Jensen, Bernard Jensen £4.95.* Includes chapters on imbalances of the intestine and the benefits of colonic cleansing. Describes specific methods of cleansing and detoxification using supplements, colonic irrigation and diet. The book also offers insights into connection between mind and body and inner cleanliness. **The Colon Health Handbook** *by Robert Gray, Emerald Publishing £5.50.* This book is written by a nutrition counsellor and covers the use of supplements, bran and psyllium husks to strip the inside of the colon of waste materials. The methods are clearly explained and also included are notes on iris diagnosis to follow the progress of benefits gained from following the plan.

CENTRES OFFERING COLONIC IRRIGATION

Brackenbury Natural Health Centre W6, Colon Health W9, Holistic Health Consultancy SW1V, Neal's Yard Therapy Rooms WC2H, Raphael Clinic NW6, Refuah Shelaymah Natural Health Centre N16, South London Natural Health Centre SW4, Violet Hill Studios NW8, Whole Health Clinic NW3, Wholeness E18, Wimbledon Clinic of Natural Medicine SW19.

Colour Therapy

Colour therapy is the use of colour or coloured light for therapeutic purposes.

On the most basic level most people are aware that if the rooms they live in are painted different colours they will have a different affect on their moods. Research has shown that blue light lowers blood pressure and has a calming effect while red light puts blood pressure up and excites the nervous system. It has also been shown that some forms of depression may be due to the light deprivation we suffer either during winter, or in offices where there are only fluorescent lights. Daylight bulbs have been invented to correct this deficiency.

The use of colour as an aid to healing is a very subtle art, and the whole spectrum of colours is used. Colour therapists may diagnose what colour someone needs by noting what colours they like and dislike, or by looking at them to see what colour their 'aura' is, or by taking a medical history. The diagnosis of exactly what colours someone lacks is a complex matter, and self-treatment is not as easy as one might think.

There a many ways in which the colour may be administered. The colour therapist may advise you to eat certain foods which have the desired colour, or ask you to drink water which has been placed in coloured containers and exposed to sunlight, or you may be bathed in coloured light. Some colour therapists concentrate on colour in clothes, and help you to discover which colours are best for you to wear because they suit your physique and temperament.

Colour therapy is perhaps best used as a supplement to other forms of treatment, and has been used for a variety of complaints, from physical disorders to depression and anxiety states. Colour visualisation can also be used as a method of self help.

The Luscher Colour Test, devised by Dr Max Luscher is a personality test which can be self administered. Here, colour preferences are used to uncover psychological make up, and this is an interesting way to find out how colour reflects one's personality.

READING

Healing Through Colour by Theo Gimbel, C.W. Daniel £7.95. A complete book on colour therapy. The author explains the historical background to the use of colour and the use of healing in the ancient temples. In addition the modern approach to colour is discussed in detail including uses in decoration, clothing, stage illumination and as a supplementary therapy in medical work. **The Healing Power of Colour** by Magda Palmer, Thorsons/Aquarian £3.99. This book examines what colour does to us, how it can be used in magic and dream interpretation and how we can use it to improve our behaviour and our health. It will help you to gain an expanded understanding of the nature of colour and how it can be used to enhance your life.

CENTRES OFFERING COLOUR THERAPY

Aetherius Society SW6, Brackenbury Natural Health Centre W6, Bretforton Hall Clinic WR11, Healing Fields Practice N7, Hygeia College of Colour Therapy GL8, Kingston Natural Healing Centre, Living Colour NW3, Natureworks, Neal's Yard Therapy Rooms WC2H, Pearl Healing Centre CR7, South London Natural Health Centre SW4, Violet Hill Studios NW8, Westminster Natural Health Centre SW1V, Women and Health NW1.

TRAININGS IN COLOUR THERAPY

Hygeia College of Colour Therapy *Title of Training:* Hygeia Colour Therapy

Training Course ending with professional Certificate & Diploma. *Duration:* Six Foundation Courses of 9 hours teaching twice yearly and one two week Advance Course (70) hours with Examinations. All fully residential. *Entry requirements:* Interview and first course assessment. *Fees:* Refer to organisers *Comments:* College was founded after 12 years research into colour and illumination effects on health patterns. Have been training in Colour Therapy since 1968, have trained most heads of other schools, and written several books on Colour Therapy, some in their seventh edition and translated into 6 other languages.

Living Colour *Title of Training:* The Living Colour Training Programme. *Duration:* Part time for about a year, 4-6 hours per week, and one year's endorsement. *Entry requirements:* The 'Colour Your Life' foundation course. Must have enthusiasm and committment to the living colour system. *Fees:* £4,200, which includes colour instruments, coloured drapes, personal therapy and support. *Comments:* Personal therapy is included in the training, and supervision is given to students giving colour therapy. The course is aimed at those wishing to persue a career in in colour therapy.

Pearl Healing Centre *Title of Training:* Healer or Therapist *Duration:* Introductory course 20 hours, over a weekend or one day per week. Advanced course as above but also includes practical and written work. *Entry requirements:* No set requirements. *Fees:* £150 per course. *Comments:* The courses are very holistic, with specialist techniques, knowledge and hands on experience. NVQ orientated.

Cranial Osteopathy

Cranial osteopathy is a spin-off from conventional osteopathy which uses cerebro-spinal fluid in the skull and pelvic area to diagnose and treat illness. It may be used in conjuction with osteopathy, or as a treatment on its own, but the treatment is very different from osteopathy.

It was originally developed by William Sutherland, an osteopath, at the end of the nineteenth century. He experimented with the theory that he could diagnose and treat disorders by using his hand to explore a patient's skull.

A Cranial Osteopath feels the palpitations of the cerebro-spinal fluid, similar to the way a doctor might take a pulse. These palpitations make slight expansion and contraction movements; the feeling and symmetry of these gives the therapist information on the health of the cranial tissues. Touching the pelvic area also gives information on the bones and muscle tone of the pelvic and lower spine. The therapy relies heavily on intuition as well as training and knowledge.

Following diagnosis the therapist manipulates the cerebro-spinal fluid to make changes in pressure which lead to benificial changes in the patient. Cranial Osteopaths can treat similar disorders to osteopaths, but also head problems such as sinuses and giddiness. The treatment is particularly suitable for babies suffering problems related to difficult birth. Therapists have also claimed success in treating epilepsy, deafness and migraine. However, the treatment is not restricted to head and spinal problems, and is seen as a treatment for the entire body.

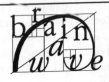

CENTRES OFFERING Cranial osteopathy
Bexleyheath Natural Health Clinic DA7, Bodywise E2, Bumblebees Natural Remedies N7, Chelsea Complementary Natural Health Centre SW10, Clapham Common Clinic SW4, College of Cranio-Sacral Therapy ME16, College of Centre NW8, Natureworks, Neal's Yard Therapy Rooms WC2H, New Cross Homoeopathy Clinic SE13, Cranial Osteopathic Association EN1, Forty Hill Natural Therapy Centre, Heath Health Care NW3, Holistic Aromatherapy Practice W12, Lavender Hill Homoeopathic Centre SW11, Lotus Healing Natural Therapy Centre , Primrose Healing Centre NW1, Raphael Clinic NW6, South London Natural Health Centre SW4, Sunra SW12, Violet Hill Studios NW8.

Training in Cranial Osteopathy
Cranial Osteopathic Association *Title of Training:* Cranial osteopathy. *Duration:* Five days. *Entry Requirements:* For osteopaths, chiropractors and manipulative therapists. *Fees:* Refer to organisers *Comments:* Limited to twenty persons.
Primrose Healing Centre *Title of Training:* Training in Cranial Osteopathy. *Duration:* One and two year courses.

Crystal/Gem Therapy

This is the therapeutic use of semi-precious and precious stones in a number of different ways.

Gemstones have been used for healing, or revered as having special powers through the ages. The Chinese have used jade to treat kidney and bladder complaints for at least 5,000 years. The American Indians were given personal stones at birth which had special powers and significance. These would be carried around in pouches worn on the owners' body.

Each variety of stone is believed to have specific therapeutic properties, though the same stone can have different effects on different people. Quartz and amethyst crystals are both used for general healing and are believed to magnify healing energies so that they become more effective, whether transmitted by some mechanical means or by a human being. The crystals or gems can be worn, carried and used as an adjunct to massage, or sometimes to focus thoughts and wishes for healing.

They can also be used in conjunction with colour therapy, using a crystal light box. This is a box with a light inside it and a hole on the outside covered with different coloured filters or gels through which the light is projected. Crystals are placed on the filter to intensify the energy of the light emitted.

Electro-crystal therapy has also been developed. This involves the transmission of different pulses of high frequency electromagnetic energy through crystals and onto the part of the body which needs to be treated. Gem elixirs are another way in which the healing energy of crystals and gems are believed to be absorbed.

Many people like to have crystals in their homes, because they feel they have a positive effect on the atmosphere. Prices for these 'domestic' crystals can range from 50p for a very small one, to five thousand pounds for a very large cluster.

READING

The Healing Power of Crystals by *Magda Palmer, Arrow £3.99.* In this book the author reveals how we can forge a link through crystals and gems to the energies of the solar system and lists a number of stones appropriate to each birthsign. Also included are the particular healing properties of specific stones and the ailments most susceptible to crystal healing. **The Power of Gems and Crystals** by *Soozi Holbeche, Piatkus £7.95.* This charming book, now in paperback, is written by one of Britain's pioneers in crystal healing. The book is packed with the most interesting historical facts and illustrated exercises. It also offers information on dowsing and healing. Just about everything you would want to know about gems and crystals.

CENTRES OFFERING CRYSTAL/GEM HEALING

Care-Healing Centre W9, Crystal 2000 FY8, Pearl Healing Centre CR7, School of Electro-Crystal Therapy HA4, Violet Hill Studios NW8, Wholistic Health and Life Extension LA5.

TRAINING IN CRYSTAL/GEM HEALING

School of Electro-Crystal Therapy *Title of Training:* Electro-Crystal Therapy *Duration:* Part time 10-15 months. 6 x two day workshops + home study. *Entry requirements:* None. *Fees:* £90 for each two-day course plus £598 for basic treatment equipment. *Comments:* Courses start March and September each year. This is the only training body for electro-crystal therapy.

Spiritual Venturers Association *Title of Training:* Crystal Healing: A Certificated Crystal Healing Course *Duration:* Part time: 6 weekends or three four day tutorials with home study. Entry requirements: An interest in healing and crystals. *Fees:* Refer to organisers *Comments:* The course is designed to give the student a basic grounding in healing techniques, knowledge of subtle energies, protection for healer and patient and information on crystals and gemstones. Licenciate membership for one year after successful completion the course. Full membership is granted one year later. Teaching Diploma Course after a further year. Membership to Affiliation of Crystal Healing Organisations (ACHO).

Alpha Clinic *Title of Training:* Crystal Awareness Part I Crystal Healing Part II Crystal Enlightenment Part III *Duration:* All courses are weekend attendance, part time, with home study with at least 3 months between each weekend course.

Entry requirements: An open mind, desire to grow spiritually, desire to heal self before healing others. *Fees:* Refer to organisers *Comments:* Course tutor trained by Katrina Raphael in New Mexico. Course content includes physiology, anatomy, disease states and drug effects.

Feldenkrais Method

In the Feldenkrais method gentle sequences of movement are taught so that students can learn how to reorganise patterns of action.

Moshe Feldenkrais was a Russian born Jew who escaped to England in 1940 from Nazi occupied France where he was working as an atomic physicist. When a knee injury prevented him from playing football he started to explore the dynamics of movement in the human body.

As with the Alexander technique much of the work involves letting go of ways of moving and holding the body which are habitual and restrictive. The process of re-learning freer movement is facilitated by slow exercises which should involve no strain or pain at all. They resemble the ways in which babies and young children learn to move. To release the 'pupil' from the pressure of gravity which puts added strain on the body, the lessons are at first carried out lying on the floor. By becoming more relaxed and more aware of how the individual body moves, the pupil has more freedom to choose a range of movements.

The Feldenkrais method is taught in two ways. 'awareness through movement' is taught in classes with a teacher verbally leading the class through a lesson. 'Functional integration' is a term used for an individual session where the teacher will guide the pupil's body through touch and gentle manipulation. These individual sessions are especially useful for those with disabilities or painful injuries.

The benefits of the method are not confined to the body. Feldenkrais felt that physical movement and posture can have a profound effect on the mind and emotions. The body not only reflects mental and emotional states but can also in turn affect them. Feldenkrais felt that by changing negative physical patterns the state of mind that produced them could be changed too.

Anyone can benefit from the Feldenkrais method. It has been used with those who have disabilities, including stroke patients and children with cerebral palsy and stiffness or injuries. The gentleness of the method makes it particularly suitable in such cases. People whose professions involve skilful, expressive movement such as dancers, singers, actors and athletes can also benefit.

CENTRES OFFERING THE FELDENKRAIS METHOD

Bodywise E2, Brackenbury Natural Health Centre W6, Feldenkrais Guild UK N10, IBISS TW7, Open Centre EC1V, Playspace NW1, Silver Birch Centre NW10.

TRAININGS IN THE FELDENKRAIS METHOD

Somatics *Title of Training:* Feldenkrais Professional Training Programme. *Duration:* 4 year training, meeting for eight weeks full time per year (three in Spring and five in Summer). *Entry requirements:* Experience in classes, and individual lessons in the Feldenkrais Method. *Fees:* Refer to organisers *Comments:* This is an internationally accredited training programme and is one of 3 on-going training centres in Europe.

Floatation Tank Therapy

A floatation tank is a bath or pool containing a concentrated saline solution of about a foot's depth, enclosed in a sound proof and light proof capsule or cubicle. The water is maintained at body temperature, and supports the body because the high concentration of Epsom salts makes the water extremly buoyant, and prevents the crinkling of the skin normally caused by prolonged immersion in water.

Floating in such an environment, where stimulation of the senses is reduced to a minimum, promotes relaxation. Some studies have shown that floating can lower blood pressure and reduce levels of stress-related biochemicals in the body. It can also help to alleviate pain, because it stimulates production by the body of endorphins - hormones which act to reduce pain.

Before floating it is necessary to wash or shower the whole body and shampoo the hair, so that body oils are not deposited in the pool. Vaseline should be applied to any wounds or scratches because the saline solution can sting on contact with breaks in the skin, although it is perfectly safe and can even promote healing. Floaters are also instructed not to touch their eyes during floating, because the water will sting these also, though once again it will not harm them. Once floating in the water on his or her back, the floater should be able to choose whether to be in total darkness, or whether to have a low level of light for reassurance. Those who suffer from claustraphobia are usually able to keep the door of the tank ajar, and the floater is able to leave the tank at any time, simply by opening the door. During the float, many floaters report feeling able to let go of tensions and anxiety, a sense of relaxation and peacefulness, and the sensation of being cosy. After the float it is common for this sense of relaxation to endure. Floats can last from fifty minutes to two hours.

One benefit of floating is that while other relaxation methods require effort to relax, floating is passive and may be an easier way to relax for those who find other methods such as meditation or biofeedback more difficult.

Floating can also be used as an aid to learning. Audio or visual tapes can be played to the floater while in the tank, and this can accelerate learning. Some people choose to listen to subliminal tapes to bring about therapeutic change.

CENTRES OFFERING FLOATATION TANK THERAPY

Float Centre NW8, Raphael Clinic NW6, South London Natural Health Centre SW4, Women and Health NW1.

Flower Remedies

These are herbal remedies derived from the flowers of plants. They are prescribed to treat the underlying negative emotional states which are seen as the cause of disease.

This system was devised by Dr Edward Bach, a doctor who practised at the beginning of this century. Working first as a pathologist and bacteriologist he found that different diseases seemed to be linked to the different temperaments of his patients, and classified these character types into seven categories which can be recognised by a predominant emotional state. These states are: fear, uncertainty or indecision, lack of interest in the present, despondency and despair, over concern for the welfare of others, loneliness and over-sensitivity. While he saw each type as possessing positive qualities which could be developed, it is the characteristic negative emotions of each which become apparent in illness.

Each category is further sub-divided for the prescription of the various flower remedies, so that for instance under the heading of 'over-sensitivity' there are four remedies: Agrimony for anxiety and mental torment hidden under a brave face; Centaury for weak will and a 'doormat tendency'; Walnut for major life changes and Holly for jealousy and suspicion.

There are no 'official' practitioners of Bach flower remedies. There are a few doctors who will prescribe them. Since they are completely safe most people who use them will select a remedy for themselves by self diagnosis, using the *Handbook of Bach Flower Remedies* which is available from the Edward Bach

Healing Centre and some health food shops. The remedies themselves are available from these two sources. Bach himself discovered the remedies by intuition, often working himself into the same state of mind for which a remedy was required and, walking among the flowers and plants growing locally, he would feel drawn to the one which offered some relief. Prescribing the appropriate remedy for yourself can also be done in this intuitive way, especially since it can be difficult to decide among the long list of mental symptoms described in the handbook which ones are really at the root of your condition. To do this some people use radiesthesia - dowsing with a pendulum (q.v.).

An invaluable item for the first aid kit is 'Rescue Remedy' which is a mixture of five of the flower remedies and can be used after a shock, or in any emotional crisis. To take the remedies, put two or three drops in a glass of water or fruit juice.

More information about Bach Flower Remedies can be obtained from the **Dr Edward Bach Centre.**

READING
A Guide to the Bach Flower Remedies *by Julian Barnard, C.W. Daniel £1.50.* A thorough and straightforward guide to the remedies in pocket size for instant reference. **Bach Flower Therapy** *by Mechthild Scheffer, Thorsons £6.99.* This is the most popular of the Bach Flower books and has a chapter on each of the remedies and also describes how to choose the right remedy. It is suitable for practitioner's reference but clear and simple enough to be of benefit to the layman.

CENTRES OFFERING BACH FLOWER REMEDIES
Aetherius Society SW6, Augenblick Centre, Bennett & Luck N1, Brackenbury Natural Health Centre W6, Clapham Common Clinic SW4, Dr Edward Bach Centre OX10, Healing Fields Practice N7, Heath Health Care NW3, Helios N1, Homoeopathic Centre W13, Kingston Natural Healing Centre, Naturecare SW16, Natureworks, Neal's Yard Therapy Rooms WC2H, New Cross Natural Therapy Centre , Pearl Healing Centre CR7, Primrose Healing Centre NW1, Shirley Goldstein, Silver Birch Centre NW10, South London Natural Health Centre SW4, Therapy Made Unique E18, Violet Hill Studios NW8, Yoga Dham HA2.

Healing
Though the technique of the 'laying on of hands' is in practice the same for many healers who see themselves as mediums for a healing force, there is often a great difference in the way they see their role in this process, and experience the force or energy itself.

This kind of healing has a long history in the Christian tradition and some spiritual healers believe that it is the power of God working through them which brings about a cure. Another kind of spiritual healer would best be described as a spiritualist healer, and believes that this power is mediated by a spirit guide or guides. Some healers are secular in their approach and do not regard their power as divine in origin, but more as a natural manifestation of their own, or universal psychic energies. However individual healers may see it, healing is usually seen as involving the transmission of energy in some form from the healer to his or her client.

A session with a healer may or may not involve them physically laying hands on you. Some work off the body, and all follow their intuition in treating each individual patient. Subjects report feeling heat or cold under the healer's hand, or pins and needles, or tingling sensations, but everyone's reactions will be different. Some people feel better immediately, others may need repeated treatments. Sessions will probably last about 30 minutes. Some spiritual healers offer 'absent healing' where healing thoughts are 'sent' to the person wishing to be healed, without any physical contact being made. Some healers have extended their work and use guided imagery and visualisation, counselling and a variety of other techniques.

Reputable healers stress that there are few 'miracle cures', and much depends for a permanent improvement of the condition on the patient's attitude and efforts to get well.

Although some healers are ambivalent about charging for their work, particularly if they feel that their ability to heal is a gift, and as such something which in turn needs to be given to others, they have to eat and pay overheads like anyone else. Some may ask for a donation rather than a fixed fee, which can be a little confusing to the client, but does offer him or her the opportunity to make their own evaluation of the treatment. Healers are now allowed to visit patients in some hospitals, at patients' request, especially those who are gravely ill.

READING

The Seven Levels of Healing *by Lilla Bek and Philippa Pullar, Rider £5.99.* The two authors describe how healing capacities can be trained and developed by applying an understanding of the seven levels of energy to the process of healing, by training and forms of self-discipline including meditation, visualisation an relaxation. **Peace, Love and Healing** *by Bernie Siegel, Rider £6.99.* This new book by the author of *Love, Medicine and Miracles* teaches how to be receptive to the messages the mind gives the body through dreams and symbols. Supported by inspiring stores of patients who have achieved remissions and miraculous cures, Dr. Siegel shows how love, hope, joy and peace of mind have strong physiological effects just as powerful as those of depression and despair.

CENTRES OFFERING HEALING

Aetherius Society SW6, Alternative Therapies Centre N16, Brackenbury Natural Health Centre W6, Care-Healing Centre W9, Centre for Personal & Professional Development N17, Changes NW3, College of Healing WR14, College of Psychic Studies SW7, Confederation of Healing Organisations HP4, Dancing Dragon Massage N16, Dancing on the Path, Greater World Christian Spiritual Association W1P, Hampstead Healing Centre NW3, Harry Edwards Spiritual Healing Sanctuary GU5, Healing Centre NW6, Healing Workshops NW5, Helios N1, Kingston Natural Healing Centre, Living Colour NW3, National Federation of Spiritual Healers TW16, Natureworks, Neal's Yard Therapy Rooms WC2H, Pearl Healing Centre CR7, Primrose Healing Centre NW1, Raphael Clinic NW6, Shirley Goldstein, Silver Birch Centre NW10, Spiritualist Association of Great Britain SW1X, St James Centre for Health and Healing W1V, Sunra SW12, Universitas Associates SM2, Violet Hill Studios NW8, White Eagle Lodge W8.

TRAININGS IN HEALING

Dancing Dragon Massage *Title of Training:* Healer Training Course *Duration:* One weekend a month over a year. *Entry requirements:* None. *Fees:* Refer to organisers *Comments:* Also introductory massage courses plus psychic development. Advanced massage training also.

Cheirological Society *Title of Training:* Diploma in Cheirological Analysis *Duration:* One-Five years depending on the level of course taken, and the emphasis is on self-motivated study. *Entry requirements:* Students should be interested in psycholgical analysis or health diagnosis, and interested in understanding and helping people. They also need dedication, committement and energy. *Fees:* Basic course fee is £100. Membership of the society is £22 per annum and the cost of books and equipment is not included. *Comments:* Courses take place at varying times of the year. Students are also recommeded to practice related subject such as meditation or yoga. This is the only organisation in Europe to offer this training.

College of Healing *Title of Training:* Diploma Course from the College of Healing *Duration:* Three part course, each part of the course consists of a six day intensive workshop plus coursework, minimum completion time is one year. *Entry requirements:* Minimum age of 20. Admission to the course is by questionaire. *Fees:* £1485 for the full course. *Comments:* The longest established healing college in Britian.

Herbalism

The use of herbal remedies to cure disease must be one of the oldest and most widespread of medical arts, and formed the basis of much of modern pharmacology. But while modern drugs which derive from plants are made by separating out the 'active' ingredient and concentrating it, herbal remedies use the whole plant. Supporters of herbal medicine say that the natural chemical balance present in the entire plant means that its effects on the body are in turn

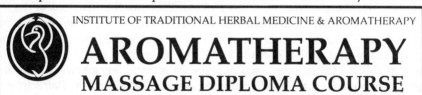

more balanced, and so the side effects caused by many modern drugs are avoided.

A herbalist may follow the western tradition and use herbs from this country and Europe, or he or she may be a Chinese herbalist and use traditional Chinese herbs.

A herbalist is not usually medically trained, though they should have undergone a training course lasting a few years. As with homoeopathy, the herbalist will take a detailed medical history and perhaps focus particularly on your diet to see whether you may be suffering from any allergies. However, unlike homoeopathic treatment, the remedies are usually prescribed for a particular complaint, rather than through building up a picture of your personality and symptoms.

Herbs are prescribed in different forms. They can be taken as an infusion, and prepared in a similar way to tea. Sometimes they need to be boiled for quite a long time. Some herbs are prescribed in tinctures, where they are suspended in alcohol, and they can also be prepared as lotions, tablets, liquids, poultices and suppositories. Often a combination of different herbs is prescribed, so that if one herb does not effect a cure, another might.

Many people take herbal remedies as a method of self-help. If you do, you can go to a specialist herbal shop (see below in the 'Resources' section) to ask advice, though it is possible to find out which herbs work for you by trial and error. Treating yourself involves infusing the plants as tea, and of course pre-prepared herbal remedies for such things as insomnia, stress and menstrual pain are available at chemist shops. One word of warning - some herbs can be toxic, especially if taken in large quantities, so if experimenting with a new herb, it is best to take advice.

READING

The Holistic Herbal by *David Hoffmann, Element £8.95.* Illustrated with original line drawings and photographs, this book places herbs in the context of Gaia, the living earth, and offers a practical, comprehensive look at the use of herbs. It includes a detailed look at the systems of the body; circulation, respiration, digestion and nervous systems. There are sections on herb gathering, preparation and herbal chemistry. As well as being a complete traditional herbal, this is a fascinating practical guide for maintaining a healthy body and soul. **Complete Herbal Handbook for the Dog and Cat** *Juliette de Bairäcli Levy, Faber & Faber £4.95.* One of a series of herbals by this author covering herbal treatment for different types of patient. Cats and dogs respond well to natural medicine and this book, divided into three parts, concentrates first on the care and rearing of young animals, secondly on the use of herbs to cure disease. The third part is a general section focusing on disease prevention.

CENTRES OFFERING HERBALISM

Acumedic Centre NW1, African Herbs Ltd TW3, All Hallows House EC3R, Alternative Medicine Clinic NW15, Bodywise E2, Brackenbury Natural Health Centre W6, British School of Oriental Therapy and Movement SE21, C.H.I Clinic SW6, Chelsea Complementary Natural Health Centre SW10, CHI Centre SW6, Chinese Clinic W1V, City Health Centre EC1Y, Clapham Common Clinic SW4, Clinic of Herbal Medicine, Clissold Park Natural Health Centre N16, Edgware Centre for Natural Health HA8, Fook Sang Acupuncture and Chinese Herbal Practitioners Training College UK NW11, Haelan Centre, Haelen Centre, Hale Clinic W1N, Heath Health Care NW3, Helios N1, Herb Society SW1W, Holistic Health Consultancy SW1V, Hong Tao Acupuncture and Natural Health Clinic HA5, Islington Green Centre of Alternative Medicine N1, Kingston Natural Healing Centre, London School of Acupuncture and Traditional Chinese Medicine (Clinic) EC1Y, London School of Acupuncture and Traditional Chinese Medicine EC1Y, Lotus Healing Centre NW8, Marigold Treatment Centre HA8, National Institute of Medical Herbalists EX1, Natural Healing Centre HA4, Neal's Yard Therapy Rooms WC2H, New Cross Natural Therapy Centre , Northwood Hills Acupuncture Clinic HA6, Notting Hill Traditional Acupuncture Clinic W11, Pearl Healing Centre CR7, Primrose Healing Centre NW1, Putney Natural Therapy Clinic, Refuah Shelaymah Natural Health Centre N16, Silver Birch Centre NW10, South London Natural Health Centre SW4, St James Centre for Health and Healing W1V, Thames & Ganges Trading Co, Traditional Chinese Medicine Clinic UB5, Wimbledon Clinic of Natural Medicine SW19, Women and Health NW1, Wood Street Clinic EN5.

TRAINING IN HERBALISM

London School of Herbology and Aromatherapy *Title of Training:* Herbal Medicine/Medical Armoatherapy Diploma Course. *Duration*: 3 years part-time (500 hours). *Entry requirements:* None: students are trained in all aspects of required knowledge. *Fees:* Refer to organisers *Comments:* Training in both Chinese traditional approach, and western medical approach.

Fook Sang Acupuncture and Chinese Herbal Practitioners Training College UK *Title of Training:* Chinese Herbal Practitioners Training Course. *Duration:* Three years part time training, weekend attendance. *Entry requirements:* Preferably degree level or vocational training. Minimum A level standard. Mature students must show enthusiasm and desire to learn. *Fees:* Refer to organisers *Comments:* Successful graduates eligible for membership of Acupuncture Practitioners Association and Hong Kong Chinese Acupuncture Association. They offer their graduated students the opportunity to join their clinical practice in order to further their skills.

London College of Chinese and Oriental Medicine *Title of Training:* Training in Chinese Herbal Medicine and Acupuncture. *Duration:* Four years. 48 days per year. 9.30-5pm. *Entry requirements:* The main criteria is an intention to help others. *Fees:* Refer to organisers

Herbalism Traditional Chinese Medicine Clinic *Title of Training:* Acupuncture and Chinese Herbal Medicine *Duration:* One to two years. *Entry requirements:* Graduate or equivalent in medical or biological science. *Fees:* Refer to organisers

Clinic of Herbal Medicine *Title of Training:* 1) Diploma of Herbal Medicine/ Phytotherapy 2) Certificate of Phytotherapy *Duration:* 1) Four years full time 2) Four years tutorial *Entry requirements:* A Level passes in at least two subjects, one must be scientific. *Fees:* On Application *Comments:* The only school offering membership to The National Institute of Medical Herbalists and The College of Practitioners of Phytotherapy. CACC accredited.

Homoeopathy

Homoeopathy is a system of medicine which is based on the idea that an illness which produces certain symptoms can be cured by a substance or drug which produces the same symptoms.

Homoeopathic remedies are substances which have been diluted sometimes up to tens of thousands of times. In their undiluted form they would produce similar symptoms to those for which they are prescribed. While conventional medicine treats with drugs which produce contrary, suppressive effects (for instance aspirin to suppress a temperature), homoeopathy follows the treatment of like by like. A simple parallel can be drawn to illustrate this contrast: if one had cold feet, one could either plunge them into hot water which would alleviate the feeling of cold for a while, or put them in cold water which might make them feel colder at first, but would then stimulate the circulation so that the body would be working to heat itself up. In the same way, the homoeopathic remedy, by aggravating the symptoms very minutely, stimulates the body's own defences or 'vital force'. The concept is also similar to that of innoculation.

Critics of homoeopathy claim that the substances are so highly diluted (sometimes as if one were putting one drop of a liquid into the Baltic sea) that the original cannot be found in the remedy. Supporters claim that even highly diluted remedies still contain the energy of the substance, though they cannot be detected by existing chemical methods.

The founder of this system was Samuel Hahnemann, a German doctor who practised in the early 19th century. He tested hundreds of drugs on healthy volunteers or 'provers' as he called them (some of whom must have been dedicated since many of the substances produced unpleasant symptoms) and catalogued the effects they had. Since many of the drugs were poisons, when Hahnemann prescribed them for his patients he tried diluting them as much as possible, and through this he discovered that in fact the more he diluted them, the stronger they became in their curative effects.

Diagnosis in homoeopathy has to be made very carefully and precisely to find the right remedy not only for the disease, but also for the individual patient. On visiting a homoeopathic doctor, he or she will take a detailed history, not just about your complaint, but also about the sort of person you are, your likes and dislikes and your physical and emotional temperament. He or she will take important events in your life into consideration and your family's medical history. For this reason the initial consultation is usually the longest.

When the remedy has been prescribed the homoeopath will tell you when and how to take it. The remedies have to be stored and taken carefully to preserve their properties. Since conventional drugs work in a way which is directly contrary to the way in which homoeopathic remedies take effect, you may decide to stop taking ordinary medicines, although it is worth discussing this with your homoeopath if this will be difficult. Some homoeopaths also recommend that you do not drink coffee, eat sweets or consume peppermint around the time you take the remedy, but this varies with the practitioner.

Homoeopathic remedies can be used to treat most reversible illnesses. On the whole they are not suitable for diseases requiring surgery, though dedicated homoeopaths would probably disagree. Useful to have around the house is the 'homoeopathic first aid kit' since all the remedies are safe enough to be self-administered. Homoeopathy has even be used with success on animals.

READING
Everybody's Guide to Homoeopathic Medicines *by Stephen Cummings and*

Dana Ullman Gollancz £4.95. The authors explain in clear terms how to treat yourself and your family with safe and effective remedies. Learn about 'casetaking' and how to prescribe for ailments such as colds, digestive problems, headaches and cystitis. Remedies for first aid use are also described as well as instructions for when it is necessary to seek outside help. The book begins with a brief outline of the fundamental ideas behind homoeopathy. **The Science of Homoeopathy** *by George Vithoulkas Thorsons £7.99.* Written by one of the world's leading homoeopaths, this work outlines both theory and practice of homoeopathy. The clear, concise language, inclusion of case histories, references and illustrations make it an excellent reference work for physicians and an informative introduction for the lay reader.

CENTRES OFFERING HOMOEOPATHY

Acupuncture and Osteopathy Clinic SW1V, Aetherius Society SW6, Alternative Medicine Clinic NW15, Alternative Therapies Centre N16, Association of Natural Medicines CM8, Bayswater Clinic W2, Bexleyheath Natural Health Clinic DA7, Bodywise E2, Brackenbury Natural Health Centre W6, British Homoeopathic Association W1N, Bumblebees Natural Remedies N7, Centre for Health and Healing W1V, Chelsea Complementary Natural Health Centre SW10, City Health Centre EC1Y, Clapham Common Clinic SW4, Clissold Park Natural Health Centre N16, College of Homoeopathy Clinic SE13, College of Homoeopathy NW1, College of Practical Homoeopathy E2, Drakefield Homoeopathic Centre SW17, Edgware Centre for Natural Health HA8, Equilibrium Therapy Centre SW18, Faculty of Homoeopathy WC1N, Gerda Boyesen Centre W3, Gestalt Centre London EC1Y, Haelan Centre, Haelen Centre, Hahnemann College of Homoeopathy E13, Hahnemann College of Homoeopathy UB1, Heath Health Care NW3, Helios N1, Hillside Practice, Holistic Health Consultancy SW1V, Homoeopathic Centre W13, Homoeopathic Health Clinic HA3, Insight Care N1, Islington Green Centre of Alternative Medicine N1, Kingston Natural Healing Centre, Lavender Hill Homoeopathic Centre SW11, Life Works NW1, Living Centre SW20, London College of Classical Homoeopathy SE1, London Lighthouse W11, London Natural Health Clinic W8, Marigold Trust WC1N, Natural Healing Centre HA4, Natural Health Clinic HA3, Natural Medicine Centre BR2, Nature Cure Clinic W1M, Natureworks, Neal's Yard Therapy Rooms WC2H, New Cross Natural Therapy Centre , Notting Hill Traditional Acupuncture Clinic W11, Portobello Green Fitness Centre W10, Private Health Centre E7, Putney Natural Therapy Clinic, Raphael Clinic NW6, Royal London Homoeopathic Hospital, Sayer Clinic: Chelsea SW6, South London Natural Health Centre SW4, Spectrum N4, Sunra SW12, Therapy Made Unique E18, Violet Hill Studios NW8, Westminster Natural Health Centre SW1V, Wimbledon Clinic of Natural Medicine SW19, Women and Health NW1, Wood Street Clinic EN5.

TRAININGS IN HOMOEOPATHY

College of Homoeopathy *Title of Training:* Licentiate of the College of Homoeopathy. *Duration:* 1) 3 years full time 2) 4 years part time. *Entry requirements:* 2 'A' levels, one being Human Biology. However, all applications are considered individually. *Fees:* Refer to organisers

Faculty of Homoeopathy *Title of Training:* Postgraduate Training in Homoeopathy *Entry requirements:* Applicants must be qualified MB or BS (Batchelor of Medicine or Surgery). *Fees:* Refer to organisers *Comments:* Refer to organisers for details

Hahnemann College of Homoeopathy *Title of Training:* (1) Beginners course (2) Paramedics course (3)Postgraduate *Duration:* Generally courses are two weekends a month, but a combination of full time and part time study is possible. (1) 3 years, (2) 2 years, (3) 1 year. *Entry requirements:* (1) Four GCE passes which must include one 'A' level in a science subject. (2) Must be qualified, registered paramedical practitioner with sufficient knowledge of anatomy, physiology and diagnosis. (3) Applicants myst be qualified homoeopathic pracititioners from abroad or from recognised institutes. *Fees:* Refer to organisers *Comments:* Fees may be paid in instalments. Exceptional cases not meeting entry requirements may be admitted, subject to an interview by the education committee.

London College of Classical Homoeopathy *Title of Training:* Four Year Full Time Professional Training Course *Duration:* Three years full-time, four years part-time *Entry requirements:* If under 21 then 5 'O' levels and 3 'A's. Otherwise 'O' level or equivalent in human biology. *Fees:* Refer to organisers *Comments:* Discretionary grants are available from many boroughs.

School of Homoeopathy *Title of Training:* Correspondence and part-time Diploma in Homoeopathy. *Comments:* This course leads to registration with The Society of Homoeopaths.

Iridology

Iridology is a method of diagnosis in which the eyes, especially the iris, indicate the physical and psychological condition of the patient. Iridologists claim that the whole body is reflected in the eye, because this is where the entire nervous system comes to the surface.

Dr Bernard Jensen, in developing this technique, has mapped the iris and correlated different segments with parts of the body. If a segment has an unusual colour or markings, or is flecked, this is an indication that the corresponding part is not functioning properly. As a diagnostic technique, Iridologists claim that not only past disorders can be recognised, but tendencies towards disease in the future can be spotted and remedied before developing. The eyes are also examined for their condition: bright or dull, coarse or fine.

Iridologists may employ a magnifying glass to examine the eyes, or take photographs and make slides from which a diagnosis can be made.

Iridology can be used as a diagnostic aid in conjunction with any other therapy.

READING

Iridology - Personality and Health Analysis through the Iris by *Dorothy Hall, Angus & Robertson £4.95.* Dorothy Hall, an experienced practitioner, introduces the way to use this diagnostic technique by detailing how to recognise the signs shown in the iris. Using this book you can attempt to find your own pattern of good health and well-being, a pattern as distinct as a fingerprint for each one of us. **The Science and Practice of** Iridology by *Bernard Jensen, Bernard Jensen £20.00.* The classic textbook for serious students of iridology. The colour photographs clearly illustrate the diagnostic techniques and the comprehensive text aids the development of skills in the student's powers of diagnosis. There is also a second volume of this work which is in even greater detail and costs approximately £80.

CENTRES OFFERING IRIDOLOGY

Alternative Medicine Clinic NW15, City Health Centre EC1Y, College of Opthalmic Somatology N1, Community Health Foundation EC1V, Helios N1, Holistic Health Consultancy SW1V, Insight Care N1, Islington Green Centre of Alternative Medicine N1, Kingston Natural Healing Centre, Life Works NW1, Natureworks, Neal's Yard Therapy Rooms WC2H, Women and Health NW1.

TRAININGS IN IRIDOLOGY

College of Opthalmic Somatology *Title of Training:* 1) Certificate Course in Ophthalmic Somatology 2) Diploma Couse in Ophthalmic Somatology *Duration:* 1) 1 year part time 2) 2 years part time on completion of certificate course *Entry requirements:* 'A' level or equivalent Anatomy & Physiology 1) and 2) can be studied concurrently *Fees:* Refer to organisers *Comments:* Training is based 'upon recognition and interpretation of the predominant miasm, leading to considerable fine tuning of iris analysis'.

Kirlian Photography

This is high-frequency photography used to produce a photograph of the 'aura' of energy around the body, and from this some people believe that diagnosis of illness can be made, whether manifest or latent.

It was discovered by Semyon and Valentina Kirlian, from the Kuban in the Soviet Union. They found that photographs made using this technique would show differences in the energy field of healthy and diseased subjects.

A Kirlian photograph is usually taken using the two hands of the subject. A furry or hairy effect can be observed in the photographs, following the outline of the palm and fingers. This is believed to be the energy emitted from the hand. However, while in strictly controlled conditions Kirlian photography can be used to diagnose certain illnesses, in normal conditions the photograph can be affected by many extraneous factors such as the condition of the film, humidity of the air and so on. It is also not at all clear whether a Kirlian picture can accurately diagnose *potential* illness, as some enthusiasts claim.

CENTRES OFFERING KIRLIAN PHOTOGRAPHY
Aura Vision TW9.

Massage

Massage is a way of working on the soft tissues, the muscles and skin, to relieve tension held in the body. There are many different massage techniques and individual practitioners may use or have been influenced by different body therapies like shiatsu, rolfing, physiotherapy or hand healing. Some masseurs (masculine) or masseuses (feminine) may rely very much on a technique, and others may use 'intuitive' massage. In 'intuitive' massage the practitioner is guided by the way the client's body feels to apply basic techniques where they are most needed - in areas where there is a build-up of tension.

A masseur/se might come to the home of the client if they are elderly or bedridden, but usually the client will visit them in their home or a health centre. Some work with the client lying on the floor but most will use a massage table. The room should be kept very warm or the cold will make the recipient of the massage tense up. The masseur/se will use oil to help their hands move smoothly over the skin and will use a variety of strokes, such as kneading, rubbing, pummelling, circling, or stroking using fingertips, thumbs or the whole hand. You may not realise how tense your muscles are until the masseur/se begins to touch them, because tension gives rise not only to feelings of pain or stiffness, but sometimes shows itself just in numbness.

Individual practitioners have different ideas on pain. A few feel that a certain amount of pain in necessary if the massage is to be effective in releasing tension.

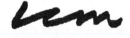

Most would feel that while working on areas which have become very tense can give rise to a feeling of discomfort, they would be careful to keep this to a minimum. While a muscle may be sore to the touch, there is also a feeling of relief which usually overrides any discomfort. Individual clients have different tastes too; some prefer a vigorous massage while others may want something more soothing. The most important thing as a client is to feel that you can discuss this with the masseur/se and they will be responsive to your needs.

Having a massage is a pleasant experience. It is a way of being nurtured, it is relaxing and, in releasing energy which has become stored up in tension, it can also be invigorating. Massage is useful as part of a programme for combating stress.

Self-massage is also possible, although it is not as effective as being massaged by someone else. Relieving a friend's stiff neck can be a very satisfying way of giving and receiving physical contact - something which can be neglected. Most people can learn how to do the basic strokes and there are many weekend courses for beginners who want to learn to use massage on family and friends. The centres listed below may offer individual massage, courses for those who want to learn to give massage or both.

READING
The Massage Book *by George Downing, Penguin £5.99.* This well known simple manual of massage has been recently republished, a testament to its popularity. Massage is an art of healing and a powerful means of communicating without words. In order to convey the full range and effect of the art, the author outlines its wider philosophy and its links with oriental cults. Included are chapters on meditation, zone therapy and massage for lovers. **The Book of Massage** *by Lucinda Lidell, Ebury Press £7.95.* A classic guide to the relaxing and healing skills of the hands. It is beautifully illustrated with drawings and photographs and includes step-by-step instructions with authoritative advice on all aspects.

144

This book teaches the effects of the power of human touch.

CENTRES OFFERING MASSAGE

Abshot Holistic Centre PO14, Alternative Medicine Clinic NW15, Alternative Therapies Centre N16, Augenblick Centre, Bates, Carrie N4, Belgravia Beauty SW1X, Bennett & Luck N1, Bluestone Clinic W1N, Body Clinic NW11, Bodywise E2, Brackenbury Natural Health Centre W6, Bretforton Hall Clinic WR11, Bumblebees Natural Remedies N7, Cabot Centre NW1, Centre for Health and Healing W1V, Centre for Personal & Professional Development N17, Changes NW3, Chelsea Complementary Natural Health Centre SW10, Chiron Centre for Holistic Psychotherapy W5, Chiropractic Clinic NW11, Churchill Centre W1H, City Health Centre EC1Y, Clapham Common Clinic SW4, Clare Maxwell Hudson NW2, College of Homoeopathy Clinic SE13, Community Health Foundation EC1V, Cortijo Romero UK LS7, Creative and Healing Arts W11, Dancing Dragon Massage N16, Edgware Centre for Natural Health HA8, Equilibrium Therapy Centre SW18, Food and Chemical Allergy Clinic CR0, Gerda Boyesen Centre W3, Green Wood College W6, Haelan Centre, Haelen Centre, Hale Clinic W1N, Hampstead Healing Centre NW3, Healing Centre NW5, Healing Fields Practice N7, Health in Action E8, Health Management IG10, Heath Health Care NW3, Helios N1, Highbury Centre N5, Homoeopathic Health Clinic HA3, Hong Tao Acupuncture and Natural Health Clinic HA5, IBISS TW7, Institute of Holistic Massage, Islington Green Centre of Alternative Medicine N1, Ken Eyerman School of Bodywork and Movement SW2, Kingston Natural Healing Centre, Lever Clinic EN1, Life Resources NW7, Life Works NW1, Living Centre SW20, London College of Massage W1P, London Lighthouse W11, London Natural Health Clinic W8, London School of Acupuncture and Traditional Chinese Medicine EC1Y, Lotus Healing Centre NW8, Massage Training Institute N5, Mehta Method of Therapeutic Head Massage N1, Muswell Healing Arts N10, Natural Health Clinic HA3, Natural Medicine Centre BR2, Nature Cure Clinic W1M, Neal's Yard Therapy Rooms WC2H, New Cross Natural Therapy Centre, Open Centre EC1V, Pearl Healing Centre CR7, Portobello Green Fitness Centre W10, Primrose Healing Centre NW1, Private Health Centre E7, Putney Natural Therapy Clinic, Raphael Clinic NW6, Refuah Shelaymah Natural Health Centre N16, Sayer Clinic: Croydon CR0, Sayer Clinic: Marble Arch W1H, Shirley Goldstein, Silver Birch Centre NW10, Skills with People N5, South London Natural Health Centre SW4, Sunra SW12, Violet Hill Studios NW8, West London School of Therapeutic Massage W11, West London School of Therapeutic Massage W11, Whole Health Clinic NW3, Wild Goose Company NW3, Women and Health NW1, Wood Street Clinic EN5.

TRAININGS IN MASSAGE

Ken Eyerman School of Bodywork and Movement *Title of Training:* The

Eyerman technique training in massage. *Duration:* 3-year diploma course part-time. 6 weekends a year plus 6 practical days per year. *Entry requirements:* None for first year of diploma course, but for 2nd and 3rd years must have completed first year. *Fees:* Refer to organisers *Comments:* Eyerman technique is a synthesis of massage and movement utilising techniques from eastern and western massage forms. Also weekend workshops.

Churchill Centre *Title of Training:* Advanced massage course. Churchill Centre Certificate in Health Care and Relaxation with Massage. *Duration:* Basic training three weekends for ITEC certificate. Advanced course two weekends *Entry requirements:* English speaking and interested to learn about massage. *Fees:* Refer to organisers

Clare Maxwell Hudson *Title of Training:* Introductory through to advanced techniques including basic massage, reflexlogy, shiatsu, sports massage, facials, etc. ITEC. *Duration:* Vary. *Fees:* Refer to organisers

Dancing Dragon Massage *Title of Training:* Basic Massage Course *Duration:* Four weekends and four evenings. *Entry requirements:* None. *Fees:* Refer to organisers *Comments:* Also introductory massage courses plus psychic development. Advanced massage training also.

Shirley Goldstein *Title of Training:* Holistic Massage Diploma Course. *Duration:* 3 weekends. *Fees:* Refer to organisers

South London Natural Health Centre *Title of Training:* ITEC and MTI Certificates in Holistic Massage. Basic and practitioner level. *Duration:* Basic: three weekends Practitioner: five or six weekends *Fees:* Basic: £230 Practitioner: £590-£810 depending on exams. *Comments:* Extra time is spent on the self awareness of the student to develop themselves and their intuition. The course can be booked and paid for in flexible modules.

Sunra *Duration:* Five half days (20 hours). *Entry requirements:* Interest in the healing arts. *Fees:* Refer to organisers

West London School of Therapeutic Massage *Title of Training:* Training in massage, anatomy and physiology, reflex zone therapy and sports therapy. ITEC. *Duration:* Three to twelve months. *Entry requirements:* None specified *Fees:* Refer to organisers

Bodywise *Title of Training:* Bodywise Massage Diploma Course *Duration:* Three terms of three weeks each. *Entry requirements:* None. Participants must attend at least 85% of course and do 30 massages to receive Diploma. *Fees:* £500.00 total (£350.00 concessions). *Comments:* 85% attendance necessary, along with at least 30 charted massage treatments, to gain Diploma. Diploma incorporates study of Anatomy, Physiology and Healing aspects of massage. Course is taught by practising Buddhists with an emphasis on developing awareness and positivity towards others.

Institute of Holistic Massage *Title of Training:* Holistic Massage. *Duration:* Nine days. *Entry requirements:* Sufficient interest in massage. *Fees:* Refer to organisers

London College of Massage *Title of Training*: 1) Beginner Massage Certificate 2) Foundation Practitioner Certificate 3) Advanced Practitioner Certificate *Duration:* 1) 10 weeks part time evening and weekends 2) 15 weeks part time evening plus 4 weekends advanced massage 3) 12 weeks part time or 4 weekends remedial massage *Entry requirements:* 1) None 2) Completion of Beginners Course 3) Completion of Beginners and Foundation Courses *Fees:* Refer to organisers *Comments:* The London College of Massage was founded in 1987 by Fiona Harrold, 'one of the UK's leading authorities on massage'. The College intends to improve the standard of massage training throughout the country. The Massage Practitioners Certificate is recognised as an approved course by the Institute of Complementary Medicine and their Advanced Certificate includes a practical massage project.

Massage International College of Oriental Medicine *Title of Training:* Acupuncture and Masseur Course. *Duration:* Three years full-time, fourth year part-time. *Entry requirements:* Minimum of 2 'A' levels preferred, but will consider serious applicants individually. *Fees:* Refer to organisers *Comments:* Because this is a full time course it attracts local authority grants.

Essentials for Health *Title of Training:* ITEC Diploma in Massage *Duration:* 80 hours part-time over 5 weekends. *Entry requirements:* An interest in massage and working with people *Fees:* £545 inclusive

Massage Training Institute *Title of Training:* The Institute of Massage Certificate in Holistic Massage, Anatomy and Physiology. *Duration:* 100 hours practise and theory; plus 50 hours out-of-class practise over a minimum of three months,(exact format depends on individual tutors). *Entry requirements:* Depends on individual tutor. *Fees:* Between £400 - £600. *Comments:* Their trainings emphasise the Mind, Body, Spirit connection and ensure that practitioners are qualified to work to a high professional standard.

Metamorphic Technique

Metamorphic technique was originally developed from foot reflexology by Robert St John, but evolved into a completely different therapy. Rather than positing that each area of the foot corresponds to a part of the body, metamorphic techique is based on the idea that the foot from toe to heel corresponds to the pre-natal period from conception to birth. This is also seen to correspond to the spine from base to head. By massaging the foot it is believed that physical and psychological traumas incurred in the womb can be healed. For it is in the nine months of gestation, according to the theory of metamorphic technique, that all our mental, physical, emotional and spiritual patterns and responses are set.

Each foot is massaged for about half an hour, generally starting at the toe and working on the arch of the foot, down to the heel. The practitioner may also work on the hands and the back of the head.

Though it was originally devised to help handicapped children, it is a gentle technique which can be used by anyone.

CENTRES OFFERING METAMORPHIC TECHNIQUE
Jeyrani Health Centre E18, Metamorphic Association SW17, Pearl Healing Centre CR7, Violet Hill Studios NW8.

TRAINING IN METAMORPHIC TECHNIQUE
Metamorphic Association *Title of Training:* Refer to organisers.

Natural Birth Control

There are various methods of natural birth control, but they all work on the theory that the fertile period in a woman's menstrual cycle can be worked out, either on certain principals, or by observing signs and changes in the body. During this time, the couple can either abstain from penetrative sex or use barrier methods of birth control (e.g. condom or diaphragm with spermicide). Couples wanting to conceive can also use them to indicate when it's likely, and, according to some theories (still unproven) can try to determine the sex of their child by making love just before ovulation (for a girl) or just after ovulation (for a boy).

Natural birth control doesn't involve taking substances or putting devices into the body, nor does it have the side effects sometimes associated with orthodox methods of birth control. However, they do require a degree of commitment by both the woman and her partner if they are to be effective. Though perhaps somewhat time consuming, natural birth control methods may provide a woman with the opportunity to get to know her own body and natural cycles more, to share responsibility for contraception and for both partners to communicate more with each other about sex. A combination of methods outlined below should be used, and *it is very important to get an expert in natural birth control to teach you.* Contacts for this are listed at the end of this section.

In general with all these methods you are more likely to avoid conceiving if you have unprotected intercourse only in the time after ovulation (a woman's fertile time) up to the next period, than if you have unprotected sex in the time after a period up to ovulation. They are only suitable for those in a long-term, monogamous relationship since they offer no protection against AIDS and sexually transmitted diseases.

Mucus Method
This involves observing the changes in quality and quantity of the mucus in the vagina throughout the menstrual cycle.

During menstruation this mucus (called 'cervical mucus') can't be observed easily, so these are not necessarily safe days. After menstruation, there may be a couple of days of no mucus, and a sensation of dryness in the vagina (however, if yours is a short cycle, you may have mucus straight away). Then the mucus will start to become more profuse, starting off whitish or yellowish, thick and tacky and becoming clearer, more slippery and stringy like raw egg white (you can stretch a strand of it between two fingers). These changes start about five days before ovulation and on the most fertile days you may have a sensation of slippery wetness and lubrication. Unprotected intercourse should be avoided from the first time you see or feel the mucus until four days after the slippery, wet sensation has gone. After this, the mucus will resume a whitish, yellowish, cloudy appearance and tacky consistency. A properly trained natural family planning teacher will enable you to learn the difference between these different kinds of mucus.

Basal Body Temperature

Just before ovulation, a woman's temperature drops slightly, and after ovulation it rises. By taking your temperature every day at the same time on waking with a basal fertility thermometer which can measure minute temperature changes, you can tell when you have ovulated. When you have recorded a temperature for three days in a row which is higher than all the previous six days the fertile time is over. Charts can be obtained from the Family Planning Association to note these temperature changes.

Because many things affect body temperature (even taking aspirin), expert help is needed to interpret the chart. This method by itself does not predict which are the infertile days before ovulation.

Calendar method

This should only be used as a cross-check with the above two methods. Before using this, you need to keep a chart of your periods for at least 6 consecutive cycles. Work out the number of days in the shortest cycle and subtract 19 - this gives you the probable first fertile and therefore unsafe day after the first day of your period. Then work out the number of days in the longest cycle and subtract 10 - this gives the probable last day of the fertile time after which it is safer to have sex again. If your cycle changes you will need to alter your calculations.

Astrological birth control

This method cannot be recommended unless you are happy to get pregnant, since there is no proof at all that it works! The fertile time, according to this method is when the sun and moon are the same distance apart in degrees as they were when the woman was born. This happens once every twenty nine and a half day lunar cycle. It is calculated with an ephemeris (an astrological table of the planets' positions).

Centres offering Natural Birth Control
   Clapham Common Clinic SW4, Family Planning Association W1N, IBISS TW7.

Naturopathy

Fundamental to the practice of naturopathy is the idea that if provided with favourable conditions, nature itself can heal the body. Illness is a result of toxins accumulating in the system and symptoms of disease are the attempts of the body to throw off these harmful waste products. We need only co-operate with this process to establish and maintain good health because nature itself is always striving for the good of the organism. While animals are in tune with this and will instinctively fast or eat foods which contain medicinal substances when they are ill, human beings, according to Naturopathy, have lost contact with this instinct for health.

   Naturopaths use different methods to restore the body to a natural state. Fasting is an important way of clearing out the substances which cause disease, and maintaining a healthy, natural diet afterwards consolidates the benefits gained from fasting. Naturopaths often use osteopathy (q.v.) as well, and hydrotherapy which is treatment with water such as the taking of hot and cold baths or showers, taking spa waters and so on.

   Naturopathy is essentially a self-help therapy. Though the naturopath can prescribe a regime which will suit the individual, it requires work on the part of the patient to stick to it. While fasting can have unpleasant side-effects at first, naturopaths stress that these are the results of the body throwing off harmful waste and are part of the healing process. The fast may not be total, fruit juice or fruit may be recommended, and the naturopath will take into account your age and disposition when advising you of how to go about it. He or she may suggest ways to ease in and out of the fast so that the exercise is not too much of a shock to the system. Diets may be rigourous at first, but once the system becomes sensitive to what it really needs, healthy eating becomes more instinctive.

   Naturopathy emphasises the importance of maintaining good health by eating well and exercising rather than taking action when symptoms develop and a cure is harder to achieve. Increasingly orthodox medicine is also now emphasising that prevention is better than cure.

READING

   Natural Therapeutics *by Henry Lindlahr and Jocelyn Probyn* Volume 1 Philosophy of Natural Therapeutics *£12.00* Volume 2 Practice of Natural Therapeutics *£8.95.* Volume 3 Dietetics *£6.50* Volume 4 Iridiagnosis *£8.75.* These four volumes are concerned with laying down the general principles of natural therapeutics and go on to give guidance and directions on the application and combination of the methods which can be used to prevent disease, promote health and help to bring about cure.

CENTRES OFFERING NATUROPATHY

Bennett & Luck N1, Body Clinic NW11, Bodywise E2, Brackenbury Natural Health Centre W6, British College of Naturopathy and Osteopathy NW3, Bumblebees Natural Remedies N7, Camden Osteopathic and Natural Health Practice NW5, Clapham Common Clinic SW4, Equilibrium Therapy Centre SW18, Forty Hill Natural Therapy Centre, General Council and Register of Osteopaths, Gerda Boysen Clinic W3, Hale Clinic W1N, Heath Health Care NW3, Helios N1, Hocroft Clinic NW2, Holistic Health Consultancy SW1V, Life Works NW1, Natureworks, Neal's Yard Therapy Rooms WC2H, Primrose Healing Centre NW1, Putney Natural Therapy Clinic, Raphael Clinic NW6, South London Natural Health Centre SW4, Violet Hill Studios NW8, Westminster Natural Health Centre SW1V, Wimbledon Clinic of Natural Medicine SW19.

TRAININGS IN NATUROPATHY

British College of Naturopathy and Osteopathy *Title of Training:* Diploma Course in Osteopathy and Naturopathy *Duration:* 4 years full time. *Entry Requirements:* Two 'A' Levels preferably including a biological sceince and chemistry plus minium 2 GCE/GCSE 'O' level passes including at least 1 of English Language, Physics, Maths or Science or Biological Science BTech or equivalent. *Fees:* Refer to organisers *Comments:* The college is applying for degree status in the near future.

Holistic Health Consultancy *Title of Training:* Naturopathic Iridology Course *Duration:* 2 Year correspondance course with periodic seminars and individual training. *Entry Requirements:* An ability to understand people and handle one's own, as well as others', problems and re-education. *Fees:* £1130 p.a. incl. Vat. Seminars and textbooks extra. *Comments:* Course work is taylored to individual pace.

Osteopathy

Osteopathy uses manipulation of the spine and joints to restore the bones, muscles, ligaments and nerves to their proper alignment and thus the patient to health.

The founder of osteopathy, Dr Andrew Taylor Still, had studied engineering as well as medicine. In developing osteopathic techniques, he approached the human body as if it fitted together like a machine, and found that disease was caused by the spinal vertebrae slipping out of position. When this happens 'lesions' appear where the muscles round the displaced vertebrae are so stressed that they pass on inaccurate information to the central nervous system, or the nerves around them become over sensitive and affect the surrounding tissue. This then affects the circulation of the blood. Since the blood was seen by Still as carrying the substances which protect us from disease, illness is then the result of blocked circulation.

On a visit to an osteopath, he or she will take your medical history, and will also be looking at the way you walk, sit and stand to see where the vertebrae may be out of alignment. Examination is also carried out with the hands, and the osteopath will feel the bones and joints. Some may also use X-rays. Treatment itself is very active and physical and may involve you in taking a variety of positions while the osteopath pulls, pushes or applies pressure to your head, arms, legs or back in a number of ways. While this may sound alarming, the treatment is usually painless. A session may last 20-30 minutes and how long you have to keep going back for depends on the severity of the problem. However, since most osteopaths are inundated with patients, they are unlikely to need to prolong your treatment unnecessarily for their own benefit! Sometimes the osteopath may give exercises to be done at home as a back up to the treatment sessions.

Osteopaths are rarely medically qualified, but should have undergone a thorough training of at least three years and be able to recognise medical conditions which lie outside their field of practice. Since osteopathy is one of the best organised therapies of the complementary medicines it is easy to get registers of qualified practitioners.

People usually go to osteopaths for 'bad backs'. and it is of course a good treatment for this ubiquitous complaint as well as for migraines and painful joints. The treatment was evolved to have a wide ranging application and can be helpful with other less obviously suitable complaints.

READING

Osteopathy - is it for you? *by Chris Belshaw, Element £5.95.* A simple worded guide to osteopathy for the patient which includes explanations of the technical terms. It explains how this manual therapy can influence the physiological mechanisms in the body that lead to healing and freedom from pain.

CENTRES OFFERING OSTEOPATHY

Acupuncture and Osteopathy Clinic SW1V, Alternative Therapies Centre N16, Aromatherapy Associates SW6, Bennett & Luck N1, Bluestone Clinic W1N, Body Clinic NW11, Bodywise E2, Brackenbury Natural Health Centre W6, British and European Osteopathic Association, British College of Naturopathy and Osteopathy NW3, British Osteopathic Association NW1, British School of Osteopathy SW1Y, Bumblebees Natural Remedies N7, Camden Osteopathic and Natural Health Practice NW5, Centre for Health and Healing W1V, Chelsea Complementary Natural Health Centre SW10, City Health Centre EC1Y, Clapham Common Clinic SW4, Clissold Park Natural Health

Centre N16, College of Homoeopathy Clinic SE13, College of Osteopaths Education Trust KT7, Creative and Healing Arts W11, Equilibrium Therapy Centre SW18, European Shiatsu School, Fook Sang Acupuncture and Chinese Herbal Practitioners Training College UK NW11, General Council and Register of Osteopaths, Gerda Boyesen Centre W3, Gerda Boysen Clinic W3, Haelan Centre, Haelen Centre, Hale Clinic W1N, Heath Health Care NW3, Helios N1, Hocroft Clinic NW2, Islington Green Centre of Alternative Medicine N1, Jeyrani Health Centre E18, Kingston Natural Healing Centre, Lavender Hill Homoeopathic Centre SW11, Lever Clinic EN1, Living Centre SW20, London College of Osteopathic Medicine NW1, London Natural Health Clinic W8, Lotus Healing Centre NW8, Maidstone College of Osteopathy ME16, Mehta Method of Therapeutic Head Massage N1, Natureworks, Neal's Yard Therapy Rooms WC2H, New Cross Natural Therapy Centre , Primrose Healing Centre NW1, Private Health Centre E7, Putney Natural Therapy Clinic, Raphael Clinic NW6, Sayer Clinic: City EC2M, South London Natural Health Centre SW4, St James Centre for Health and Healing W1V, Sunra SW12, Violet Hill Studios NW8, Westminster Natural Health Centre SW1V, Wimbledon Clinic of Natural Medicine SW19, Women and Health NW1, Wood Street Clinic EN5.

TRAININGS IN OSTEOPATHY

Andrew Still College of Osteopathy *Title of Training:* Diploma in Osteopathy *Duration:* 5 years part time, weekends *Entry Requirements:* Minimum of 5 GCEs, 2 of which should be A levels, preferably in a science subject. For mature students with sufficient experience these may be waived. *Fees:* Refer to organisers

College of Osteopaths Education Trust *Title of Training:* Diploma in Osteopathy *Duration:* 6 years part-time mostly weekends. *Entry Requirements:* 'O' levels and 'A' levels in basic sciences. A science review course of six months part time is available to those not suitably qualified. *Fees:* Refer to organisers *Comments:* Graduates of the Diploma in Osteopathy course are equipped to practice Naturopathy as well.

London College of Osteopathic Medicine *Title of Training:* Membership course MLCOM. *Duration:* Thirteen months of 3 days per week. *Entry Requirements:* (1) Reigstered medical practitioner (2) 6 years at least post qualification (3) Must pass entry examination. *Fees:* Refer to organisers

London School of Osteopathy *Title of Training:* Diploma Course in Osteopathy *Duration:* 5 years part-time (18 weekends per yr). *Entry Requirements:* 3 'A' levels in science subjects. *Fees:* Refer to organisers *Comments:* Exceptions to the above entry requirements may be made in the case of mature students.

British School of Osteopathy *Title of Training:* BSc in Osteopathy. *Duration:* 4 years full-time. *Entry Requirements:* 2 science A levels, preferably biology and chemistry. There are special provisions for non standard entry - offer two bridging courses (intensive short courses) fee in anatomy, physiology and chemistry. *Fees:* Refer to organisers *Comments:* Since this is an academic course discretionary awards may be available from local authorities. Write to the Registrar for further details. Graduates are eligible to apply for membership of the General Council and Register of Osteopaths.

British College of Naturopathy and Osteopathy *Title of Training:* Diploma Course in Osteopathy and Naturopathy *Duration:* 4 years full time. *Entry Requirements:* Two 'A' Levels preferably including a biological science and chemistry plus minium 2 GCE/GCSE 'O' level passes including at least 1 of English Language, Physics, Maths or Science or Biological Science BTech or equivalent. *Fees:* Refer to organisers *Comments:* The college is applying for degree status in the near future.

Polarity Therapy

In polarity therapy the body is seen as a made up of the universal energy which forms both the material and spiritual universe. It uses a variety of techniques including manipulation, stretching postures, and adjustment of diet to remove blocks in the flow of this energy through the body and to bring about the state of balance and health.

Randolph Stone, its originator, studied osteopathy, naturopathy and chiropractic and spent the last ten years of his life in India with his spiritual teacher.

He saw the body as having five energy centres which correspond to the elements of earth, water, fire, air and ether (ether is the fifth of five elements which according to Indian philosophical systems make up the universe). Specific exercises of 'polarity yoga' are prescribed to release and harmonise the energy of these centres, which may have become blocked through early emotional traumas, bad living habits or environmental influences. It is important that the energy is not only released, but also balanced between centres. The body's energies are seen as flowing in polarity between positive and negative poles. Good health is achieved when this flow reaches a point of equilibrium called 'neutral'.

Most of the work in polarity therapy is manipulation to balance the energies. This is sometimes done by the therapist by placing each hand on different parts of the body to facilitate the flow of energy between them. The body can be massaged in a clockwise or anti-clockwise direction or on the right or left side as is appropriate to the energy pattern of the recipient. Three types of pressure can be applied: positive, which makes the energy move, negative, which unblocks energy and can involve deep work on tissues, and neutral which is soothing. The therapist may also discuss the feelings which arise in the course of treatment, and any problems the client has.

The nutritional approach in polarity therapy usually begins with a cleansing programme. Natural, cleansing foods are eaten to purify and strengthen the body's own resources by expelling toxins from the system. Different foods are then reintroduced into the diet and monitored for the effects they have on the client's mental and physical well-being. Then a healthy eating programme is worked out for the individual client which will help to maintain this state of balance and health for life.

Polarity therapy requires some effort on the part of the client to change habits which are harmful, and for him or her to work on their own using the postures. Stone himself stressed that the achievement and maintenance of good health requires that we make this effort. It also asks for a positive attitude and willingness on the part of the client to change.

READING

The Polarity Process by Franklyn Sills, Element £8.95. This is a detailed explanation of how the theory of 'universal energy' can be understood and applied. Based on Dr. Randolph Stone's work in facilitating the free flow of life's finer energies. Franklyn Sills also provides a study guide to Dr. Stone's original writings, offering a new clarity to the subject. **Your Healing Hands** by Richard Gordon, Wingbow £9.95. This introduction to Polarity Therapy is well written and clearly illustrated and provides a practical hands-on approach to the therapeutic touch and natural healing. The book reinforces the feeling more than the intellect for those who want to practise polarity.

CENTRES OFFERING POLARITY THERAPY

Abshot Holistic Centre PO14, All Hallows House EC3R, Bodywise E2, Brackenbury Natural Health Centre W6, Edgware Centre for Natural Health HA8, Helios N1, Jeyrani Health Centre E18, Neal's Yard Therapy Rooms WC2H, Primrose Healing Centre NW1, Raphael Clinic NW6, Refuah Shelaymah Natural Health Centre N16, Shirley Goldstein, South London Natural Health Centre SW4.

Radionics

Radionics (in some cases known as radiesthesia or psionic medicine) is diagnosis and treatment which is carried out at a distance using particular instruments to aid the healer's own psychic faculties.

The principle involved is similar to dowsing, where a stick held by the dowser will twitch to show the hidden presence of water, oil or minerals underground, or can be used to find missing articles or persons. In radionics, a pendulum (a weight on the end of a lenght of thread) is often used. After getting the patient to fill in a detailed questionnaire, a 'witness' - a drop of blood on a piece of blotting paper or a lock of hair - is taken. This 'witness' is believed to act as a link between the practitioner and the patient. Diagnosis can then be carried out in a number of ways. The practitioner may ask questions about the patient's condition and the pendulum will indicate either a positive or negative answer depending on the way it swings. The pendulum may be used over diagrams of the body, to indicate which parts need treatment, and further questions will indicate how severely affected these parts are and what has caused them to malfunction. The pendulum may be used with special charts to show, on a scale of 0-100, how well or how feebly an organ is working. Practitioners vary in how much equipment they use; some prefer to use only a pendulum, while others may use boxes with dials, and an array of electronic equipment.

Once diagnosis has been made, a similar process is used to find the right treatment. Once again, different practitioners may use different methods, so that a wide range of treatments, and methods of 'transmitting' them to the patient may be used. Some will simply write and recommend that patients take a particular remedy or course of treatment. Others may perform a kind of 'distant healing', by focussing on the patient and their particular complaint mentally.

Radiesthesia's beginnings were fraught with difficulty, largely because of the hostility of the medical establishment towards what they saw as 'quackery'. It was developed by a distinguished American neurologist, Dr Albert Abrahams. At the beginning of this century, Abrahams made a curious discovery while using the standard medical technique 'percussion' - tapping the body of a patient to determine the condition in the internal organs. He found that if the patient was facing west, the same sound would be given consistently by patients suffering the same disease, as long as they were tapped in the same area. Developing this, Abrahams then found that if a healthy person held a sample of blood from a diseased person, the sound given when he tapped them was characteristic of the disease suffered by the owner of the blood. Believing that the reaction was caused by electromagnetic force, he devised and marketed a box device to measure resistances from the patient's sample. However, results from 'the box' as it was called, were not always consistent, and it was even banned in some states in America. Ruth Drown, a Californian chiropractor in the 1930s developed her own kind of box and was prosecuted by the Food and Drug Administration. The pioneer of Radionics in the UK, George de la Warr narrowly escaped prosecution by someone who had bought his version of 'the box' .

The problem for exponents of radionics had been that they believed that the force involved was electromagnetic and could be measured under test conditions. In fact, results of such tests tended to be patchy except in one notable case. In 1924 a committee was set up to investigate a British version of the box, headed by Sir Thomas Horder. A Scottish homoeopath was asked to identify substances using the box, and to the surprise of the committee his results were almost completely correct.

Radionic theory is now less concerned with electromagnetic energy exclusively,

156

but sees all life forms as part of and affected by a common field of energy which includes, in its grossest form, electromagnetic energy. It is by influencing this field that the healing is performed.

Radionics can be used for any condition, mainly because it does not interfere with any other form of treatment. It is best perhaps with chronic, mysterious complaints which conventional medicine has failed to diagnose. It is also frequently used by those with terminal illness to ease pain and provide psychic support. It is also used in agriculture to increase crop yields, and animals respond well to radionic treatment.

READING

Spiritual Dowsing by Sig Lonegren, Gothic Image £4.95. This is a book for all who approach dowsing in a spirit of openness and sincerity. A new and dynamic approach which makes explicit the link between this ancient art and inner growth. The approach is extremely practical, guiding the beginner into both usage and philosophy, empowering the reader to take personal responsibility in his or her action in dowsing either the earth's energies or for healing. **Radionics and the Subtle Anatomy of Man** by David Tansley C.W. Daniel £2.95. David Tansley believes that the time is ripe for radionics to bear witness to an energy field of a more subtle nature and to this end wrote an examination of the wider influences of radionic energy with regard to the probability of underlying force fields which may affect the health of the physical form.

CENTRES OFFERING RADIONICS OR RADIESTHESIA

Gerda Boyesen Centre W3, Natural Healing Centre HA4, South London Natural Health Centre SW4, Violet Hill Studios NW8. Mill Hill Health Care NW7.

Reflexology

This is a technique in which particular areas on the soles and sides of the feet are seen to correspond to the organs of the body. These are massaged to promote the health of the organs. Reflexology can also be used as a diagnostic tool.

Reflexology is an art the origins of which stretch back to ancient China. It was Dr William Fitzgerald, an Ear, Nose and Throat specialist interested in acupuncture who started using it in the West. His ideas were developed and exported to the United States by Eunice D Ingham whose book, *Stories the Feet Can Tell,* was published in 1932.

Treatment is carried out with the patient lying bare footed on a couch. The reflexologist will feel for tiny lumps under the surface of the skin which are believed to be crystalline deposits. The place on the foot where these are found indicates which organ is not functioning properly. For instance, the big toe corresponds to the top of the head and brain, and various parts of the heel to the bladder, sciatic nerve and sexual organs. The reflexologist will massage these spots which can be surprisingly sensitive when touched, so it is not uncommon to feel some pain. Most people feel the discomfort is worth it to achieve the therapeutic results, and at least the very sensitivity of the spot convinces patients that the reflexologist is really 'onto' something. Treatments continue until the spot is no longer sensitive. A session may last from 15 to 45 minutes and a course of treatment a few weeks.

READING

Reflexology Today *by Doreen Bayly, Thorsons £3.99.* A well loved introduction to the practice of reflexology which is one of the most pleasant of all holistic therapies. This book is valuable for student and layman alike and includes charts of the feet and the body zones. **Better Health with Foot Reflexology** *by Dwight Byers, Ingham Publishing £10.95.* This book combines the use of both hand and foot reflexology and is the most accurate and complete guide to the subject. It has become the standard reference for the International Institute of Reflexology

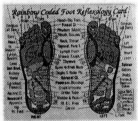
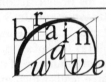

and is extensively illustrated with methods of treatment as well as the organs of the body and other functions. **Holistic Reflexology** *by Avi Grinberg Thorsons £20.00.* An authoritative and detailed fully illustrated guide designed to meet the need for in depth treatment. Mainly for therapists and their students, including case histories and the understanding of holistic treatment of patients. New and highly recommended.

CENTRES OFFERING REFLEXOLOGY

Acupuncture and Osteopathy Clinic SW1V, All Hallows House EC3R, Alternative Medicine Clinic NW15, Alternative Therapies Centre N16, Association of Natural Medicines CM8, Association of Reflexologists WC1N, Bayly School of Reflexology WR6, Bennett & Luck N1, Bodywise E2, Brackenbury Natural Health Centre W6, British School - Reflex Zone Therapy of the Feet (Ann Lett Ltd) HA9, British School of Reflexology CM17, Bumblebees Natural Remedies N7, Central London School of Reflexology, Centre for Personal & Professional Development N17, Chelsea Complementary Natural Health Centre SW10, Churchill Centre W1H, Clapham Common Clinic SW4, Clissold Park Natural Health Centre N16, College of Homoeopathy Clinic SE13, Edgware Centre for Natural Health HA8, Equilibrium Therapy Centre SW18, Falcons SW11, Food and Chemical Allergy Clinic CR0, Forty Hill Natural Therapy Centre, Gerda Boysen Clinic W3, Green Wood College W6, Haelan Centre, Hampstead Healing Centre NW3, Heath Health Care NW3, Helios N1, IBISS TW7, Institute of Clinical Aromatherapy SE6, Islington Green Centre of Alternative Medicine N1, Janice Ellicott School of Reflexology SW6, Jeyrani Health Centre E18, Kingston Natural Healing Centre, Living Centre SW20, London College of Massage W1P, London Lighthouse W11, Lotus Healing Centre NW8, Mill Hill Health Care NW7, Natural Healing Centre HA4, Natural Medicine Centre BR2, Naturecare SW16, Natureworks, Neal's Yard Therapy Rooms WC2H, New Cross Natural Therapy Centre, Portobello Green Fitness Centre W10, Primrose Healing Centre NW1, Private Health Centre E7, Putney Natural Therapy Clinic, Raphael Clinic NW6, Sayer Clinic: Chelsea SW6, Sayer Clinic: Covent Garden, Silver Birch Centre NW10, South London Natural Health Centre SW4, Sunra SW12, Therapy Made Unique E18, Violet Hill Studios NW8, West London School of Therapeutic Massage W11, Westminster Natural Health Centre SW1V, Wholeness E18, Women and Health NW1, Wood Street Clinic EN5, Yoga Dham HA2.

TRAININGS IN REFLEXOLOGY

British Reflexology Association *Title of Training:* Reflexology. *Duration:* Attendance at 3 weekends and 1 full day. Minimum 2 month interval between courses. Home study and practise required. Minimum length of training 8-9 months. *Entry Requirements:* None. *Fees:* Refer to organisers

British School - Reflex Zone Therapy of the Feet (Ann Lett Ltd) *Title of*

Training: (1) Introductory and (2) Advanced Training in Reflex Zone Therapy of the Feet. (3) Midwives course (4) Reflex Zone Therapy of the Nervous System. *Duration:* Courses are three days each. *Entry Requirements:* Applicants should have previous medical training, or training in nursing, physiotherapy, midwifery, acupuncture, osteopathy or naturopathy. *Fees:* Refer to organisers

British School of Reflexology *Title of Training:* Reflexology training courses. *Duration:* 8 months part-time. *Fees:* Refer to organisers

Reflexology Centre *Title of Training:* Basic and advanced course in reflexology. *Duration:* Weekend courses. Details on request. *Fees:* Refer to organisers

Janice Ellicott School of Reflexology *Title of Training:* Intensive Reflexology course to practitioner level. *Duration:* Six days tuition and two months of home study and practice. *Entry Requirements:* None *Fees:* £250 *Comments:* It includes the use of aromatic oils on the feet as an extended massage after the pressure-point treatment.

West London School of Therapeutic Massage *Title of Training:* Training in massage, anatomy and physiology, reflex zone therapy and sports therapy. ITEC. *Duration:* Three to twelve months. *Entry Requirements:* None specified *Fees:* Refer to organisers

Churchill Centre *Title of Training:* Basic and advanced trainings in Foot Reflexology. *Duration:* Basic training two weekends or four days. Advanced training is two weekends. *Entry Requirements:* English speaking and interested to learn about massage. *Fees:* Refer to organisers

Association of Reflexologists Refer to organisers

Raworth Centre Refer to organisers

Central London School of Reflexology Refer to organisers

Bayly School of Reflexology *Title of Training:* The Bayly School of Reflexology Introductory and Advanced Courses. *Duration:* Part time, attendance at three weekends and examination day. Home study between courses. Average length of training 8-9 months. London and regional venues. *Entry Requirements:* None *Fees:* Whole course (including examination fee) £297.87 + VAT - £350. *Comments:* Students of the school can join the I.C.M. Register and the Association is affiliated to the B.C.M.A.

Rolfing

Rolfing is a technique evolved by Ida Rolf, which is also sometimes called structural integration. It seeks to realign the body by manipulation of the connective tissue.

A useful rule of thumb in looking at body alignment is that the body should show a symmetry between the right side and the left, looking face on. Looking side on, one should be able to draw a straight line from the bottom of the ear to the ankles which should pass through the middle of the shoulders and middle of the hips. If the body is not in alignment extra energy is needed to maintain equilibrium. For instance if the head is protruding forward (sticking one's neck out) then the muscles in the back of the neck must work at holding the head in position. Whereas if the head is sitting centrally, balanced directly over the spine, little energy is needed to hold it in place. Thus if one's body is out of alignment, one is using more energy when simply standing than if the body were not out of alignment.

The experience of being rolfed is like having a very deep and sometimes painful massage. The rolfer uses not only his or her hands but elbows too.

There are a standard ten sessions of one hour duration. Each session builds on the last one and works on a different part of the body. Some rolfers take before and after photos to keep a record of the changes that happen and let you have duplicates.

Fritz Perls the founder of gestalt therapy swore it helped him reduce the pain of angina. However, like the Alexander technique, it is not a treatment for any particular disorder, but a system aimed at prevention.

In this country, rolfing usually comes under the umbrella of 'structural bodywork' which includes other techniques such as structural integration.

READING

The Power of Balance by Brian Fahey, *Metamorphous Press £13.95*. Dr. Fahey is a fine worker in the interdisciplinary effort to enhance mutual co-operation between rolfing, medicine and chiropractic. This book reflects his comprehensive philosophy and provides dynamic information for all health professionals concerned with improving their patients' level of well-being. **Rolfing** *by Ida Rolf, Healing Arts Press £15.15*. This is the classic text on Ida Rolf's therapy which attempts to align and balance the physical body within its gravitational field. Rolfing is a system of massage of the connective tissue which releases physical and emotional stress and leaves the patient with both physical and emotional well-being. **Rolfing** is intended for the interested but untrained lay-person as well as the professional in need of specific technical information. Well illustrated with both photographs and line drawings.

CENTRES OFFERING ROLFING

Neal's Yard Therapy Rooms WC2H, Rolfing Centre, Violet Hill Studios NW8, Westminster Natural Health Centre SW1V.

Shiatsu and Acupressure

Shiatsu is a massage technique which involves stimulating or relaxing the acupuncture points and meridians. The word shiatsu means 'finger pressure' in Japanese. It is like a form of acupuncture which does not use needles. The principle is the same: to release and balance the flow or ki (ch'i in Chinese) or

BODY THERAPIES

life energy at points where it may have become blocked or over stimulated.

In Japan shiatsu is practised widely, often as a form of self help by one member of the family on another. The Chinese version is called acupressure, and in practice is virtually the same as shiatsu.

After the completion of the case history, diagnosis is usually carried out by palpation of the abdomen and observation of any abnormalities in the skin or muscles. Sometimes the practitioner may take the pulses, as in an acupuncture session (see section on acupuncture for an explanation of 'pulses'). In this way the practitioner decides which points and meridians need work to balance the energy flow. The massage itself is a mixture of general strokes over particular parts of the body to promote the harmonious flow of ki energy, and direct pressure on the acupuncture points with the fingertips or elbows. The intensity of the pressure also varies between gentle massage to a very strong pressure, but the recipient should not have to experience any more pain than is involved in the pleasurable release of tension. The practitioner may also use gentle manipulation to loosen joints and stretch the meridians, the energy pathways.

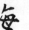
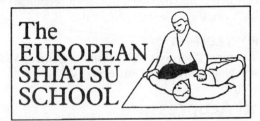

A session may last from 45 minutes to an hour and a quarter.

Shiatsu helps to maintain health by toning up the body's energy, and can be used to treat a variety of complaints, such as tension, low vitality, pre-menstrual tension, lower back pains, stiffness in the neck and shoulders, digestion problems, asthma, headaches and insomnia. It can also help to promote greater emotional tranquillity. As will some other alternative therapies, there are contra-indications for some conditions.

If you know the right pressure points to use, you can practise shiatsu on yourself for first aid to relieve pain or cramps, and some people become so adept at this that they use it on trips to the dentist.

READING

Shiatzu by *Yukiko Irwin, Arkana/Penguin £7.99.* The line drawings and clear concise instructions in this book are intended to help anyone learn and use the shiatsu points to the best advantage. Aches and pains of everyday living can be relieved by this therapy at the hands of almost any sympathetic layman. **The Natural Healer's Acupressure Handbook** by *Michael Blate, Henry Holt £6.80.* This book illustrates how 'acupuncture without needles' can be used by the lay-practitioner as a alternative to aspirin and other commonly used drugs to alleviate pain and discomfort. Problems for which treatment is suggested include headaches, anxiety, nosebleeds, stagefright, cramps and exhaustion. Also included are first-aid treatments while awaiting medical attention. **Soft Tissue Manipulation** by *Leon Chaitow, Thorsons £19.95.* This is a practitioner's guide to the diagnosis and treatment of soft tissue dysfunction and reflex activity. The book provides students with a working knowledge of the diagnostic and therapeutic use of neuro-muscular, muscle energy and strain-counterstrain techniques. It also covers systems involving reflex points and trigger points.

CENTRES OFFERING SHIATSU

Abshot Holistic Centre PO14, Acumedic Centre NW1, Acupuncture and Osteopathy Clinic SW1V, Bennett & Luck N1, Bodywise E2, Brackenbury Natural Health Centre W6, British School of Oriental Therapy and Movement SE21, British School of Shiatsu-Do NW3, Bumblebees Natural Remedies N7, Changes NW3, Chelsea Complementary Natural Health Centre SW10, City Health Centre EC1Y, Clapham Common Clinic SW4, Clare Maxwell Hudson NW2, Clissold Park Natural Health Centre N16, Community Health Foundation EC1V, Creative and Healing Arts W11, Edgware Centre for Natural Health HA8, Equilibrium Therapy Centre SW18, European Shiatsu School, European Shiatsu School, Green Wood College W6, Haelan Centre, Haelen Centre, Health in Action E8, Heath Health Care NW3, Helios N1, Hillside Practice, IBISS TW7, Islington Green Centre of Alternative Medicine N1, Ki Kai Shiatsu Centre, Kingston Natural Healing Centre, Lavender Hill Homoeopathic Centre SW11, London College of Shiatsu, London School of Chinese Massage Therapy

N10, Natural Health Clinic HA3, Natural Medicine Centre BR2, Natureworks, Neal's Yard Therapy Rooms WC2H, New Cross Natural Therapy Centre, Nine Needles Health Care Centre TW9, Notting Hill Traditional Acupuncture Clinic W11, Portobello Green Fitness Centre W10, Primrose Healing Centre NW1, Putney Natural Therapy Clinic, Raphael Clinic NW6, Refuah Shelaymah Natural Health Centre N16, Sayer Clinic: Marble Arch W1H, Shiatsu Clinic, Shiatsu College, Shiatsu College NR2, Shiatsu Society RG11, South London Natural Health Centre SW4, Sunra SW12, Violet Hill Studios NW8, West London School of Therapeutic Massage W11, Westminster Natural Health Centre SW1V, Women and Health NW1.

TRAININGS IN SHIATSU

British School of Oriental Therapy and Movement *Title of Training:* 1) Certificate Course in Shiatsu. 2) Advanced Course in Shiatsu. *Duration:* 1) One year consisting of 4 terms (twelve weeks each), 12 classes per term (Saturdays 2-6.30pm). *Entry Requirements:* None specified. *Fees:* Refer to organisers *Comments:* Study background, philosophy and aetiology of traditional Chinese medicine. Students must complete a number of ongoing treaments for practical assessment, and taught Kitaiso (a 'movement system') to facilitate student's own healing powers. A self development ingredient is added to the course through the movement and Ki.

British School of Shiatsu-Do *Title of Training:* Diploma Couse in Shiatsu-Do. *Duration:* Three years part-time. Evening, weekend or daytime timetables. 650 hours in total to become a practitioner. *Entry Requirements:* Open to everyone. *Fees:* £2576 plus VAT, £435 for foundation course. UB40 places available. *Comments:* Weekend only, or weekend and evening courses commence throughout the year. It is the longest established school of its kind in the country, offering Classical Meridian system plus Zen Shiatsu, Seitai and Cranio-Sacral Techniques.

European Shiatsu School *Title of Training:* 1) Shiatsu Foundation Course 2) Shiatsu Practitioner Course. *Duration:* 1) 4 weekends (part time) 2) 3 years (14 weekends per year) part time. *Entry Requirements:* No entry requirements for the Foundation course. Practitioner Diploma courses requires completion of Foundation course. *Fees:* Refer to organisers *Comments:* Branches in London, Bath, Brighton, Bournemouth, Devon, Canterbury, Oxford, Marlborough, Reading, Wiltshire, Portugal and Spain. Most of the teaching staff have paramedical qualifications, mainly chartered physiotherapists. Have now introduced an intensive 18 month training taking place every Friday excluding summer holidays.

Healing Shiatsu Education Centre *Title of Training:* Professional training course in Healing-Shiatsu. *Duration:* 3 years training part time. Three 5 day residential workshops per year, excluding the introductory weekend. *Entry*

Requirements: Non-residential introductory weekend held in Bristol. *Fees:* Refer to organisers *Comments:* Wholistic training offering students ability to work on themselves using meditation and self healing practices as well as developing professional skills as practitioners.

Ki Kai Shiatsu Centre *Title of Training:* Diploma Course in Shiatsu and Oriental Meditaion. *Duration:* 1 year part time and 3 years part time, 500 hours in total. Courses during weekdays and weekends. *Entry Requirements:* None *Fees:* £790.00 per annum, with no extras. *Comments:* Intakes in October, January and March. Classes are kept small for a caring and supportive environment. Much emphasis is placed on the student's self deveopment. The wide range of fully qualified teachers give a broad based, comprehensive training in Shiatsu.

Nine Needles Health Care Centre *Title of Training:* (1) 1 year evening course in Shiatsu (2) 3 year course in Oriental Medicine including acupuncture, shiatsu, moxibustion, etc. *Duration:* Evenings part-time, three days a week. *Fees:* (1) £1,410 or £1,100 on lump payment. (2) First and third years as above, second year £2,800 or £2,500 on lump payment.

Shiatsu College *Title of Training:* Shiatsu training to professional standard, beginners classes and post graduate workshops, held in London. *Duration:* Professional training 2 years weekdays, or 3 years weekends. Refer to organisers for full details. *Entry Requirements:* Application forms considered individually. *Fees:* Refer to organisers *Comments:* College has a new venue in London, W10. Teaching team of 'unique, leading Shiatsu teachers!'

London School of Chinese Massage Therapy *Title of Training:* Professional training in Traditional Chinese Massage/Tui Na and An Mo. *Duration:* Three years. *Entry Requirements:* Ability and commitment are essential. *Fees:* Refer to organisers

Shiatsu London College of Shiatsu *Title of Training:* Training in Shiatsu.

Tai Chi Chuan

Though tai chi is often bracketed with the martial arts, it is more akin to moving meditation. In tai chi slow, flowing movements which follow a set pattern enable practitioners to harmonise mind, body and spirit and become more deeply centred in themselves. Its applications can be as form of healing, for self-defence and as a spiritual discipline.

Legend has it that tai chi was originated by Chang Sanfeng, a thirteenth century Chinese Taoist monk, who adapted an earlier martial art form used by the monks for protection. The story goes that observing the movements animals make, Chang Sanfeng saw that they comprised of circular movements which he then formalised into a set of postures. These were then joined together and became the ritualised, dance-like movements or 'forms' of tai chi. The practice of tai chi lies within a whole spiritual and philosophical tradition which is largely

Taoist, but which also incorporates some aspects of Buddhism.

The emphasis in performing the movements is not on strength or exertion, but on relaxation, concentration and balance. The knees are kept bent and movement is achieved by shifting the greater part of the body's weight slowly from one foot to the other while the hands make careful and gentle pushing and circling gestures. Attention is also paid to correct breathing. Physically the aim is to develop muscle control, fluidity and grace. After mastering the techniques and much practice, the practitioner should become one with the movements to the extent that they are no longer exercising deliberate control, but letting the movements happen through them. This can occur if the practitioner has been able to open themselves up sufficiently to the chi energy, which in Chinese philosophy is the lifeforce present in everything.

As a form of self-defence the idea is that aggression can be neutralised through yielding. If one does not meet an attacker's force head on but instead gives way, the aggression will exhaust itself. Most people however do not take up tai chi primarily for self-defence, since one would probably have to be very experienced to use it successfully in this way.

Tai chi is often recommended therapeutically to those who suffer from tension and anxiety, high blood pressure and heart complaints because of its relaxing effect. It can promote and maintain good health both physically and mentally.

READING

Embrace Tiger, Return to Mountain by *Chungliang Al Huang, Celestial Arts, USA £9.95.* A popular classic first published in the USA, beautifully produced and illustrated with photographs and calligraphy. Not a martial arts manual, but a unique exploration of the basic principles. Al Huang writes: 'I remain interested less in the structure of exact positions, but more in the content and the spirit of dance in the form' and describes himself as a 'Tai Ji dancer'. **Way of Harmony: A Guide to the Soft Martial Arts** by *Howard Reid, Unwin Hyman £7.95.* Written by the producer of the 1983 BBC TV series *Way of the Warrior*, this book is a practical guide to Chi Kung, Tai Chi Chuan, Hsing I and Pa Kua systems of exercises which cultivate inner strength and vital energy and increase self-knowledge. It also includes a section on oriental paths to balance: diet, breathing exercises, meditation and therapeutic techniques. The book is aimed at those who want to combine the physical skills of the martial arts with a deeper mental approach. Profusely illustrated with colour photographs and drawings. **Tai Chi for Two: the Practice of Push Hands** by *Paul Crompton Shambala £11.95.* 'Push Hands' is a basic exercise for two partners practiced by Tai Chi students. This book presents it as a means of training oneself to relax under physical and mental pressure and to improve one's interactions with others in everyday life. Includes step-by-step instructions and photographs demonstrating the movements, plus chapters on Taoist philosophy and the concept of Tai Chi energy. Paul Crompton has been teaching Tai Chi in Britain since the early 1970s.

CENTRES OFFERING TAI CHI CHUAN

Bodywise E2, Community Health Foundation EC1V, Croydon Buddhist Centre CR0, Healing Centre NW5, Health in Action E8, Helios N1, IBISS TW7, Life Resources NW7, London School of T'ai Chi Chuan (The) W4, Lotus Healing Centre NW8, Martial Arts Commission, Refuah Shelaymah Natural Health Centre N16, School of T'ai-chi Ch'uan - Centre for Healing WC1H, Spiral W12, Studio E NW6, Violet Hill Studios NW8, Women and Health NW1.

TRAINING IN TAI CHI CHUAN

School of T'ai-chi Ch'uan - Centre for Healing *Title of Training:* T'ai Chi Ch'uan Foundation Training. *Duration:* 3 years, weekly classes, 3 terms per year. *Entry Requirements:* Genuine interest and commitment. *Fees:* Refer to organisers *Comments:* The aim of this training is to help students understand the principles of T'ai Chi, 'by connecting with centre of peace and light'. An holistic training incorporating philosophy, symbolism, and 'chi-king'.

Yoga

Yoga is a means of self help towards physical and mental health. It has been practised in India for over 3000 years, and can be used as a way of relaxing and keeping fit, as well as a kind of meditation technique.

Yoga comes from a Sanskrit word meaning 'union' which has the same root as the English word 'yolk'. The aim of yoga is union with the divine, with life. Though in the west we are most familiar with the form of yoga which involves physical postures ('hatha' yoga) the word yoga is used to describe many different disciplines which can be used to develop spiritual potential. For instance, there is karma yoga which is service to others through work and bhakti yoga which is union with the divine principle through religious devotion.

There are different systems of hatha yoga teaching too. However, all involve basic postures which have names like 'Cobra', 'Praying Mantis', 'Tree' and 'Corpse' pose. The poses are designed to stretch and strengthen muscles and ligaments, and to stimulate the internal organs and circulation. Though encountering the body's stiffness can be uncomfortable at times, yoga teachers stress that there should not be too much strain involved, and one should not try to push one's body beyond its limits. The temptation to push the body into the pose, rather than relaxing into it can be strong, and can even lead to injury. For this reason it is advisable to attend a yoga class, where the teacher will be able to show you the best way to do the pose.

Hatha yoga also involves attention to the breath. Proper breathing is seen as crucial to good health and to developing mental and emotional clarity. Breathing exercises are usually part of yoga practice, and the aim is to let go of the tension, particularly in the diaphragm, which leads to tense, shallow breathing and an overall sense of restriction. After a yoga session, the practitioner should relax fully. This may also involve some sort of meditation.

The benefits of yoga are increased relaxation, greater strength and suppleness, and better posture. Yoga has also had beneficial effects in the treatment of diseases, notably high blood pressure, multiple sclerosis, arthritis, asthma, backache (but care should be taken not to strain the back), painful periods, constipation and other chronic conditions. Some places hold classes specifically for handicapped people.

READING
Book of Yoga *by the Sivananda Yoga Centre, Ebury Press £7.95.* This classic guide to yoga is clear and comprehensive, superbly illustrated with full colour photographs. There are easy to follow instructions for working into the postures book examines a modern approach to the discipline of yoga. The photographs include examples of bad posture and how to correct it. The yoga courses start at beginner's level and progress to an advanced standard. Included is a chapter on working in pairs and groups and some explanation of the way yoga practice helps the muscular system.

CENTRES OFFERING YOGA
3HO Kundalini Yoga Foundation NW4, All Hallows House EC3R, Alternative Therapies Centre N16, Bhratiya Vidya Bhavan (Institute of Indian Culture) W14, Bodywise E2, British School of Shiatsu-Do NW3, Chelsea Complementary Natural Health Centre SW10, Community Health Foundation EC1V, Creative and Healing Arts W11, Croydon Buddhist Centre CR0, Edgware Centre for Natural Health HA8, Health Management IG10, Heath Health Care NW3, Helios N1, Hillside Practice, Holistic Yoga Centre MK19, IBISS TW7, Iyengar Yoga Institute W9, Jeyrani Health Centre E18, Kingston Natural Healing Centre, London School of Chinese Massage Therapy N10, Lotus Healing Centre NW8, Mushindokai NW1, Natureworks, Pearl Healing Centre CR7, Satyananda Yoga Centre, Shanti Sadan W11, Silver Birch Centre NW10, South London Natural Health Centre SW4, Sunra SW12, Violet Hill Studios NW8, West London Buddhist Centre W11, Yoga Dham HA2.

TRAININGS IN YOGA TEACHING
Iyengar Yoga Institute *Title of Training:* Teacher Training Course in Yoga. *Duration:* 2 years part-time. *Entry Requirements:* Candidates must have studied with a qualified Iyengar teacher for 2 years previously, have a good grounding in the basic postures, and be able to maintain headbalance for 5 minutes. *Fees:* £300 per annum. *Comments:* In addition to the basic Yoga teaching qualification,

the Institute runs courses for teachers wishing to progress and gain higher certificates. The training follows the method of BKS Iyengar and is recognised worldwide.

Synthesis of Light Holidays (SOL) *Title of Training:* Yoga Teacher Training *Duration:* One Month. *Fees:* Refer to organisers *Comments:* Held at the ashram of Swami Satchidananda, Virginia, USA. Food and accomodation included.

London School of Chinese Massage Therapy *Title of Training:* Professional training in Chinese Massage Therapy, Tui Na and An Mo and Shiatsu. *Duration:* Three years, part time. *Entry Requirements:* Strong academic ability absolutely essential, paper qualifications not necessary. *Fees:* Refer to organisers *Comments:* Affiliation with Nanjin College of Traditional Chinese Medicine as practised throughout the Peoples' Republic of China. unabridged TCM for A thorough training encompassing many principles of Traditional Chinese Medicine including basic theory, functions of the Zangfu (organs), Jingluo (the channels and collaterals), aetiology (cause of disease), diagnosis, pathology, yoga, meditation, yoga therapy, anatomy and physiology, psychology.

International Sivananda Yoga Vedanta Centre *Title of Training:* Yoga 1 - Beginner Yoga 2 - Beginner/Intermediate Yoga 3 - Intermediate Yoga 4 - Intermediate/Advanced Yoga 5 - Advanced 1 Yoga 6 - Advanced 2 Meditation 1 - 3 *Duration:* 2 classes weekly, one and a half hours each, for 4 weeks or 1 class weekly for one and a half hours on Saturday for 8 weeks. *Entry Requirements:* None for beginners courses. Previous courses must be attended prior to advancing to next courses. Those who have experience of Yoga considered individually for appropriate classes. Meditation 1 - Graduates of Yoga 1. *Fees:* Refer to organisers *Comments:* Sivananda Vedanta Centre is part of an international Yoga organisation, headquarters of which are in Canada. Founded by Swami Vishnu Devananda in 1970. Non-profit charity its purpose is to propagate the ancient science of Yoga, which is a means of achieving physical, mental and spiritual well-being. Other activities include Indian cooking, diet and nutrition, vegetarian cooking, fasting weekends, open classes, pensioners classes, pregnancy classes, children's classes, private classes. Retreats are arranged periodically in UK, and Yoga vacations (ashrams) available in Quebec, Bahamas, India, California and New York. Teacher Training Courses (TTC) given at various Ashrams throughout the year.

Yoga British School of Yoga *Title of Training:* 1) Teacher Diploma Hatha Yoga 2) Yoga Therapy Diploma *Duration:* 1) 1 year 2) 2 years *Entry Requirements:* Refer to organisers for full details. *Fees:* Refer to organisers *Comments:* Also run workshops and other courses covering hypnosis, massage, aromatherapy, meditation, relaxation, stress consultant, and audio and video cassettes for use at home.

British Wheel of Yoga *Title of Training:* British Wheel of Yoga Teaching Diploma. *Duration:* Two and a half years, plus one further year to complete written syllabus. *Entry Requirements:* At least two years Yoga experience with a recognised Yoga teacher. *Fees:* Refer to organisers *Comments:* One of two qualifications recognised by Local Education Authorities in England and Wales, Adhere's to syllabus guidelines prepared by European Union of National Federations of Yoga. Comprehensive study course dealing with the synthesis of Yoga without being restricted by the teachings or method of any one particular discipline.

Yoga Satyananda Yoga Centre *Title of Training:* Yoga Teacher Training courses.

OTHER BODY APPROACHES

Active Birth
Active Birth Centre NW5, Dick Read School for Natural Birth, Highbury Centre N5, Splashdown Birth Pools HA1, Welcome Home Birth Practice N8.

Aston Patterning
Institute of Structural Bodywork WD4, Pearl Healing Centre CR7.

Bioenergetic Medicine
Wimbledon Clinic of Natural Medicine SW19.

Chiropody
Alternative Therapies Centre N16, Body Clinic NW11, Central London School of Reflexology, Chelsea Complementary Natural Health Centre SW10, Clapham Common Clinic SW4, Edgware Centre for Natural Health HA8, Equilibrium Therapy Centre SW18, Hale Clinic W1N, Heath Health Care NW3, Homoeopathic Health Clinic HA3, Living Centre SW20, Marigold Trust WC1N, Natural Health Clinic HA3, Natureworks, Private Health Centre E7, Putney Natural Therapy Clinic, Sayer Clinic: Chelsea SW6, Sayer Clinic: Marble

Arch W1H, Wimbledon Clinic of Natural Medicine SW19.

Complementary Medicine (misc.)

Bluestone Clinic W1N, British School of Oriental Therapy and Movement SE21, Craniosacral Therapy Education Trust N3, Naturemed Partnership GL5.

Diet Therapy

All Hallows House EC3R, Alternative Medicine Clinic NW15, Bayswater Clinic W2, Bennett & Luck N1, Brackenbury Natural Health Centre W6, Centre for Health and Healing W1V, Changes NW3, Chessington Hypnotherapy Clinic, Clapham Common Clinic SW4, Clinic of Herbal Medicine, Colon Health W9, Edgware Centre for Natural Health HA8, Equilibrium Therapy Centre SW18, Falcons SW11, Hayes Hypnotherapy Centre UB4, Heath Health Care NW3, Holistic Health Consultancy SW1V, Homoeopathic Health Clinic HA3, Institute for Optimum Nutrition SW6, Kingston Natural Healing Centre, Life Resources NW7, Natural Health Clinic HA3, Nature Cure Clinic W1M, Natureworks, Neal's Yard Therapy Rooms WC2H, New Cross Natural Therapy Centre, Primrose Healing Centre NW1, Putney Natural Therapy Clinic, Raphael Clinic NW6, South London Natural Health Centre SW4, Therapy Made Unique E18, Traditional Chinese Medicine Clinic UB5, Violet Hill Studios NW8, Westminster Natural Health Centre SW1V, Women and Health NW1.

Hellerwork

All Hallows House EC3R, European Hellerwork Association HP5, Institute of Structural Bodywork WD4, Pearl Healing Centre CR7.

Macrobiotics

Community Health Foundation EC1V, London School of Macrobiotics EC1V.

Magnetic Therapy

Pearl Healing Centre CR7, Wimbledon Clinic of Natural Medicine SW19.

Pulsing

Open Centre EC1V, Wholeness E18.

Rebalancing

Institute of Structural Bodywork WD4, Pearl Healing Centre CR7, Violet Hill Studios NW8.

Reiki

Alternative Therapies Centre N16, Kingston Natural Healing Centre, Neal's Yard Therapy Rooms WC2H, Primrose Healing Centre NW1, Radiance

Education Unlimited NW3, Violet Hill Studios NW8.

Tibetan Medicine
IBISS TW7, Tibet Foundation WC1A.

Traditional Chinese Medicine
CHI Centre SW6, Clapham Common Clinic SW4, Life Works NW1, Natureworks, Sayer Clinic: Chelsea SW6, Sunra SW12.

OTHER TRAININGS

Active Birth
Active Birth Centre *Title of Training:* The Active Birth Teacher's Training Course. *Duration:* Two years part-time and can be done largely through correspondence if you wish. Twelve study days per year. *Entry Requirements:* None. Mostly for women. *Fees:* Refer to organisers *Comments:* Certificate given by the association. Intake in September of each year. Would welcome Scottish applicants!

Jeyrani Health Centre *Title of Training:* Jeyrani Way: Self Hypnosis for Enjoyable Birth. *Duration:* Part-time for 6 months. *Entry Requirements:* Qualified practising midwife or nurse. Also psychologists and others with an interest in childbirth are considered. *Fees:* Refer to organisers *Comments:* Intensive 1:1 coaching ensures excellent results, with birth time being reduced to possibly less than 6 hours.

National Childbirth Trust (NCT) Refer to organisers

Chiropody
Edinburgh School of Chiropody Refer to organisers

Cardiff School of Podiatry *Title of Training:* BSc (General Honours) University of Wales. *Duration:* Three years full time. *Entry Requirements:* Two 'A' levels, plus English Language and two sciences at 'O' level/GCSE. Mature students are welcome to apply, consideration given on basis of qualifications and experience. *Fees:* Refer to organisers *Comments:* 'It is the only course in Podiatry/Chiropody in the Principality of Wales leading to State Registration under the Professions Supplementary to Medicine Act 1960'.

Birmingham School of Chiropody and Podiatric Medicine Refer to organisers

Northern Ireland School of Chiropody Refer to organisers

Complementary Medicine (misc.)
Association of General Practitioners of Natural Medicine *Title of Training:* 1) Foundation Course of Comprehensive Training in Natural Medicine. 2) Post graduate Diploma Specialist Courses *Duration:* 1) One year foundation course 20 hours per week. 2) Three-four year Post Graduate Diploma specialist courses

- 20 hours weekly of formal study. *Entry Requirements:* 1 and 2: A reasonable standard of English and an aptitude for learning. All applicants will be interviewed by the Principlal of the College. 2) Must be a graduates of Foundation Course or have recognised training in natural medicine. *Fees:* Refer to organisers *Comments:* Prospectus £1 available from the Registrar.

Association of Natural Medicines *Title of Training:* Association of Natural Medicines Training in:- Acupuncture, Naturopathy, Homoeopathy, Aromatherapy, Counselling, Massage, Reflexology. *Duration:* Acupuncture, Homoeopathy, Naturopathy three years part time. Others, approximately 9 months part time. *Entry Requirements:* Acceptance by interview. *Fees:* Refer to organisers *Comments:* Teaching is broad based, incorporating many topics, as described, allowing the student to choose their therapy from an enlightened position and one of knowledge.

London College of Chinese and Oriental Medicine *Title of Training:* Diploma in Chinese Herbal Medicine and Acupuncture. Diploma in Chinese Herbal Medicine. *Duration:* 4 years part time - acupuncture and chinese herbal medicine. 2 and a half years part time - chinese herbal medicine. *Entry Requirements:* Acu/chm - 5 'O' levels and 2 'A' levels. May be waived in life experience extensive and/or mature students. Chm - must be qualified acupuncturists or have completed the year ground course in traditional chinese medicine. *Fees:* Refer to organisers *Comments:* Guru Dharam Singh Khalsa, the principle tutor, trained in Vietnam from boyhood and his 25 years experience is unique in this country. Other activities that take place at the Lotus Healing Centre, the College's clinic, include anatomy courses, kundalini yoga practitioner courses, healing courses, Yoga, oriental dance and many more.

Craniosacral Therapy Education Trust *Title of Training:* Craniosacral Therapy. *Duration:* One year. Course is held over nine 3-day seminars and one five day seminar. *Entry Requirements:* This is a post graduate course for practitioners of complementary or orthodox medicine and therapy. A good grounding in anatomy, physiology, medical diagnosis and clinical experience is required. *Fees:* Refer to organisers *Comments:* Successful graduates are eligible to join the Craniosacral Therapy Association, a professional body set up to maintain standards, provide insurance and give support to practising therapists. 'It is the most comprehensive training available in the UK, with attention being placed on a whole person approach to therapy'. Practising craniosacral therapists may attend advanced courses run yearly.

Hellerwork

European Hellerwork Association *Title of Training:* Hellerwork Practitioner Training. *Duration:* 1,250 hours of study spread over four seperate phases of residential training, home study and in-the-field working. *Entry Requirements:* Over 21 years old, high school graduate or equivalent, must have completed the entire Hellerwork series of body balancing sessions as a client. *Fees:* £8,000 in total, inclusive of 9 weeks room and board for residential element, all books and supervision. *Comments:* Physical, emotional and financial maturity is assessed at a selection panel prior to accepting the students onto the training. Some students may be provisionally accepted pending completion of other courses e.g. psychotherapy or massage training.

Macrobiotics

Community Health Foundation *Title of Training:* Kushi Institute Certificate Course *Duration:* Level 1: 6 weekends and 6 day intensive or 4 weeks daytime. Level 2: 4 weekends and 9 day intensive or 6 weeks daytime. Level 3: 5 weeks daytime. *Entry Requirements:* Ideally completed an introductory Shiatsu or cooking course. *Fees:* Refer to organisers *Comments:* Emphasis is on teaching students the deeper understanding behind macrobiotics and shiatsu, along with practical skills.

INTRODUCTION TO SPIRIT

What is Spiritual?

The word spiritual must be one of the most difficult to define in the English Language. The dictionary definition of 'spirit' alone ranges across the whole gamut of soul, ghost, animation, courage, breathing, mind and alcohol. The meaning it has for an individual tends to vary according to their particular values and beliefs. However, though the word may take different forms for different people, it is usually used to denote whatever is of greatest, highest or deepest value for that person, and how this is expressed in their lives.

The groups included here fall under the category of spiritual because their practices and beliefs all aim to take the practitioner beyond their normal, limited sense of themselves. Specifically they aim to take people beyond their sense of themselves as separate egos or selves, isolated from other people, from the world and the universe in which we live. In some way they aim directly to facilitate contact with the 'transpersonal'; that experience of the self as being part of a greater whole, and of partaking of what is spoken of in traditional religious systems as the divine, something which exists both within and beyond time and the particular. They may seek to do this in many different ways.

The Difference between Religion and Spirituality

Religions are one way in which spirituality can be expressed. They represent a system of beliefs and practices which have become recognisable as a particular tradition. Religion and the spiritual are *not* synonymous, and spirituality can be expressed and developed in many ways outside of religion.

The Search for a New Spirituality

In many people's minds the emergence of 'alternative' spiritual movements is associated with the sixties and the search of many people at that time for deeper, more lasting values than those offered by what seemed to them to be an over-materialistic society. Disaffected with a society which seemed to be obsessed with consumerism, achievement and conformity, and with orthodox religions which appeared irrelevant and stultified, some people turned to drugs, some to politics and others to religion, while some turned to all three.

The seeds of this collective change in consciousness were sown much earlier however. It was in 1893 that The League of Liberal Clergymen of Chicago, Illinois set up the World Parliament of Religions, a forum where followers of faiths from East and West could meet together and share perspectives. This assembly of Christians, Jews, Muslims, Buddhists, Hindus, Taoists, Confucians and Spiritualists led to the creation of the first centres of Hinduism, Buddhism and Islam in the U.S.

But it was not until 1965 when the U.S. government ended the restrictions on Asian immigration which had been in force for nearly fifty years that the dialogue between East and West was opened on a massive scale. Though this move was intended to allow refugees from Maoist China to take up residence in the U.S., many Asian teachers and holy men took the opportunity to make their voices heard in the heart of the West.

It was not only to the East that those in search of spiritual nourishment turned. At the same time Christianity experienced a revival in the form of 'born again' sects, who sought to rekindle enthusiasm for the religion that many Americans and Europeans had grown up with. There has also been a revival in interest in western occult traditions, and pre-christian or 'pagan' belief systems. At the turn of the century groups were formed which took some of their inspiration from the esoteric Judaic Kabbalah, and in some cases this was blended with the practice of ritual magic - notoriously in the case of Aleister Crowley. Today there are still practitioners of the 'old religion', witches and warlocks, who adhere to the folk religion of Europe which went underground with the advent of Christianity, but was never quite eradicated by it. Recently too there has been a growing interest in the religious beliefs and practices of the American Indians.

East meets West

Originally it was Europeans who went out to colonise what were then thought of as the less 'civilised' countries of the east, Africa and the 'New World 'of the Americas, or to convert their people to Christianity. Subsequently a strange reversal has taken place. Now the west is benefiting from a counter-colonisation and the ideas and philosophy of these countries seem to offer many people a different perspective. It seems as if

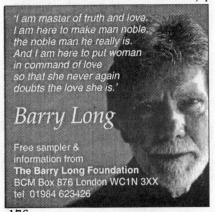

many of the attitudes and beliefs which underpin the culture and religion of these countries are not only as valid as ours, but also offer an outlook which may complement the traditional emphasis of western culture. In the west a high value tends to be placed on individual achievement and activity, on science and the intellect, and on technical ability. Broadly speaking, the outlook of eastern religion speaks more of what is collective, and stresses the importance of looking inwards, of experience rather than mental knowledge. In addition to this, 'native' or pagan religions offer a profound sense of connection with the natural world of which we are a part - a sense which we urgently need to recapture if we are to avert ecological disaster. Broadly speaking, while the west strives, the 'new religions' accept and open to what is. The influx of these new ideas perhaps offers an opportunity for a balance between these two poles.

Some people in the West have been attracted to this complementary attitude and have found it an expansive, holistic way of being. However, perhaps there can be a danger here of rejecting western culture wholesale, which not only has a great deal of value within it, but also represents an integral part of a westerner's whole outlook and response to life.

Gurus and spiritual teachers

The guru-disciple or teacher/apprentice relationship has been important in many spiritual traditions. In the west however we tend to be sceptical about gurus and people who might be purporting to know more than we do. This scepticism may be by no means a bad thing sometimes as there are some teachers who have shown themselves to be simply more charismatic than wise. We are also very wary of leaders because while they can do great good they can also do great harm.

A common image of the guru is perhaps of an Indian swami, bearded and loinclothed who probably lives in a cave and holds forth to hundreds of faceless, adoring disciples. The whole idea seems very foreign. Most gurus are not in fact like this, and the mystique which surrounds them, not always of their own making, may obscure the wisdom they might have to offer. The only way to determine if a particular teacher has something for you is to follow your instinct about him or her.

Though the guru is in the main an eastern concept, there have been and still are western teachers in the same vein. Gurdjieff, the native Russian teacher who gathered a number of followers round him at the beginning of this century, and who is still influential, is an example.

There are also spiritual groups who do not emphasise the importance of a teacher or leader. Sometimes they take their inspiration from the writings of a teacher who is dead, or simply from a particular faith or set of beliefs.

Cults
One fear often expressed about spiritual groups is that they are cults designed to take away people's autonomy. Stories of dubious recruitment tactics and brainwashing techniques hit the headlines a few years ago. In some cases there have even been allegations of physical force being used on troublesome group members.

While some of these reports may be true, it is this kind of scandal which tends to get publicised. The groups which have operated in this kind of way represent a very small number indeed of the total. Perhas what has not been publicised as much is the very real benefits many people have derived, and satisfaction they have gained from their involvement with *bona fide* spiritual groups. If you come up against dogmatism, intolerance or authoritarianism it is to be hoped that you will recognise it, though of course this is sometimes easier with hindsight than when faced with a teacher, group or leader who seems to have it all worked out.

Different types of Groups
The groups included in this book have different beliefs and ways of organising themselves. They employ different practices and are organised differently, and some are large, some small. In some the emphasis is on community and there may even be residential communities associated with the group. In others importance may be placed on individual study and practice; in fact in some groups there are few or even no meetings at all. Some of the centres we have listed are less like groups but are individuals or organisations running courses and workshops with a strong spiritual dimension.

Another variable is the level of commitment seen as ideal by different groups. Some groups offer an alternative lifestyle to those deeply involved, and others are more informal. Some are much more closely knit as groups and others are much looser in structure. The centres range from those with residential communities, offices and commercial enterprises on the premises, to those which meet in members' own homes.

Some of these groups are religious in the traditional sense of the word. They follow a recognisable set of religious teachings such as Sufism, Buddhism, Hinduism or Christianity. Others may have a spiritual framework in the sense that they emphasise a universal perspective and the divinity present in humanity, perhaps using traditional religious terminology, but not subscribing to any one particular traditional religious philosophy. A group like the Theosophical Society is an example of this. Then there are others which are much more secular, and which do not have any religious context at all, but which see themselves as addressing the spiritual perspective. Enlightenment Intensives are an example of this approach.

What they do

Once again a very wide range of activities constitute the practices of spiritual groups in London.

Meditation: This came from the east and to a greater or lesser extent usually forms part of the practice of those groups which hail from the eastern tradition. However, meditation has also been practised in western traditions. In Christianity it usually takes the form of contemplation of a particular subject, though some people have also incorporated a less directed style into the traditional forms of Christian worship. Secular groups are also using meditation since it adapts itself well to a non-religious framework. More information about the different kinds of meditation is given in the section on the subject in this book.

Ritual and devotional practices: While meditation has gained a great deal of credibility with many people in the west and even some sections of the medical profession recognise its therapeutic value, ritual is often still regarded with a great deal of suspicion. Some people find such activities weird or esoteric, and others feel uncomfortably reminded of their own religious upbringing, especially if they have

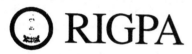

rejected it. Some people fear they will be taken over in some way if they let themselves get involved in rituals. Perhaps this is because we live in a society in which the rituals have to a certain extent lost the meaning they originally had. Weddings and funerals though they do in fact serve a useful purpose, socially, psychologically and spiritually, rarely act now as a way in which we can recognise and demonstrate the significance of important events in our lives. But ritual is an important way of focussing on feelings and values, and giving them a communal context.

Spiritually, ritual is used in this way. It serves to enable the participants to get in touch with their highest values and express these communally. It also places personal experience and emotion in the wider context of universal human experience. Many people enjoy ritual from the outset, finding that they recognise and respond to its use of the imaginative faculties. Others find they they prefer to know what is going on first before they engage.

Rituals are used by some Christian, Buddhist and Hindu groups, and in Paganism and Shamanism.

Chanting and prayer: Sound has been used in both east and west to express the spirit. The repetition of mantras (short phrases with spiritual significance or meaning) focuses the mind and also calls up deeper levels of energy. It can unite the physical (because singing, chanting or praying is a physical act), the emotional (because music evokes a strong emotional response) and the mental (especially if words are involved). Prayer is traditionally central in Christianity. Mantras are often used by Buddhist and Hindu groups. Music and chanting is important in the Sufi tradition.

Study: Some groups particularly emphasise study, talks and discussion. They may discuss the writings of a teacher or teachers and philosophers. They may have programmes of lectures by people on various topics. Taped lectures are becoming increasingly popular as a way in which people can make more contact with a teacher or lecturer, and absorb his or her teachings more fully by repeated listening. In some cases these methods are the only ones used by a particular group or association

Other methods: There are many other ways in which particular groups facilitate growth and communication. Some adapt therapeutic techniques, some meet together in different ways, some emphasise the importance of the arts and so on. This all points

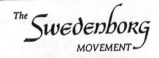

to the fact that the definition of what is spiritual is widening to include different aspects of culture.

Spiritual Groups in London

There are many spiritual groups in London practising in different ways. The decision to investigate the possibility of a spiritual path is very much a matter of instinct, of the heart. People usually become interested in a particular group because they have read something which seems to make sense to them, or because they have met someone involved in some sort of spiritual path, or because they feel attracted to a practice, like meditation or chanting. If you are drawn to this kind of search, don't be put off too soon by the vast array of groups which you may feel are not for you. As it says in the bible - 'seek, and ye shall find'!

Spirituality versus Psychology

Psychology has been called the modern religion. Freud's work exposed for the first time to much of the western world the depths of the human psyche, the inner world. What he saw there was the dark underside of experience, the unregenerated primitive instincts which had remained throughout the long process of civilisation seemingly untouched and merely pushed into unconsciousness. The resistance which Freud encountered in the course of publicising his work and ideas is a measure of how deeply his picture of human nature threatened the image of what it was to be human at the time. Yet paradoxically in many ways Freud's view echoed assumptions of the time - that man is essentially 'sinful', and his lower nature needs to be kept in check by society and religion. But while the orthodox solution was salvation by God and good works, Freud's was that knowledge of unconscious functioning through analysis would set the patient free of his or her own 'demons'.

With the development of Freud's original ideas, some psychologists and therapists have attempted to redress the balance, and in different ways have stressed that as well as hiding problems and complexes, the psyche also has hidden heights. While we may be largely unconscious of our instincts and repressed desires and hates, we are also unaware of our potential for joy and loving participation in the universe.

The question of when psychology and spirituality are similar, and when they are different is still being hotly debated as some psychologists turn to meditation and mysticism, and some gurus incorporate therapeutic techniques into their teachings. Both seek to offer practices and techniques which bring about individual growth, and both aim to free people from restrictive habitual ways of acting and being.

However, while it may often be difficult to distinguish the difference between spiritual and psychotherapeutic practice, it may be possible to distinguish different levels within both disciplines. Various theorists have suggested that it may be important to build a mature sense of one's individuality before going beyond the individual self. Some psychotherapies may concentrate more on developing a sense of 'who I am', and regard this as the limit of their work. Others have sought to include a more spiritual dimension into their work, or may have been founded on the premise that the spiritual quest is the most important one from a psychological point of view.

However, while there may be a great deal of overlap in practice, many psychologists and therapists are still quite wary of what they may see as an attempt to avoid painful feelings by going off into a cosmic 'bliss-out' in religion. Spiritual teachers too can be suspicious of therapy, feeling that it is simply equivalent to putting an elastoplast on the mortal wound of human suffering. It seems that the dialogue between psychology and spirituality has only just begun. It may take a long time for the two to settle their differences. However, in general more people are beginning to question what they see as an artificial division between what has in the past been called 'spiritual' and what has been called 'worldly'.

The 'New Age'
The last two decades has seen a growth in what has become known as 'New Age' activity and thinking. Even some sections of the media have hailed the 1990s as an era when society will turn away from the hard-edged, money-making 1980s and adopt caring, green, spiritual values.

The term 'New Age' can be used to cover a diverse number of attitudes, beliefs and activities, to the extent that it can be difficult to see what they have in common. As the name suggests, the central idea in New Age thinking is that humanity has reached a critical stage in its evolutionary development which will lead to a change in people's outlook and consciousness. New Age philosophy is characterised by various concerns:

1) The mystical nature of the universe: the fundamental reality of the universe is seen as love, and the universe is seen as ultimately benign and purposeful.

2) Global conciousness: belief in the oneness of humanity, and the importance of community and sharing.

3) Non sectarian spirituality: all religions are seen as expressions of the same vision, and great importance is placed on the individual's right to choose their own path, whether this takes a traditionally religious form or the form of secular spirituality.

4) Abundance rather than scarcity: the belief that that there are enough resources for everyone in the world both material and immaterial. 'Scarcity' mentality is seen as responsible for scarcity.

5) The importance of preserving natural environment, an ecologically sound lifestyle and a respect for nature.

6) Human potential and personal development: human beings have more potential than they realise, and are, in essence, divine. It is seen as our responsibility to develop this potential.

7) Human beings as creators of their own reality: the individual is seen as responsible for his or her own life, and as creating that reality through attitudes, thoughts, feelings etc.

8) Importance of the feminine: belief that it is necessary to redress the balance caused by over-valuing what is seen as the 'masculine' in our culture by reasserting the value of the 'feminine' and questioning the power of men.

9) 'Holistic' model in science, medicine etc: the belief that the universe is not a mechanism made up of randomly functioning parts but is a living organism which works as an indivisible whole.

In general, humanity is seen as progressing into a time of greater spirituality and world harmony.

There is much overlap between the New Age movement and the 'Human Potential' movement, which grew out of humanistic psychology in the 1960s. This is more psychotherapy and 'personal growth' oriented and less mystical in outlook, though in practice there are ideas, approaches and methodology common to both.

Critics of New Age philosophy have claimed that it concentrates too exclusively on the positive aspects of the universe, and therefore attempts to ignore, or at least deals inadequately with, the presence of suffering and evil in the world. New Agers have been criticised for being too credulous and subjective, and of attempting to dispense with reason and logic. Whatever the pros and cons of the movement, it is proving to have a steady following as evinced by the continuing popularity of New Age events.

Meditation

There are so many different kinds of meditation that it can seem hard sometimes to define what it is they all have in common. The benefits of meditation are being recognised in the west, though it is still sometimes seen as something strange or eccentric. However, it is more down to earth than going into some sort of psychedelic trance, or 'contemplating one's navel'.

Meditation is turning the attention inwards, away from all the external things which demand our attention. It involves focussing the mind, usually on one particular object or idea. In meditation the mind is cleared of all the extraneous thoughts which take up a lot of our energy, or for a little while at least our involvement with all those thoughts is suspended, so that a clearer, calmer experience of oneself is possible.

There are various ways of achieving this, depending on the particular meditation practice. Different kinds of meditation may be useful for different purposes, or temperaments. There are practices in which the meditator concentrates on the breath as it comes in and out of the body, without trying to change it in any way. This focuses the attention, and helps to bring together the awareness of mind and body. There are meditation techniques where a colour, shape or form is pictured and held in the attention. This 'visualisation' technique has been used in a very particular way to help in the treatment of illness, especially by cancer sufferers. Here the meditator will visualise his or her illness, and then see the body fighting that illness and suppressing it. Some yogic forms of meditation involve concentrating on an actual object such as a candle or a stone, and some use a 'mantra' or phrase repeated over and over again. There are meditation practices where there is no one object of concentration at all, and the meditator just tries to sit and be aware of all the changing thoughts and feelings passing through his or her mind. This is the Zen 'sitting' meditation.

Usually these kinds of meditation are done sitting down, often cross-legged or kneeling while sitting on cushions. However, this is by no means essential if it is difficult for you to do, and they can be done sitting in a chair. However, some practices involve movement. There are 'walking meditations' where concentration is on the body as you walk, and the processes involved in moving. The 'Dynamic Meditation' practised by followers of the Bhagwan Shree Rajneesh involves very vigorous whirling and dancing movement.

The benefits of meditation are just as diverse as the practices. One of the most immediate effects can be that the meditator feels more calm and relaxed. Many people take up meditation initially as a way of combating stress. It can also increase one's ability to concentrate, and helps the meditator develop a sense of a still, calm centre from which they feel more able to direct their lives creatively. It can also help to generate a greater sense of self-acceptance and warmth towards others. It can also be a way of achieving higher states of consciousness and heightened awareness.

Although there are quite a few books on the subject, as with learning any other skill, it is important to find a teacher who has experience themselves and can give you direct instruction and help. Centres which teach meditation are listed below, and will offer an explanation of their particular practices.

CENTRES OFFERING MEDITATION
Abshot Holistic Centre PO14, Alternative Therapies Centre N16, Barry Long Foundation WC1N, Bhratiya Vidya Bhavan (Institute of Indian Culture) W14, Biomonitors, Brahma Kumaris World Spiritual University NW10, British Buddhist Association W9, British School of Oriental Therapy and Movement SE21, British School of Shiatsu-Do NW3, Buddhapadipa Temple, Cabot Centre NW1, Centre for Personal & Professional Development N17, Changes NW3, College of Healing WR14, College of Psychic Studies SW7, Cortijo Romero UK LS7, Croydon Buddhist Centre CR0, Foundation for International Spiritual Unfoldment E7, Fountain London N14, Gaia House TQ12, Graigian Community NW5, Healing Voice TW10, Healing Workshops NW5, Health Management IG10, Helios N1, Heruka Buddhist Centre NW11, Holistic Yoga Centre MK19, Homoeopathic Health Clinic HA3, Hong Tao Acupuncture and Natural Health Clinic HA5, IBISS TW7, Jamyang Meditation Centre N4, Ki Kai Shiatsu Centre, Life Resources NW7, Living Colour NW3, London Buddhist Centre E2, London Serene Reflection Meditation Group, London Shambala Centre, London Sufi Centre W11, London Zen Society NW1, Lotus Healing Centre NW8, Lucis Trust SW1, Mushindokai NW1, Pearl Healing Centre CR7, Psychosynthesis and Education Trust SE1, Raphael Clinic NW6, RIGPA Fellowship N1, Satyananda Yoga Centre, School of Meditation W11, School of T'ai-chi Ch'uan - Centre for

Healing WC1H, Shanti Sadan W11, South London Natural Health Centre SW4, St James Centre for Health and Healing W1V, Studio E NW6, Sunra SW12, Transcendental Meditation Baker Street Centre NW1, Transcendental Meditation National Office LU7, Transcendental Meditation SW1P, Violet Hill Studios NW8, White Eagle Lodge W8, Wild Goose Company NW3.

TRAINING IN MEDITATION

Foundation for International Spiritual Unfoldment *Title of Training:* Meditaion *Duration:* Three months *Entry Requirements:* None *Fees:* Refer to organisers *Comments:* This annual residential course offers a uniqe form of mediation.

Lucis Trust *Title of Training:* Arcane School *Duration:* Correspondence course which requires daily meditaion, monthly reports and study papers. If continued the course can last over ten years. *Entry Requirements:* None. *Fees:* No fees as the Trust is funded by donation. *Comments:* This is training for world service, using meditation and esoteric philosophy, with a special focus on the teachings of Alice Bailey.

SPIRIT

THE TRADITIONS

Buddhism

Buddhism has been dubbed 'Britain's fastest growing religion' by Arnold Toynbee. It has in fact been in existence for over 2,500 years. Its founder, the Buddha, saw suffering as central to the human condition, and his teaching concerned the ways in which people could transcend this suffering. These are the practice of an ethical lifestyle, and of meditation which then leads to insight into the nature of existence and the causes of human suffering.

Suffering is caused because according to Buddhism everything is impermanent. Human beings seek everlasting happiness by trying to hold onto what must fade or die. When this happens we experience pain, and try to avoid this pain by seeking another object of happiness in the world. Buddhist practices seek to take the practitioner beyond this cycle of holding on and running away, and to cultivate not a state of indifference, but one of joyful acceptance of the impermanent nature of existence. This understanding is not intellectual but a profound experience which leads to complete freedom. This state is called 'Nirvana'.

Buddhism emphasises the importance of the individual's own growth towards greater consciousness of him or herself. The development of 'mindfulness' is an important part of much of Buddhist meditation. Mindfulness starts with awareness of oneself - of one's body, one's feelings and emotions, and one's mind - and of other people and the world around one. It develops ultimately into awareness of absolute reality.

Alongside the emphasis on individual development, concern for other people and for life - the development of compassion - is also seen as crucial. In the later developments of Buddhism especially, Nirvana is not seen simply as a neutral state of being without passion or desires, but more positively as a dynamic state of joy, contentment and compassion.

As it spread to different countries from India where it started (and from where it has now virtually died out), Buddhism adapted itself to different cultures. This gave rise to very different approaches to the original teachings. The groups listed below reflect these approaches. The Theravada tradition emphasises morality, the monastic lifestyle and the original Pali scriptures. Tibetan Buddhism is part of the 'Vajrayana' or tantric tradition which is colourful, ritualistic and emphasises psychic energy and often visualisation meditations. Zen Buddhism is perhaps the form that most people in the West have heard of through pithy Zen stories or the cryptic sayings which abound in the tradition. Zen's approach is anti-rational with an emphasis on zazen (meditation) and direct experience.

READING
What the Buddha Taught by Walpola Rahula, Evergreen/Grove Weidenfeld £7.15. Addressed to the 'educated and intelligent reader' and written by Dr Rahula, himself a Buddhist monk and scholar, this is a lucid and comprehensive introduction to Buddhism. The new revised and expanded edition also contains selected texts from sutras and the Dhammapada. With sixteen black and white illustrations. **The Buddhist**

186

Handbook: a Complete Guide to Buddhist Teaching and Practice by John Snelling, Rider £6.95. John Snelling is the editor of the Buddhist journal *The Middle Way* and uniquely placed to offer this overview of a vast subject. This is the first basic introduction to help the newcomer orientate him or herself to the many different schools, doctrines and organisations which comprise the world of Buddhism, as well as a useful addition to the library of the practising 'western' Buddhist. **A Buddhist Bible** *by Dwight Goddard, Beacon Press U.S.A. £11.95.* First published in 1932, this is one of the books which originally stimulated western interest in Buddhism. Goddard's preface states that his collection of major texts: 'is not intended to be a sourcebook for critical, literary and historical study; it is only intended to be a source of spiritual inspiration designed to awaken faith, and to develop faith into aspiration and full realisation'.

CENTRES OFFERING BUDDHISM

British Buddhist Association W9, Buddhist Society SW1V, Croydon Buddhist Centre CR0, Gaia House TQ12, Heruka Buddhist Centre NW11, London Buddhist Centre E2, London Serene Reflection Meditation Group, London Shambala Centre, London Zen Society NW1, Nichirin Shoshu of the United Kingdom, RIGPA Fellowship N1, West London Buddhist Centre W11.

Christianity

Christianity is the majority and official religion of this country. Central to Christian belief is the importance of love (expressed in Christ's axiom 'love thy neighbour as thyself') which is seen as a divine attribute made manifest by god sending his son to earth to become man. This symbolises for Christians the possibility of humanity also expressing this love of god. The worship of the creator god in prayer and ritual is also central to Christian practice.

Acting in the world to help others is also stressed, and for this reason Christians have traditionally been involved in medical and charitable work, both in their native countries and abroad, often in Third World Countries.

As well as this emphasis on good works, there is also a strong mystical tradition within Christianity where solitary communion with, and personal experience of, god enables the believer to become receptive to the divinity, and thus enter a deeper union with him/her.

Some Christian groups today seek to re-interpret the original doctrines in a way which is relevant to modern life. One of these is Matthew Fox, proponent of 'creation spirituality' (see 'Reading' below). This is founded on the belief the human condition is not one of 'original sin' (implying that we are basically bad or separated from God), but one of 'original blessing' (implying that we are basically good and in harmony with God).

Christianity is rich in myth and symbol, and this has inspired many artists, writers and composers through the centuries.

READING

Meister Eckhart - The Man from whom God hid Nothing by Ursula Fleming, Fount

£2.95. "God is a light shining in itself in silent stillness." These are words from the great German mystical theologian, Meister Eckhart (1260-1329). Ursula Fleming's incisive exploration into his teaching sheds light on this remarkable man who is one of the most controversial figures of Christian history. This is a selection from his writings which are as relevant today as they were six centuries ago. **A Lesson of Love: The Relevations of Julian of Norwich** Edited and translated by Fr. John-Julian OJN, Darton Longman and Todd £6.95. At the age of thirty, Dame Julian of Norwich (14th Century) was granted a series of sixteen mystical revelations of the crucified Christ. She devoted the next twenty years to prayer and contemplation, and described her visions and her understanding of them in The Revelations of Divine Love, the first book written in the English language by a woman. **Original Blessing: A Primer of Creation Spirituality** by Matthew Fox, Bear & Co £8.50. Matthew Fox is a Dominican scholar and spiritual teacher, an eloquent advocate of Creation Spirituality. Original Blessing is an empowering and necessary book which leads us back to our own creativity and that deep ecstatic centre which resides beneath any fear of death.

CENTRES OFFERING CHRISTIANITY
Christian Community W6.

Hinduism

Hinduism is not a homogenous religious system in itself. It is more a collection of different ideas, schools and cults. The word 'Hindu' is Persian for Indian, and was used by outsiders to lump together all the indigenous cults and religions of the Indian sub-continent.

It is difficult to isolate any one belief or practice which all Hindus have in common. For instance, though most Hindus believe in a creator god in some way, there are some who don't. Some are vegetarian, while others will eat meat. Most accept the authority of the Veda scriptures, which have been written over the 5,000 years of Hinduism's development.

However, the struggle for personal salvation is common to all Hinduism. The spirit or true self, Atman as it is called, is present in each individual. The Atman is the god within us, and is identified with Brahman, the Absolute, the origin and cause of all that exists. Maya, or human ignorance, keeps us from understanding our real nature, and realising our identity with this ultimate principle, and so we identify more with the phenomenal, ever changing world. The soul is seen as passing through countless births because it is attached to this world of appearances. Release from the cycle of incarnation is possible when the individual reaches a full realisation that the real self is one with Brahman. This release is called moksha.

Because Brahman is seen as indefinable and unknowable, Hindus have traditionally worshipped the divine principle in more accessible forms. There are many more personal gods who are believed to be manifestations of Brahman, and who are worshipped because they are more human and act as a bridge between the relative world of human experience and the Absolute or god.

There are many different schools within Hinduism. Some have a very devotional approach, some see asceticism as a path to liberation, and others emphasise the importance of working in society for the collective good. Meditation, chanting and ritual are all practices employed by Hindu groups. The practice of Yoga is central in Hinduism. This is not just the Hatha Yoga we are familiar with in the West, which is the physical discipline of perfecting poses or Asanas (see 'Yoga' in Body section). Yoga means yoke or union, and it is a discipline which unites one with the universal or divine. Other forms of Yoga practised by the groups below include Bhakti Yoga, the discipline of devotion or love, Mantra Yoga, the chanting of Mantras, and Karma Yoga which is work as a spiritual practice.

In the personal struggle towards freedom, the teacher or guru is of great importance. Most modern Hindu groups centre around a teacher and their interpretation of the Hindu vision.

READING

Hinduism by K M Sen, Penguin £4.50. This book is an introduction to Hinduism and its sacred texts, the *Vedas*, the *Upanishads* and the *Bhagavad Gita*. Included is also a discussion of the three Hindu religious paths — the path of knowledge *(jnana)*, the path of work *(karma)* and the path of devotion *(bhakti)*. While giving insight into the caste system, the history of Hinduism and its nature and function, it also provides a look at current trends and customs and festivals. **Training the Mind through Yoga** by M V *Waterhouse, Shanti Sadan £3.00*. This collection of fourteen lectures introduces the general reader to the traditional methods of training the mind used in the spiritual science of *Adhyatma Yoga* and the 'yoga of self knowledge'. Beginning with an introduction to the *Bhagavad Gita* the lectures cover various aspects on refining the mind and emotions through discussing the stages in meditation the training of the yogi, awakening the higher consciousness and training and discipline. **Autobiography of A Yogi** by *Paramahansa Yogananda, Rider £5.95*. An authoritative introduction to the science of yoga, this book is a classic in its field, revealing the scientific foundation underlying the great religious paths of both east and west. It is an account of Yogananda's own search for truth which includes explanations of the laws governing miracles and recounts his meeting with many saints and sages throughout the world.

CENTRES OFFERING HINDUISM

Bhratiya Vidya Bhavan (Institute of Indian Culture) W14, International Society for Krishna Consciousness (ISKON), Satyananda Yoga Centre, Shanti Sadan W11.

Paganism

The word 'pagan' derives from the Latin 'pagus' which simply means an inhabitant of the countryside. However, since the fourth century AD it has been used in a derogatory sense to denote those who subscribe to a creed other than the majority religion. In former times, the word inspired fear, hatred and the zeal to convert those who, in their primitive ignorance, did not know any better.

In reality Paganism is the natural religion, the native spirituality of the country, and it has been practised in Britain ever since the end of the last Ice Age 11,000 years ago. Any indigenous cult specific to a land and its culture may be called 'pagan'. British paganism was influenced by successive waves of pagan invaders over the centuries - Celtic, Scandinavian and Teutonic. Under its umbrella can be included the Celtic Druids, the Scandinavian godi, the medieval witchcult, Renaissance hermeticism and alchemy. Paganism still survives in the succession of 'New Age' cults and sects today.

The sense of continuity in Paganism derives from the magic of place, of myth and of music. It comes from the heart rather than the head, and a central feature of it is the celebration of Mother Earth and of nature. One expression of this is in the rituals which acknowledge the year's turning. These take place ideally at ancient sites such as Stonehenge and Glastonbury, which were specifically built to harness the stellar, lunar, solar and human energies in one harmony.

Modern British paganism is a revival of the old beliefs and practices, and today in many parts of the country there are cults of the Goddess, the Wicca, Odinism and Druidism. Imported varieties of paganism have also made their impact over the last decade (e.g.the shamanism of the North American Indians).

Common to all pagan cults are 'green' values - the promotion of an ecologically sound environment and the celebration of a transpersonal spirit through rite, dance, song and music. Paganism also explores the possibilities for empowering the individual through getting into a right relationship with the cosmos.

READING
Life and Times of a Modern Witch by Janet and Stewart Farrar, Headline £2.95. This book is written by two well known witches, as a result of a worldwide survey conducted to answer the many questions concerning their beliefs and rituals. Read this book to discover what kind of people become witches, what powers they possess, whether or not they worship Satan and a host of other things. **The Spiral Dance: A Rebirth of the Ancient Religion of the Great Goddess** by Starhawk, Harper and Row £9.95. A classic resource book for the women's spirituality movement, including rituals, invocations, exercises and magic. It is a brilliant overview of the growth, suppression and modern day re-emergence of witchcraft as a Goddess worshipping religion. This is a book of tools, continually in the process of renewal in response to changing times. **Wicca: the Old Religion in the New Age** by Vivianne Crowley, Aquarian/Thorsons. Vivianne Crowley here explains the 'way of the witch', the quest for the self, showing how wicca

— rapidly regaining its former popularity — has relevance in today's world. Included are the subjects of black and white magic, nudity, the God and Goddess within, the future of witchcraft and more. Additionally there is an explanation of the relationship between Witchcraft and Jungian psychology.

CENTRES OFFERING PAGANISM

Acca and Adda WC1N, Asatru Folk Runic Workshop, Centre for Pagan Studies SW2, Eagle's Wing Centre for Contemporary Shamanism NW2, House of the Goddess SW12.

Qabalah

The Qabalah (alternatively spelt Kabbalah or Cabala) is primarily based on esoteric Jewish teachings and is at the heart of the western esoteric tradition. It is a philosophy and psychology of great theoretical and practical depth, its essential doctrine being that each individual person has the potential to realise their inner divinity and express this in all walks of life. There is evidence in the Old Testament of the existence of the Quabalah in pre-Christian times. It was not committed to writing until the Middle Ages, however, and most development has taken place in the nineteenth and twentieth centuries.

The Qabalah uses the 'Tree of Life' as a complete map of different levels of consciousness. There are may ways to use the Tree of Life. Being easy to both visualise and memorise, it can serve as a guide to personal development.

The Tree of Life is composed of eleven spheres, which represent everything from the body and the physical world through to the most central, or deepest aspect of our spiritual being, the place where individuality blurs into union with all other consciousness. In learning to have practical experience of these different spheres, so the individual can add to his/her knowledge of the different parts of him/herself.

In the Qabalah, each individual is believed to have their own Tree of Life inside them which has to be directly experienced rather than believed as a matter of dogma. Just as human beings have experiences common, so there are also group or collective Trees. It can thus be seen as relevant to both the evolution of the individual, and through the individual, the whole planet. *(Will Parfitt)*

READING

Kabbalah and Psychology by *Z'ev ben Shimon Halevi, Gateway £6.95.* The author examines psychology as the study of the archetypal world which hovers between Earth and Heaven. Psychology here is set against the scheme of Kabbalah which takes into account the divine origin of the human being, reincarnation, mystical experience as well as madness. The Tree of Life is studied in relation to both Freudian and Jungian psychology. **The Mystical Qabalah** by *Dion Fortune, Aquarian/Thorsons £7.95.* Of the books that Dion Fortune wrote, this one stands out as a seminal work in the development of the Qabalah and its incorporation into the Western Mystery Tradition. This is a useful reference book for those involved in the esoteric philosophy of the West and the study of the psychology of mystical experience. **The Living Qabalah: A Practical and Experiential Guide to Understanding the Tree of Life** by *Will Parfitt,*

Element £8.95. Fully understood, the Qabalah offers a unique system of personal exploration and development, allowing us to examine all aspects of ourselves - our personality, soul and spirit. Using practical and experiential exercises designed for newcomer and expert alike, this illustrated manual provides a new way of using Qabalah in daily life.

Shamanism

This is found as part of the native cultures of many different societies all over the world, for instance among the Aborigines of Australia, Lapplanders, American Indians and the Bon Po priests of Tibet. Traditionally the shaman uses rhythmic drumming and chanting, or more rarely, hallucinogenic drugs to alter consciousness and journey into 'non-ordinary reality' (as Carlos Castaneda called it in his popular Don Juan shamanic books) in order to gain insight, heal the sick or make contact with guides or teachers. Ritual and mask-making may also be used by modern shamans to facilitate this dialogue with what, in modern psychological terms, might be called the unconscious. It is largely the shamanism of the North American Indians which has made the most impact here, with their *sweat lodge* tradition (a sort of do-it-yourself sauna in which participants chant for long periods) and the *medicine wheel* teachings. This tradition particularly stresses the importance of nature as teacher, healer and guide.

Shamanic ritual and journeying to 'non-ordinary reality' has also been taken up for psychotherapeutic purposes, notably by Stanislav Grof in his *holotropic therapy*. Grof uses various techniques to induce hallucinations in his clients, and has evolved a system of psychotherapy around their experiences.

READING
Way of the Shaman *by Michael Harner Bantam (U.S.A.) £3.60.* Written by an experienced healer and widely travelled field worker, the Way of the Shaman is the most popular guide for the beginner on the shamanic path. Clearly explained practical techniques lead us up to the the understanding and practice of deep physical and spiritual healing, as practised by shamans everywhere. **Medicine Woman** *by Lynn Andrews, Penguin £5.99.* Neither Lynn Andrews nor Carlos Castaneda have escaped controversy in their books but the value of their accounts grows out of the potential for personal transformation they demonstrate which is available to us all. Andrews' first book describes her initiation by Agnes Whistling Elk. In later books she goes on to work with shamans and medicine people all over the world. **Shamanic Voices** *by Joan Halifax , Dutton U.S.A. £9.55.* This anthology allows shamans from as far afield as Australia, Africa and Alaska to speak for themselves about the rituals they guard and the experiences they have undergone. Their altered states of consciousness act as a bridge for those they serve between everyday life and the eternal. Dr. Halifax provides an excellent introductory essay and brief prefaces to every individual account.

CENTRES OFFERING SHAMANISM
Acca and Adda WC1N, Asatru Folk Runic Workshop, Centre for Pagan Studies SW2, Eagle's Wing Centre for Contemporary Shamanism NW2, House of the Goddess SW12.

TRAINING IN SHAMANISM
Eagle's Wing Centre for Contemporary Shamanism *Title of Training:* "Elements of Shamanism" *Duration:* One Year part-time residential (26 days in all). *Entry Requirements:* Interview or Introductory workshop. *Fees:* £875 in instalments. *Comments:* Intake in October or January.

Spiritualism

Spiritualism is centred round the belief of the survival of the personality after death, and that there can be communication between the living and those 'on the other side'. This communication takes place through 'mediums', or 'sensitives' as they are sometimes known, who channel the messages of the dead. The messages may take the form of words of comfort or advice to friends or relatives, and spiritualists believe that this proves that they are still in existence, but in another 'plane' or world .

Many spiritualists are also involved in spiritual healing, which involves either the laying on of hands (hand healing) or absent healing where the patient undergoes treatment at a distance (see 'Healing' in the Body section). Spiritualism in this country usually has a Christian context, although orthodox Christianity tends to regard it with suspicion.

There are a number of spiritualist churches throughout London, where services are held. These involve a service similar to a church service, but at a paticular point a medium will give messages from the 'other side' to particular members of the congregation.

Spiritualism is an organised religion, and is therefore distinct from other forms of psychism, where mediums contact what they believe are spirits in order to make predictions and/or give advice. Another example of psychism is the 'channelling' of books or philosophical or religious teachings through someone who belives themselves to be in touch with a spirit guide.

READING
The Wanderings of a Spiritualist *by Sir Arthur Conan Doyle, Ronin £5.95.* This is a personal account of spiritualism or communication with the dead by the popular writer of the Sherlock Holmes stories. It includes meetings with remarkable people, geographical accounts and political musing from a spiritualist perspective. **The Book on Mediums** *by Allan Kardec, Weiser £9.95.* Although over a century has passed since its original publication, the Book on Mediums remains the most comprehensive and basic text on spiritualism, revealing the fundamental principles of communication with the spirit world. The book contains instruction on the theory of manifestations, the meaning of communicating with the invisible world, the development of mediumship, the difficulties and the dangers that are to be encountered in the practice of spiritism. **Testimony of Light** *by Helen Greaves, C.W. Daniel £4.95.* This book describes the after death experience through the communication given to Helen Greaves by her former friend and teacher, the late Frances Banks, through telepathy across the veil. The message given in the scripts is that the death of the body is but a gentle passing to a much freer and fuller life.

CENTRES OFFERING SPIRITUALISM

Alternative Therapies Centre N16, Centre for Personal & Professional Development N17, Helios N1, Spiritualist Association of Great Britain SW1X, Women and Health NW1.

Sufism

Sufism originated in Persia in the sixth century AD as a reaction against what the Sufis saw as the rigidity and worldliness of orthodox Islam. After the time of Mahommed the movement became unpopular with some Muslims, who thought it heretical, and many Sufis suffered condemnation and persecution. The word itself comes from 'suf' which is Persian for the white woollen cloaks the mystics wore. The term 'sufi' is actually correctly used to describe those who have attained knowledge of the divine. An individual who is still on the path is called 'faquir', which means poor, in the sense of spiritual poverty.

Like most mystical traditions the aim of Sufism is direct experience of, and ultimately union with, God, and this is achieved through love, both of other people and of God. Sufism has been called 'the religion of the heart'. There is no dogma, nor any highly structured philosophical system which defines the beliefs of Sufism. The approach is largely devotional, and the emphasis is on intuition and feeling. It stresses the idea of equilibrium and wholeness. The human being is potentially a microcosm of the balanced unity of the universe. The ideal is not to withdraw from the world, but to bring vision and insight into the world. Achieving knowledge of God, the practitioner becomes in turn a vessel for God's knowledge to act in the world.

It is a very fluid tradition and personal communication between teacher and pupil is of central importance. The Teacher initiates the pupil into a chain of Teacher-pupil relationships, the lineage of which stretches back to Mahommed.

The Sufis have always used many different methods to develop consciousness, as the groups which exist in the West today still do. Their practices include contemplative meditation, guided visualisation, breathing exercises, music and the 'whirling' which is associated with the dervishes.

Sufism has inspired much literature. Poetry and the use of symbolism figure largely in the tradition as a means of expressing the experience of the divine. *The Rubaiyat of Omar Khayyam* is perhaps the most famous Sufi inspired text in the West, though their influence is thought to be widespread in European culture. Some claim that Gurdjieff, the Russian mystic and philosopher, was taught by Sufis.

Today Sufi groups vary a great deal. Some are still very much rooted in Islam, and others are more eclectic in their approach. Some advertise their activities while others maintain the traditional secrecy about their activities, believing that those who are truly seeking will find them.

READING

What is Sufism? *by Martin Lings, Mandala/Unwin Hyman £4.95.* An eloquent and authoritative introduction to the mystical dimension of Islam. Martin Lings writes from his own personal experience and deep understanding of Arabic culture and religion: nine concise and powerful chapters convey the essence of Sufism. **Rumi and Sufism** by Eva de Vitray-Meyerovitch, Post-Apollo Press, U.S.A. £9.95. A beautifully illustrated book exploring the life thought and background of one of Islam's greatest mystics, written by a French scholar who became a believer in Islam through her works on Sufism. A clear and approachable introduction to the subject, with fascinating material on the *Mevlevi* brotherhood to which he belonged. **The World of Sufi** by *Idries Shah and others, Octagon £12.50.* An anthology of writings about Sufis and their work, with contributions from many authors, including Idries Shah, Doris Lessing and Peter Brent. Chapters on the classical tradition of the Sufis; Sufi humour; Sufi spiritual practices; modern psychology and Sufism; Sufi literature; and current study materials.

CENTRES OFFERING SUFISM
London Sufi Centre W11, Nimatullahi Sufi Order W2.

Modern Teachers

Anthroposophical Association
Rudolph Steiner House, 35 Park Road, Regents Park , London NW1.
(0171) 723 4400
Rudolph Steiner, an Austrian living at the turn of the century, coined the term 'anthroposophy' (meaning awareness of one's humanity) to sum up his wide-ranging philosophy. Anthroposophy seeks to unite all of humanity's spiritual knowledge, covering the arts, science, philosophy and religion, and encompasses a whole social outlook emphasising the importance of human growth. Steiner applied his teaching to medicine, (see the Anthroposophical Medical Association), education (there are several Steiner Schools in the UK), science, and even agriculture where he devised a unique organic system of growing crops.

Barry Long Foundation
BCM Box 876, London WC1N 3XX.
(01984) 623426
Barry Long is an Australian, born in 1926, who lived for 20 years in London and began teaching publicly in 1983. He now teaches in Australia, New Zealand, Europe and the UK through public meetings and seminars, and through books and tapes covering various aspects of 'life and living, death and dying, love and making love, meditation and the art of being'.
There is no formal practice, but Barry Long's teaching encourages the application of greater attention and stillness to all aspects of living to bring about greater self-knowledge and love. He stresses the importance of direct experience rather than religious forms or dogma, and of realising the truth for onself, rather than relying on a guru. No groups or gatherings as such except when Barry Long gives a seminar or talk. Books and tapes available mail order.

Christian Community
Temple Lodge , 51 Queen Caroline Street , London W6 9QL.

(0181) 748 8388

Set up by Rudolph Steiner in 1922, the Christian Community seeks to re-affirm the spirit of Christianity. Central ideas are the importance of the resurrection as a symbol of individual growth; the inner meaning of the sacraments; reincarnation; freedom of thought. The arts and counselling are seen as an important part of spiritual practice.

Eckankar

8 Godolphin Road, Shepherds Bush, London W12 8JE.

(0181) 746 0131

Eckankar takes its direction from Sri Harold Klemp, with the help of whom followers aim to make contact with the Light and Sound of God which is believed to purify the consciousness, and lift the individual into heavenly states. Three principles are important: firstly that the soul is eternal, secondly that travellers on the path of ECK dwell in the spiritual planes, and thirdly that the soul has no past or future, but lives in the present. ECK spiritual aides are provided to give spiritual assistance. Also open discussion groups. Practice is through spiritual exercises (e.g. contemplation of the mantra 'HU', study of dreams and discourses, and service to life.

Lucis Trust

Suite 54, 3 Whitehall Court, Victoria, London SW1 2EF.

(0171) 839 4512

The Lucis Trust administers a number of programmes: The Arcane School, a meditation school run by correspondence; Triangles, which is a global network of individuals from different spiritual paths who use prayer and meditation to spread goodwill in the world; World Goodwill, which publishes material presenting a global spiritual perspectives on the issues facing humanity; and Lucis Press which publishes Alice Bailey's books. Free lending library of esoteric books available in London. Meetings fortnightly in the Charing Cross Hotel. Meditation meetings at the time of the full moon, and lectures on healing, ecology, development, metaphysics etc at the time of the new moon .Bi-monthly journal, The Beacon, and quarterly, World Goodwill newsletter.Established by Alice A Bailey, an author and lecturer in the first half of this century who pioneered the idea of a New Age of global co-operation and wholeness. She wrote 24 books presenting an esoteric perspective on psychology, occult meditation and the evolution of humanity, which aim to help individuals be more effective in serving humanity and the Plan of Light and Love during what is seen as a time of transition into the Age of Aquarius. She founded the Lucis Trust as an international agency in the raising of human consciousness, and it now has consultative status with the United Nations.

Thomas Troward Society

Lahaina, 24 Beresford Road, North Chingford, London E4 6EE.

(0181) 529 8097

A society based on the work of Thomas Troward, a man with a background in law who later became a judge. The society offers counselling and publications based on creative thought, spiritual psychology and 'Science of Mind'. They offer lessons in the 'Science of Mind', 'Mental Science' and spiritual counselling. Fees by donation according to arrangement. Their aim is to put people in touch with their inner creative source.

White Eagle Lodge

9 St. Mary Abbots Place, Kensington High Street, London W8 6LS.

(0171) 603 7914

Founded in 1936 on the teachings of the spirit guide and teacher- White Eagle - who channelled his message through Grace Cooke. The purpose of the teaching is to enable each individual to develop the light of the Christ spirit which is believed to be in every human heart, so that it can radiate into the world. The teaching says that the basic law which controls life is love, expressed through love for God, humanity and nature, and this love is seen as leading people, through the experience of many lives, back to total awareness of the God within them.

OTHER GROUPS

3HO Kundalini Yoga Foundation

55 Sunny Gardens Road, London NW4 1SJ.

(0181) 203 7302

3HO stands for the healthy, happy, holy organisation. They practice and teach Kundalini Yoga which seeks to awaken the dormant cosmic energy in human beings and refine it by drawing it up through the seven chakras, or centres of consciousness and energy. The practices include adopting particular positions and movement, breathing techniques, meditation, chanting of mantras and use of mudras (symbolic gestures).

Yogi Bhagan is the mahan tantric who also facilitates the white tantric yoga technique

Aetherius Society

757 Fulham Road, London SW6 5UU.

(0171) 736 4187

Founded by Dr George King who was given the command: "Prepare yourself! You are to become the Voice of Interplanetary Parliament!" According to the Society, his previous practice of Yoga enabled him to go into a trance state and make contact with a being from the planet Venus, called Aetherius. The society aims to spread the teachings of this and other interplanetary guides, including Jesus and Buddha who they believe came from Venus. This solar system is believed to be ruled by an interplanetary parliament based on Saturn. Planets are seen as classrooms where we learn various lessons through thousands of lives. A new master is to come shortly in a flying saucer to lead those who are ready into a New World. Various kinds of yoga, prayer, mantra yoga, pranayama, spiritual healing are practiced.

Baha'i Faith

27 Rutland Gate, Knightsbridge, London SW7 1PD.

(0171) 584 2566

According to the Enclyclopaedia Britannica this is the 'most widely spread independent religion in the world after Christianity'. Central to the Baha'i Faith is the belief in the oneness of mankind and of all religions. It originated in Persia through a succession of three teachers, a 'Forerunner' who prepared the way for the 'Founder', Baha'u'llah, who died in 1892. The 'Interpreter' then explained the teachings further. There are no priests or clergy, but there are local Baha'i communities practising together through prayer, meditation, service to humanity and worship through work. They have their own scriptures, holy places and parliament.

Beshara Trust
Frilford Grange, Frilford, Near Abingdon, Oxon OX13 5NX.
(01865) 391344
The Beshara Trust was set up to provide an environment where any person who wishes to establish a spiritual dimension in their life can come together with others to study and work towards this. It seeks to do this without the restrictions of dogma or religion.

College of Psychic Studies
16 Queensberry Place, London SW7 2EB.
(0171) 589 3292/3
The College of Psychic Studies - established 1884 as the London Spiritualist Alliance Ltd.- runs courses, workshops and hosts lectures on a range of subjects which include healing, psychic phenomena, psychology of past lives, channelling etc. Training in healing and psychic unfoldment given. They believe that at the human level there is no single truth, but that truth can be found in all the great spiritual traditions, and also outside of them.

Findhorn Foundation
The Park, Forres IV36 OTZ .
(01309) 690311
Residential community founded in 1962 by Eileen and Peter Caddy and Dorothy Maclean on the principles that God, or the source of all life, is accessible to each of us at all times, and that nature, including the planet, has intelligence and is part of a much larger plan. Findhorn has no formal doctrine or creed, recognising that all major world religions share the same underlying principles. They subscribe to the 'New Age' belief that an evolutionary expansion of consciousness is taking place in the world, which will infuse humanity with spiritual values. Work, sacred dance and meditation are practised, however it is daily life which is seen as the 'spiritual classroom' with an emphasis on living and working in community with others and developing a responsive relationship to the earth. A range of courses is run (see 'Residential Workshops').

Graigian Community
10 Lady Somerset Road, Kentish Town, London NW5 1UP.
(0171) 485 1646 (after 12 noon and before 6pm)
The Graigian Society grew out of the first green party, and at its core is the 'first Green monstery', a spiritual community in a house full of the creative works of its occupants. They aim to 'bring about a caring and sensitive society'. Workshops and groups are held to facilitate self development through 'natural psychology' which stresses relating to others, creativity, the arts and has elements of the philosophy of Jung and Gurdjieff.

They believe that human growth is as important as environmental measures to save the earth. Conduct local environmental campaigns and run groups on 'Being in a Group' and art therapy. Members of the community are easy to spot because of their green striped habits, friendliness and gentleness. They have a leaning towards the Celtic and medieval, and strong links with Wales where annual community holidays are held. 'Graigian' comes from 'Y-Graig' which is Welsh for 'The Rock'.

International School of the Golden Rosycross
45 Woodlands Road, Earlswood, Redhill, Surrey.
A group in the tradition of the Rosicrucian.

Open Gate
6 Goldney Road, Clifton, Bristol.
(0117) 97345952
Open Gate are not a group, but run workshops on aspects of psychology, spirituality and the arts, and longer programmes in East/West studies, process oriented psychology, Buddhist and Shamanic studies. They hold residentials and retreats, some with well known spiritual teachers.

Subud Central London
50 Shirland Road, London W9 2JA.
(0171) 286 3137
Founded by Muhammad Subud, (known to his followers as 'Bapak') an Indonesian who died in 1987. It is not a religion or teaching it itself - members are from all faiths - but aims to be a way of understanding and following the inner messages of religious teachings.This guidance is given through the 'latihan' or inner training, where an inner vibration is transmitted from person to person and causes illumination.

Theosophical Society
50 Gloucester Place, London W1H 3HJ.
(0171) 935 9261
Theosophical belief is that man is essentially a part of the all pervading spirit which energises all matter. It sees a common essence in all religion.

RESOURCES

COMMUNICATION

HOLISTIC SHOPS

The shops below are either book-shops, new age shops, whole food shops, and other similar shops that contain a large range of mind/body/spirit material. They may sell books, music tapes, astrology software, essential oils etc.

Acumedic Centre
101-105 Camden High Street, Camden, London NW1 7JN.
(0171) 388 5783/(0171) 388 6704
Shop on the main Camden High St. They sell books on acupuncture and Chinese medicine, with an assortment of alternative medicine aids such as ionisers, massage equipment, tapes and biofeedback machines.

Ainsworths Homoeopathic Pharmacy
38 New Cavendish Street, London W1M 7LH.
(0171) 935 5330/(018833) 40332
As the name suggests they sell a large collection of homoeopathic remedies.

Air Improvement Centre
23 Denbigh Street, London SW1V 2HF.
(0171) 834 2834
Sell ionisers, humidifiers and air conditioning equipment.

Atlantis Bookshop
49A Museum Street, London WC1A 1LY.
(0171) 405 2120
Mon, Tues, Wed, Fri 10-5.30, Thurs 10-8, Sat 11-5. It's the world's oldest occult bookshop, established in 1922. It covers all areas of occult, spiritualism, psychism, paganism and wicca, spirituality along with lighter subjects such as dowsing, ley lines and mythology.

Aurora
16A Neal's Yard, Covent Garden, London WC2.
(0171) 379 5972
This shop is open to the public and stocks a wide range of natural quartz crystals, dowsing pendulums, rainbow crystal

jewellery and balls, cards and posters and new age music and videos. Open Mon-Sat 10-6. Also mail order.

Back Shop
24 New Cavendish Street, London W1M 7LH.
(0171) 935 9120   14 New C.
All manner of things for the back are here including chairs, pillows, beds, shoes, exercise equipment and meditation stools which give correct support to the back, and even a 'massage pillow' — a cushion which vibrates to give you your own portable massage. Also books,

videos, mail order. 10am-6pm Mon-Sat.

Back Store Ltd
330 King Street, Hammersmith, London W6.
(0181) 741 5022
Mon-Fri 10-6, Sats 10-4. Everything for the back is here. Allow yourself some time to choose.

Bennett & Luck
54 Islington Park Street, Islington, London N1 1PX.
(0171) 226 3422
A large shop with a wide range of wholefoods and homoeopathic and herbal remedies, books, native American jewellery. There is also a lunchtime cafe with organic salads and hot food. Are very willing to give advice health issues. Friendly shop. 9-7 Mon-Fri, 9-6.30 Sat. Close to Highbury and Islington Tube

Books Etc
120 Charing Cross Road, London WC2.
(0171) 379 6838
General bookshop which has a good selection of books on Mind Body Spirit, psychology, psychotherapy, alternative medicine.

RESOURCES

Books For A Change
52 Charing Cross Road, London WC2H 0BB.
(0171) 836 2315
Jointly organised by CND, Friends of the Earth, the Unitied Nations Association and War on Want. A 'green' bookshop with books on practical and political aspects of ecology, plus recycled stationery, periodicals and some very nice postcards. Send SAE for comprehensive catalogue.

Books for Cooks
4 Blenheim Cresent, London W11 2EE.
(0171) 221 1992
Comprehensive range of cook books. Very large collection of food and wine books in print and a sizeable number of second-hand books also. Large sections on vegetarian, vegan and special diets. 9.30-6 Mon-Sat.

Bumblebees Natural Remedies
35 Brecknock Road, London N7 0AD.
(0171) 267 3884 (0171) 607 1936
A bountiful display of natural medicines, herbal and homoeopathic remedies and nutrutional supplements, aromatherapy, skin and cosmetic products. No product has been tested on animals.

Charlie's Rock Shop
Merton Abbey Mills, Wimbledon, London SW19 2RD.
(0181) 544 1207
This shop is set within a large craft market in South London and sells crystals, music tapes, video tapes, native American products, ceremonial products and figurines.

Compendium Bookshop
234 Camden High St., Camden Town, London NW1 8QS.
(0171) 267 1525 / 485 8944
Compendium, 'Britains best bookshop' (Time Out) has as an extensive range of books on self help, humanistic psychology, astrology, personal development, alternative medicine and complementary therapies, mythology, occult, women's studies, spiritual traditions and healing. Large range dealing with recovery, co-dependency and the subject of adult children of alcoholics. Large range of American imported material, a selection of self-help audio cassettes and tarot decks. Fast, efficient, mail order service, VISA and Access accepted (same day despatch on telephone orders). Special orders undertaken. Books supplied for conferences, groups etc. 'We employ specialist staff who are experts in their areas of responsibility!'. They also have a sense of humour.

Dillons Bookstore
82 Gower St, London WC1E 6EQ.
(0171) 636 1577
Very large bookshop which is easy to browse round, the books being mostly in subject order. They have a comprehensive stock of alternative medicine, psychology, psychotherapy and spirtual books.

Equinox
The Astrology Shop, 78 Neal St, London WC2.
Specialise in astrological and heavenly goods. This is also the base for Equinox, computer generated star charts. They aim to

provide goods and services connected with astrology and celebrating the glory of the heavens.

Family Planning Association
27-35 Mortimer Street, London W1N 7RJ.
(0171) 636 7866
Mon-Thur 9-5, Fri 9-4.30. Books on birth control, conception, sexuality.

Friends Book Centre
Friends House, 177 Euston Road, London NW1 2BJ.
(0171) 387 3601
Mon-Fri 9.30-5.30, except Tues opens 10.30. Open occasionally on Sats). This is a bookshop run by the Quaker Society of Friends and covers books on Quakerism and other religions, as well as pacifism, peace education, alternative business and feminist theory. Also offer a mail order service.

Gaetano Vivo
5a Devonshire Road, London W4 2EU.
(0181) 742 3305
Chiswick's premiere new age centre offering a wide variety of books and products. Also have therapies and metaphysical practices on offer such

as astrology, aurasoma, clairvoyance, graphology, healing, mediumship, palmistry, tarot and colour readings.

Genesis Books
188 Old Street, London EC1V 9BP.
(0171) 250 1868
Monday to Friday, 11.30 till 7.00, Sat 11.00 till 3.00 (sometimes till 5pm if busy). Small bookshop situated in a therapy complex, with macrobiotic cafe located in building (the East West restaurant). They specialize in alternative medicine and macrobiotics books. Massage, psychology, herbalism, religion, Buddhism etc. Also sell crystals, new age cassettes and videos and books and publications dealing with green issues. Also sell walter filters, air purifiers, incense. Mail order service for books. Situated within Community Health Foundation.

Karnac (H)
56 Gloucester Road, London SW7 4QY.
(0171) 584 3303
Mon-Sat 9am-6pm. Specialise in books on psychoanalysis, analytical psychology and psychotherapy. Also accept VISA, ACCESS, AMEX. Their noticeboard give details of meetings, seminars, conferences, in the area on subjects related to helping professions and their aim is to 'help the helpers!'

Karnac (H)
118 Finchley Road, London NW3 5HT.
(0171) 431 1075
Stock a comprehensive range of books on psychoanalysis, psychotherapy, analytical psychology (Jung). Others includes art, fiction, reference, philosophy,

poetry, drama and women's studies. Appropriately situated just round the corner from the Freud Museum (qv), and close to the Tavistock. They also publish books in the psychoanalytic and psyhcotherapy field and maintain a 'substantial list of reprints and original titles'. Mail order from the Gloucester Road Branch who can charge to credit cards against written or telephone orders. Hours of opening are Monday to Saturday 9.00 till 6.00.

Mysteries
9 Monmouth Street, Covent Garden, London WC2H 9DA.
(0171) 240 3688
Mainly a bookshop but they also sell pendulums, ritual magic candles, dakinis, pentagram rings, runes - you can make contact with the etheric just around the corner from John Le Carre's fictional home of MI5 at Cambridge Circus. It doesn't seem possible that anything else could be crammed into this lilac fronted shop - and indeed it's often so full of people it can be difficult to get inside. Though primarily a bookshop (esoteric, self help, spiritual, natural health etc), there is also music and self help tapes and videos, jewellery, tarots and crystals. Tarot and palm readings are also carried out on the premises. Mail order.

Natural Medicine Centre
87 Beckenham Lane, Shortlands, Bromley, Kent BR2 ODN.
(0181) 460 1117
This natural health centre has a bookshop on the premises covering holistic health, self healing,

complementary medicine, womens issues, personal development, family issues, ecology. They also sell herbs and herbal remedies, aromatherapy products and audio tapes. Open Mon-Sat 9.30-5.30 and some evenings.

Neal Street East
5 Neal Street, London WC2H 9UP.
(0171) 836 6252
The bookshop on the first floor of this shop selling oriental arts and crafts specialises in books on all things oriental. This includes eastern religions, meditation and oriental mythology; oriental astrology and divination; health from chinese herbs, kiatsu to macrobiotics; martial arts and yoya; oriental customs, arts and culture. They also stock calligraphic inks and brushes and can show you how to use them in their Chinese brush painting workshops. Other events hosted by the bookshop are ikebana and cookery demonstrations, and Chinese New Year Celebrations.

Neal's Yard Agency
14 Neal's Yard, Covent Garden, London WC2 9DP.
(0171) 379 0141
Their main focus is information on courses, workshops and holidays in and around London and abroad, but they also sell a select range of books and magazines in the personal development field. Are a good source of information for this field.

Neal's Yard Remedies
68 Chalk Farm Road, London NW1 9AN.
(0171) 284 2039
One of the branches of Neal's Yard set near Camden Market. They sell books, incense, aromatherapy products, herbal remedies, native American products, posters, flower remedies and herbs.

Neal's Yard Remedies
14 Covent Garden, London WC2.
(0171) 379 7222
Set in the hub of activity of Neal's Yard, this shop sell books, incense, aromatherapy products, herbal remedies, native American products, posters, flower remedies and herbs.

Paradise Farm
182A Kings Road, London SW3.
(0171) 376 5264
This shop is open to the public and stocks a wide range of natural quartz crystals, dowsing pendulums, rainbow crystal jewellery and balls, cards and posters and new age music and videos. Also mail order.

Passage Bookshop
5 Canning Cross, Grove Lane, Camberwell, London SE5 8BH.
(0171) 274 7606
General bookshop, but because it is next to the Maudsley Hospital carries titles on mostly psychiatry, but also books on psychotherapy and psychology.

Portobello Wholefoods
266 Portobello Road, London W10.
(0181) 968 9133
A wholefood shop that also sells a range of new age products: books, incense, herbal remedies, native American, magazines, herbs and original art.

Revital Health Shop
3a The Colonnades, 123 Buckingham Palace Road, Victoria, London SW1 W9RZ.
(0171) 976 6615

Silver Moon
68 Charing Cross Road, London WC2H OBB.
(0171) 836 7906
The largest women's bookshop in Europe. Centrally located and carrying a comprehensive stock of women's fiction and books about women. They stock books on

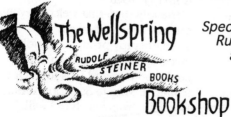

RESOURCES

health, self-help, religion and spirituality, lesbian fiction, black women's fiction, crime, poetry and education. They also sell tee-shirts, mugs, jewellery, cards and other gifts. Nearest tube is Leicester Square. They also have a fast, efficient mail order service. Mon-Sat 10.30-6.30.

Skoob
15 Sicillian Avenue, Southampton Row, Holborn, London WC1A 2QH.
(0171) 404 3063
10.30-6.30 Mon. Second hand books on psychology.

Skoob Two
17 Sicilian Avenue, Southampton Row, Holborn, London WC1A 2QH.
(0171) 405 0030
A second hand bookshop, they have a large selection of second-hand titles covering new age, alternative health, magic, divination and general esoterica as well as Buddhism, Eastern philosophy, Yoga and martial arts. Two floors. 10.30 - 6.30 Mon to Sat. 10% discount for students and UB40's.

Snapdragon
12 South Park, Sevenoaks, Kent TN13 1AN.
(01732) 740252
Snapdragon is a fantasy/new age shop; an unusual combination which has evolved out of a firm conviction that spiritual growth begins with stimulation of the imagination, especially if one can release the joyous child within us. To that end they are awash with elves, trolls, dragons, unicorns, rainbow crystals, an extensive range of earth crystals and lots of unusual and fascinating things. They offer a

mail order service (the catalogue is £1, refundable). Hours of opening are 8.30 till 5.30 Monday to Saturday.

Spiritualist Association of Great Britain
33 Belgrave Square, London SW1X 8QL.
(0171) 235 3351

Strange Attractions
204 Kensington Park Road, London W11 1NR.
(0171) 229 9646
A shop selling unusual items such as electronic lava lamps and vibrational sensors as well as the more usual items such as books, music tapes, flower essences, aromatherapy products etc. This shop is worth a visit especially to sample some of their more arcane wares.

Trading Post
Second Floor, New Building, Camden Lock, London NW1.
(0181) 888 0088
North American Indian arts/crafts centre set in the new block built in Camden market.

Treehouse
7 Park Road, Crouch End, London N8 8TE.
(0181) 341 4326
A friendly shop that welcome you to browse. They sell cards, aromatherapy products, candles, incense, oil burners, cushions, books, pottery and kids toys. Open 9.30-5.30 Mon to Sat. Closest tube is Highgate from which the walk is downhill, but you can also use Finsbury Park tube.

Verde
75 Northcote Road, London SW11 6PL.
(0171) 924 4379
This littel known shop sell only
their own brand of essential oils
which are of excellent quality.
Worth a visit.

W. & G. Foyle Ltd
*113-119 Charing Cross Road, London
WC2H OEB.*
(0171) 437 5660
Very large general bookshop.
Covers the 'mind body spirit' field.
Books are sorted by publisher so it's
often difficult to browse.

Waterstone & Co. Ltd.
*193 High Street Kensington, London W8
6SH.*
(0171) 937 8432

Waterstone & Co. Ltd.
*68-69 Hampstead High Street, London
NW3 1QP.*
(0171) 794 1098

Waterstone & Co. Ltd.
*99-101 Old Brompton Road, London
SW7 3LE.*
(0171) 581 8522

Waterstones Booksellers
*193 Kensington High Street, Kensington,
London W8 6SH.*
(0171) 937 8432
Largish bookshop with a large
'mind body spirit' section in the
basement.

Waterstones
*12 Wimbledon Bridge, Wimbledon,
London SW19.*
(0181) 543 9899

Waterstones
9-13 Garrick Street, London WC2N 7LA.
(0171) 836 6757

Waterstones
*128 Camden High Street, London NW1
0NB.*
(0171) 284 4948

Waterstones
266 Earls Court Road, London SW5 9AS.
(0171) 370 1616

Waterstones
*39-41 Notting Hill Gate, London W11
3JQ.*
(0171) 229 9444

Waterstone & Co. Ltd.
*121-125 Charing Cross Road, London
WC2.*
(0171) 434 4291
Mon-Fri 9.30-7.30, Sat 10-7. Good
general bookshop with sections on
psychology and psychotherapy, self
help, mystical, spirituality,
divination.

Watkins Books Ltd
*19-21 Cecil Court, Covent Garden,
London WC2N 4EZ.*
(0171) 836 2182
Mon-Sat 10-6 except Weds when
they open at 10.30. Watkins is
known for the breadth and depth of
its selection of books on natural
therapies, personal development,
astrology, mysticism etc. One of the
best sections in London on
spirituality and religion including
eastern and western approaches,
and the works of spiritual teachers.
Over 18,000 new titles and
extensive second hand and
antiquarian books. Offer a mail

order service. Also have a large selection of cassettes, jewelery, gemstones tarot cards, games, posters, incense etc.

Wellspring Bookshop
5 New Oxford St, London WC1A 1BA
(0171) 405 6101
Specialists in the work of Rudolf Steiner and other anthroposophical writers. Books on Christianity and esoteric subjects.

Wholefood Books
24 Paddington Street, London W1M 4DR.
(0171) 935 3924
Mon 8.30-6, Tues-Thurs 8.30-6.60, Sat 8.30-1.30. Specialises in nutrition and health, alternative therapies, natural childbirth and childreearing, organic gardening and farming, wholefood cookery. There also a wholefood shop.

Wilde Ones
Kensington Market Basement, 49-53 Kensington High St, London W8.
(0171) 376 2870

Wilde Ones
283 King's Road, London SW3.
(0171) 352 9531

Wisdom Publications
402 Hoe Street, London E17 9AA.
(0181) 520 5588
All books are Buddhist orientated, including travel, art, language, all types of Buddhism. Other products sold include meditation cushions and mats, videos, cassettes, incense, posters, postcards and notepads. They produce a free mail order catalogue which is regularly updated. Their noticeboard is strictly for Buddhist events, such as courses or fundraising. Flyers are also included in their mailouts. They are probably the largest stockist of Buddhist books in the UK and Europe. They import titles from all over the world. 'Our purpose is to promote and provide a comprehensive service of Buddhist books in the West. We are also committed to preserving Tibetan Buddhism whilst the Chinese occupation of Tibet continues.'

Wonders
31 The Market, Covent Garden, London WC2E 8RE.
(0171) 497 2992
Sell books, cards tarot, calendars, aromatherapy products, ceremonial products, clothes, crystals, figurines, food supplements, health aids, herbal remedies, incense, jewellery, magazines, native American products, original art, posters, music and spoken tapes and video tapes.

Wood Matters
12a Brecknock Road, London N7 0DD.
(0171) 700 2638
An ecological shop with some holistic stock. Specialise in recycled and chlorine free paper products, recycled products and organic 'healthy' paints. They aim to provide environmentally friendly gifts and stationary, organic household paints and varnishes, literature for a sustainable lifestyle and reclaimed wood.

World Tree
17 Station Parade, Kew, Surrey, London TW9 3PS.
(0181) 332 0162
Sell all crystals, gemrocks, fossils, runic works (with commissions take

for customized work), special horoscopes of all the planets birth stones interpretations, showing how the different stones will affect individuals in differing ways. Mail order services for runes and horoscopes. Send SAE for details. 'Our vision is to instill a magical interface between mind and nature in people's thinking and in the world of men'. They display healers cards, animal rights and rainforest campaign material on their noticeboard. Open every day from 12.00 till 6.00.

Zeitgeist
171 The Pavement, London SW4 0HY.
(0171) 622 5000
No books here, but an unusual collection of up-market gifts and new age products including calendars, an extensive collection of jewellery, crystals and original art.

PUBLISHERS AND DISTRIBUTORS

Arkana
27 Wrights Lane, London W8 5TZ.
(0171) 938 2200
Publish New Age books for Mind, Body and Spirit, psychology, transformation, health, science and mysticism, women's spirituality and astrology.

Arrow Books
Random Century House, 20 Vauxhall Bridge Rd, London SW1V 2SA.
(0171) 973 9700 ex 217
A publisher of general titles, with some New Age, health and self help titles.

Ashgrove Distribution
4 Brassmill Centre, Brassmill Lane, Bath BA1 3JN.
(01225) 425539
Promote and distribute books of various publishers. Subjects include new age, health and healing, earth mysteries, esoteric, religion and myth, psychology, philosophy and folklore.

Bantam Books
Transworld Publishers
61-63 Uxbridge Rd W5 5SA.
(0181) 579 2652/3 x442
General publishers with small range of self-help, popular psychology titles.

C W Daniel Ltd
1 Church Path, Saffron Walden, Essex CB10 1JP.
(01799) 521909
Publishers of books on natural healing, and the metaphysical and spiritual.

Dorling Kindersley
9 Henrietta Street, Covent Garden, London WC2E 8PS.
(0171) 836 5411
Range of books strong on visuals covering health (including a series from the British Holistic Medical Association on common problems), yoga and massage, childcare, vegetarian cooking.

Element Books
The Old School House, The Courtyard, Bell St, Shaftesbury, Dorset SP7 8PL.
(01747) 851448
One of the largest publishers and distributers of books on eastern and western religious traditions, spiritual teachers, psychology, modern spirituality, healing etc.

Faber & Faber
3 Queens Square, London WC1N 3AU.
(0171) 465 0045
Titles on religion, philosophy, health, medicine, nursing, midwifery and psychology.

Fontana Paperbacks
Ophelia House, Fulham Palace Road, London W6 1AA.
(0181) 741 7070
Some publication of health and green issues.

Foulsham
Yeovil Road, Slough, Berks SL1 4JH.
(01753) 526769
Publish varous self help and health titles, and have just started a new

imprint, Quantum, for 'the exploration of inner space and its practical application'.

Fowler & Co Ltd
1201 High Road, Chadwell Heath, Romford, Essex RM6 4DH.
(0181) 597 2491
Shop open Mon-Fri 9-5. Astrology specialists and mind, body, spirit titles. Also carry cassette tapes. Small shop and mail order.

Free Association Books
26 Freegrove Road, London N7 9RQ.
(0171) 609 5646/0507
Interesting range of books on psychoanalysis, psychotherapy, women & gender, social sciences

---

RIDER

BOOKS WITH SOUL

Recent bestsellers:

THE TIBETAN BOOK OF LIVING AND DYING
Sogyal Rinpoche

AGELESS BODY, TIMELESS MIND
Deepak Chopra

WOMEN WHO RUN WITH THE WOLVES
Clarissa Pinola Estes

New Titles:

ROAD TO HEAVEN: Encounters with Chinese Hermits
Bill Porter

TAMING THE TIGER: Tibetan Teachings for Improving Daily Life
Akong Tulka Rinpoche

For more informaton and catalogues contact:
Rider
Random House
Vauxhall Bridge Road
London SW1V 2SA
(0171) 973 9670

and group relations. Their journal, Free Associations, includes scholarly articles on women, race, power, group dynamics in institutions.

GAIA Books Ltd
20 High St, Stroud, Gloucestershire GL5 1AS.
(01453) 752985
Titles on natural health and living, self development and ecology, including The Gaia Atlas of Planet Management. Independently owned company.

Grafton Books
c/o HarperCollins Publishers, Ophelia House, Fulham Palace Road W16 1AA.
(0181) 741 7070
Some publications on green issues.

Piatkus Books
5 Windmill Street, London W1P 1HF.
(0171) 631 0710
Piatkus publish books in business, self-help, health, mind body spirit, popular psychology and fiction categories. Books can be sent by post on receipt of cheque. They 'aim to create the best books they can and treat each new book as something special'.

Rider Books
Random House, 20 Vauxhall Bridge Road, London SW1V 2SA.
(0171) 973 9670
Publish books on ancient mysteries, divination, health and healing, martial arts, mysticism and religion, occult and personal growth.

Shanti Sadan
29 Chepstow Villas, Notting Hill Gate, London W11 3DR.
(0171) 727 7846
Publications, books on yoga, Vedanta, poetry and the mysticism

of the far east. Translations of Sanscrit classics. Publish 'Self Knowledge', a yoga quarterly journal devoted to spiritual thought and practice. Single copy including postage £1.50

Thorsons Publishing Group
77-85 Fulham Palace Road, Hammersmith, London W6 8JB.
(0181) 741 7070 x4735
Large selection of titles in the Thorsons, Aquarian and Crucible range; health, self-help, spirituality, psychology, healing, psychic, women's interest, Eastern philosophies. Continue to expand in the field of new age and alternative health publishing.

University Associates International
45-47 Victoria Street, Mansfield, Notts NG18 5SU.
Distribution centre of books on management training, organisation development, effective leadership etc.

Wellspring Publications Ltd
46 Cyril Mansions, Prince of Wales Drive, London SW11 4HW.
(0171) 720 3541
Publishers of books in mind/body/ spirit, self-development, psychology of vision and health (inner and outer) fields. Aim to publish books which are visionary, lead the planet forward and provide prosperity and wellbeing. Also supply tapes. Accept orders for books and tapes through the post. Wellspring state that 'our customers are mostly those who want their todays and tomorrows

to be different from their yesterdays'.

White Eagle Publishing Trust
9 St. Mary Abbots Place, Kensington, London W8 6LS.
(01730) 893300
Publishing wing of White Eagle Lodge (qv). Publish the work of White Eagle, a spirit guide. Publish other books on related subjects: astrology, reincarnation spiritual unfoldment, meditation, life after death. Send SAE for catalogue. Small bookshop on the premises (phone for opening hours).

Wisebuy Publications
25 Rest Cottages, London NW6 1RJ.
(0171) 433 1121
Publish three titles on food allery, healthy eating and massage and relaxation.

FILMS

British Association for Counselling
1 Regent Place, Rugby CV21 2PJ.
(01788) 578328
Catalogue can be purchased for £1 (including p&p) describing videos and films for hire.

Concord Video and Film Council
201 Felixstowe Road, Ipswich, Suffolk IP3 9BJ.
(01473) 726012
Wide range of videos and films available for hire or purchase covering psychotherapy and counselling, alternative medicine, relationships, peace, social/global issues, the arts, environment, race relations etc. Psychotherapy videos include famous therapists in action, coverage of issues such as death and bereavement, child abuse, eating disorders, drug addiction, group psychotherapy, counselling techniques etc. A real treat is the fly-on-the-wall's view of a Californian encounter group - get all the action without taking any of the risks! Hire charges range from £1 to £20, and sale from £20 to £200. Send £3 for video catalogue (includes updates).

MAGAZINES

Achilles Heel
48 Grove Avenue, Muswell Hill, London N10 2AN.
(0181) 883 3349

Caduceus
38 Russell Terrace, Royal Leamington Spa, Warks CV31 1HE.
(01926) 451897
Articles on holistic healing, natural health, spirituality and the connection between body, mind and spirit aimed at healers, health care professionals and members of the general public with an interest in exploring holistic health. Quarterly, £2.50 per issue, 38pp.

Group Relations
152 Park St Lane, Park St, St Albans AL2 2AU.
(01727) 872010
A journal for people working in groups and teams. Published three times a year. £1.85 per issue. Sub £6.

Here's Health

Victory House, 14 Leicester Place, London WC2H 7BP.

(0171) 437 9011

Monthly national magazine specialising in holistic health: treatments and issues. Aimed at the general public who want to know more about alternative medicine, how to get healthy and keep healthy. Covers food, therapies, exercise, emotional issues, dealing with specific illnesses and leisure.

Health and Homoeopathy

Hahnemann House, 2 Powis Place, Great Ormond St, London WC1N 3HT.

(0171) 837 3297

Articles about homoeopathy, research, history, institutions and uses and treatment of particular conditions. Published by the Hahnemann Society. Quarterly, subscription £8 per annum. Apply for specimen copy. £1.20 cover price.

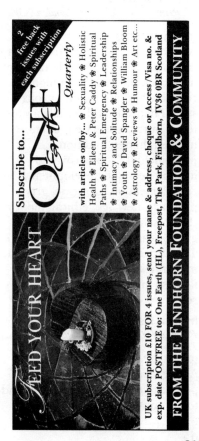

RESOURCES

Human Potential
5 Barb Mews, Brook Green, London W6 7PA.
(0171) 371 2432
The who, what, where, when and why not of the 'growth' movement. Articles cover humanistic psychology, Jungian psychotherapy, sexuality, spirituality, controversy etc. with interviews and news, book reviews, and an extensive calendar of events with all the workshops and groups you could ever want to go to in the following three months. Subs, quarterly, £8 per year. £2 per copy.

I to I Magazine
92 Prince of Wales Road, London NW5 3NE.
(0171) 267 7085
An independent alternative/new age magazine covering a wide range of important life issues in a highly readable and often humourous style. Politically and socially aware, I to I's journalistic style is open-minded, honest and non-judgemental. Topics covered include personal development, complementary medicine, green products, new age, ethical, money (LETS schemes), human rights, galleries and exhibitions and more. This is one of the few independent magazines that has managed to flourish and grow through the recession.

Insight Network
PO Box 490, Hove, East Sussex BN3 3BU.
(01273) 726970
A magazine which aims to help people to empower themselves and to encourage them to take responsibility for their own lives, health and the environment.

Journal of Alternative and Complementary Medicine
Mariner House, 53a High Street, Bagshot, Surrey GU19 4AH.
(01276) 451522
Independent magazine devoted to alternative and complementary medicine. Published monthly by Green Library - £1.95. each issue. £25 sub.

Journal Of Complementary Medicine
P.O. Box 194, London SE16 1QZ.
(0171) 237 5165
An academic publication which focuses on research and hopes to promote complementary medicine to other fields of science. £3.95 per issue. Twice a year.

Kindred Spirit
Foxhole, Dartington, Totnes, Devon TQ9 6ED.
(01803) 866686
New Age magazine covering earth energies, meditation, healing, death, spiritual experiences, crystals, scientific breakthroughs, psychology, esoterica, complementary medicine, alterantive therapies, environvmental issues. Interviews with innovative thinkers, environmentalists, spiritual teachers and therapists, plus news, book reviews, a resource directory and mail order catalogue. £2.40 per issue, £9.50 per annum subscription or £21 for three years.

RESOURCES

Planetary Connection
PO Box 44, Evesham, Worcester WR12 7YW.
(01386) 858694
Magazine with global perspective with articles on personal growth, spirituality etc. Qtly £1.85.

London and South East Connection
Laurel Cottage, Watery Lane, Donhead St Mary, Shaftsbury, Dorset SP7 9DF.
(01747) 828913
An A5 size magazine given out free in at various London venues. Aim to publicise and network a broad spectrum of activities that encourage personal development and natural and holistic therapies. Seek to provide a current guide with editorial to reflect and stimulate personal growth, alternative therapy and holistic medicine. To this end they publish advertisements, articles and profiles concerning the above.

New Humanity
51A York Mansions, Prince of Wales Drive, London SW11 4BP.
(0171) 622 4013
A politico-spiritual magazine which envisages integrating the disciplines of science, philosophy, politics, the arts, religion and the humanities to promote closer co-operation and understanding among them. 'Endeavours to clarify a direction in which humanity might evolve towards harmony and integration through diversity of knowledge.' Available bi-monthly.

Nuit Isis
Mandrake Publications, BOX 250, Oxford OX1 LAP.
(01865) 243671
A bi-annual magazine established since 1986, dealing with the occult and left hand path. It can be bought for £2.50 a copy at occult and new age bookstores, or by subscription at £5.00 per annum. The publishers welcome new writing on the occult and ask for advance information before sending books to avoid disappointment.

One Earth Magazine
The Park, Findhorn, Forres IV36 0TZ.
(01309) 691641
A magazine for those who are those interested in spiritual growth and social harmony. Print reviews of books, tapes, videos and products. Connected with the Findhorn Foundation.

Open Mind
Granta House, 15-19 Broadway, Stratford, London E15 4BQ.
(0181) 519 2122x220
Is published bi-monthly by MIND, the National Association for Mental Health. Now in it's eigth year of publication the magazine has covered topics such as psychotherapy for troubled young people, complementary medicine, the politics of poverty, who should pick up the therapy bill... It has encouraged debate among health care professionals, patients and their relatives. OPEN MIND provides a regular 'benefits' column, an update on research in mental health publications, international developments and full listings of coming events. Yearly

rates for six issues: £8 individuals, £10 organisations and institutions.

Prediction
Link House, Dingwall Avenue, Croydon, Surrey CR9 2TA.
(0181) 686 2599

Psychic News
2 Tavistock Chambers, Bloomsbury Way, London WC1A 2SE.
(0171) 405 3340
Established 1932. The world's only independent weekly Spiritualist paper containing news, reviews, events and comment. Price 24p. Obtainable from newsagents or direct subscription.

Rainbow Ark
PO Box 486, London SW1P 1AZ.
(0171) 738 4296
None profit making magazine with articles covering interesting and controversial ideas and possibilities: spiritual, ecological and humanitarian, green issues, health, new age, philosophy, esoterics, news, current affairs, reviews, 'odd thoughts spot'. Extensive diary listing holistic and green events. For free trial copy send 27p stamp to address above. Published quarterly. 50p per issue, £3 annual subs (incl p/p.).

Resurgence
Ford House, Hartland, Bideford, Devon EX39 6EE.
(01237) 441293
Perhaps the most 'literary' of the magazines devoted to holistic topics, Resurgence can boast of contributors such as Kathleen Raine and James Hillman and edited by Satish Kumar. A high standard of photography has recently been featured even more by the addition

of colour pages. Subjects covered are ecology and its spiritual roots, cultural values, holistic education, world issues, religion, the countryside etc. Substantial book reviews section and a poetry section. Bi-monthly established 1966. Cover price £2.40. Available from bookshops, health and new age shops.

Talking Stick
PO Box 3719, London SW17 8XT.
(0181) 767 3473
Run a quarterly magazine which is a forum for researches into mythology and practical magic. They also run fortnightly talks.

The Therapist
c/o European Therapy Studies Institute, 7 Chapel Road, Worthing, West Sussex BN11 1EG.
(01903) 233541
A magazine for therapists by therapists. For anyone using knowledge of human behaviour in their work.

Thomas Troward Society
Lahaina, 24 Beresford Road, North Chingford, London E4 6EE.
(0181) 529 8097
Publish 'New Light' is the in-house journal of the Thomas Troward Society. £6/issue.

Vegan Society
7 Battle Road, St Leonards on Sea, East Sussex TN37 7AA.
(01424) 427393
The Vegan magazine is the Journal of the Vegan Society. 36 pages, quarterly. News, articles, health and nutrition, recipes, young vegans pages, book and product reviews. Also publish books on aspects of veganism, including The

Cruelty Free Shopper which contains comprehensive listings of products made and tested without cruelty to animals.

Yoga and Health
21 Cadburn Crescent, Lewes, East Sussex BN7 1NR.
(01425) 616483
A monthly magazine which has been running for nearly 25 years. It covers the whole range of yoga activities in this country and abroad. It also covers a wide range of health topics and vegetarian fare. The magazine is available at most newsagents or by subscription.

LIBRARIES

Church Street Library
Church Street, Kensington, London NW8.
(0171) 798 1480
Section on religion.

Fulham Library
598 Fulham Road, London SW6 5NX.
(0181) 748 3020
Christian religious collection.

Health Information
Marylebone Library, Marylebone Road, London NW1 5PS.
(0171) 798 1039
Public lending library with special section on health and medicine, with particular emphasis on alternative therapies. They are happy to answer telephone, written or personal enquiries.

Newham Bibliographical Services Department
62A Pond Road, Stratford, London E15.
(0171) 511 1332
Section on Eastern Religion.

NETWORKS

Networks can range from highly structured organisations with strict membership criteria, to loose, informal contact groups. Some are simply information services, while others aim to help members exchange skills and resources.

RESOURCES

Association for Therapeutic Healers
Neal's Yard therapy Rooms, 2 Neal's Yard, London WC2.
(0171) 240 0176
ATH is an association for professional healers who combine healing with other therapies. Membership costs £15.00 a year, with £10.00 initial joining fee, and is open to professional healers/ therapists. Associate Membership costs £10.00 a year, and is open to students. Friend of ATH, costs £10.00 a year and is open to anyone interested in activites and philosophy of ATH. All the above receive newsletters and may attend seminars and workshops.

Breakthrough Centre
7 Poplar Mews, Uxbridge Road, Shepherds Bush, London W12 7JS.
(0181) 749 8525
An alternative business centre, providing support, training and networking for everyone seeking to combine work with personal growth and ethics. Introductory evenings twice monthly. Self-employed and career changes equally welcome.

Business Network 2000
The Breakthrough Centre, 7 Poplar Mews, Uxbridge Road, London W12 7JS.
(0181) 749 8525
The sucess of the business network (founded in 1982), BN 2000 maintains a directory of members working to introduce holistic principles to the world of work. A quarterly newsletter further encourages information between members. A grass roots national organisation. Annual subscription £35 by standing order.

Daisy Chain
25 Priory Court, Chipstead Road, Banstead, Surrey, SM7 2HJ
(01737) 370396
For people interested in holistic health and self development. Regualr talks and workshops held covering a wide range of subjects under mind, body, spirit umbrella. Also courses, day trips and weekends away.

Neal's Yard Agency
14 Neal's Yard, Covent Garden, London WC2 9DP.
(0171) 379 0141
An agency which can book you in to any of its vast range of workshops, courses, training or personal development and holidays on it's books. There is no fee to the public. Drop in and browse through the brochures on display. You can also book over the phone, credit cards accepted. Staff give informed and impartial advice.

Scientific and Medical Network
Lesser Halings, Tilehouse Lane, Denham, Nr Uxbridge, Middx UB9 5DG.
(01895) 835818
Informal international group whose 600 strong membership consists mainly of qualified scientists and doctors, with some psychologists, engineers and philosophers. It aims to extend contemporary scientific and medical thinking beyond its current materialistic way of looking at the world, and include 'non - physical possibilities' . Its main concerns include the nature of consciousness; brain/mind interface, parapsychology, causality; healing, psychoneuro-immunology; science, ecology and spirituality; values in

education and training. Publish a newsletter three times yearly. Associate membership open to those sympathetic with aims (£7.50 pa). Full membership by invitation only to scientists. Members receive members lists, and can participate in local groups, working groups and special seminars and lectures. Mail order tapes of lectures.

Whole Health Institute
Mickleton House, Mickleton, Chipping Campden, Glos GL55 6RY.
(01386) 438727
Aims to provide a focus and meeting ground for professionals and lay people interested in the

cause of health, and promote a new spirit in the healing arts, from both a traditional and non-traditional standpoint. Headquarters are in the USA.

EDUCATION

British School of Osteopathy
1-4 Suffolk Street, London SW1Y 4HG.
(0171) 930 9254
BSc in Osteopathy, 4 years full time. See 'Osteopathy' section for further details.

Centre for Continuing Education

City University
Northampton Square, London EC1.
(0171) 253 4399
They run evening classes in psychology, psychotherapy and counselling.

Holistic Early Learning School
2 Amherst Road, Ealing, London W13 8ND.
(0181) 998 2723
A school for three month to five year olds. Part-time and full-time. With health food diet, homoeopathic first-aid facility for minor ailments. A wide range of educational activities. Offers an individual approach to the care and education of young children. Have a school, nursery and prep for the young. They aim to address all aspects of development within each child so that they progress physically, socially, emotionally as well as intellectually.

School of Homoeopathy
8 Kiln Road, Llanfoist, Abergavenny, Gwent NP7 9NS.
(01873) 856872

Pan Academy
PO Box 929, Wimbledon, London SW19 2AX.
A course for social and global pioneers. The PanLife training is designed to help you develop yourself and your project to the maximum potential.

RECOGNISED ACADEMIC COURSES

Birkbeck College- Centre for Extra-Mural Studies
26 Russell Square, London WC1B 5DQ.
(0171) 631 6669
Day and evening adult education classes on psychology, psychotherapy, religion, myth etc. Typically courses on counselling, Transactional Analysis, Gestalt, Family Therapy, Co-Counselling, Psychosynthesis and Personal Construct Therapy. Ring or write for prospectus which is published yearly in June. For a ten week course of 20 hours the cost is £28.

One third of the fee for OAP's and unemployed.

Centre for Complementary Health Studies
Exeter University, Streatham Court, Rennes Drive, Exeter EX4 4PU.
(01392) 433828
(1) DPhil and (2) MPhil in Complementary Health Studies. (1) 2 years part-time. (2) 1 year full-time or two years part-time, although applicants are advised to allow at least 50% longer than these minimum requirement. (1) Applicants should be those working in complementary and orthodox medicine or other caring professions with day-to-day responsibility for patients. (2) Substantial academic study in the arts, sciences or social sciences. (1) £1,500 per annum, (2) £1,900, overseas students £5,000.
The centre also runs a research programme, and offers certain information services.

Hawkwood College
Short Residential Courses

Hawkwood College has been a centre for adult education since 1948. It is renowned for the beauty and peace of its setting in a Cotswold valley looking across to the Severn estuary. It offers courses in music, science, arts and crafts, but also seeks to foster ways and means to a spiritual foundation of life to counterbalance the materialistic values which dominate most fields of human activity today, with particular reference to the work of Rudolf Steiner.

Apart from weekend and week courses, there is a four year full-time Artistic Therapy Course. The Live Water Trust is also based at Hawkwood, which is researching into pollution treatment and the vitalisation of water. Bio-dynamic agriculture is practised, and visitors can be certain that they are enjoying fresh, nourishing food.

FOR MORE INFORMATION PHONE
Stephanie or Tony on (01453) 764607
Hawkwood College, Painswick Old Road, Stroud, Gloucestershire, GL6 7QW

Polytechnic of East London
School for Independent Study, Polytechnic of East London, Holbrook Centre, London E15 3EA.
(0181) 590 7722
Title: (1) BA/BSc by Independent Study, (2) MA/MSc by Independent Study. (1) 3 years full-time, 5 years part-time. (2) Minimum: full-time 1 year, part-time 2 years. (1) 2 A levels required, or comparable qualifications. (2) Honours degree, or equivalent. Apply to course adminstrator for details of fees.

Roehampton Institute of Higher Education
Senate House, Roehampton Lane, London SW15 5PS.
(0181) 878 8117
(1) Diploma in Psychological Counselling (2) MSc in Psychological Counselling. Duration: (1) 1 year part-time (2) 2 year part-time. Entry: (1) Appropriate academic qualifications or experience in helping professions and counselling. (2) Candidates must be 25 years old and have a degree with a pass at 2.2 level or above. Special entry may be given to those with appropriate professional qualification. Fees: Refer to organisers.Comments: also run Diploma in Counselling and Supervision Course and Certificate in Counselling in Formal and Informal Settings (mainly for those in youth or social work). Also offer Certificate in Counselling in Formal and Informal Settings (one year part-time), open to youth and community workers; Introduction to Music Therapy (ten week part-time); Diploma in Dance Movement Therapy (two years part-time).

School of Psychotherapy and Counselling
Regents College, Inner Circle, Regents Park, London NW1 4NS.
(0171) 487 7406
MA in the Psychology of Therapy and Counselling Duration: 27 months with the possibility of 12 months extension in special cases Entry Requirements: Combination of a Bachelor's degree or appropriate equivalent, some professional experience and experience of groups, self-exploration, own therapy or counselling. Candidates will be considered individually in terms of experience and may be accepted without all the formal entry requirements. Fees: £200 deposit plus six payments of £850 for the whole course. Comments: Course consists of academic seminars on Humanistic and Integrative Psychotherapy and Existential, Psychoantic and Transpersonal approahces plus a range of second year options. Training seminars. Supervised six month part-time placement and writing a thesis. Degree awarded by Antioch University and additional British validation sought.
Post Qualifying Diploma in Existential Psychotherapy once the Masters Degree (above) is obtained. Two years duration.

SERVICES

ETHICALLY SOUND INVESTMENTS

A number of ethical investment funds have sprung up over the last few years, just as 'green' products have become much more common. However, what is becoming evident is that one person's 'green' is another person's 'grey' area.

Different ethical investment funds have different criteria - some for instance are very clear on not investing in the tobacco industry, others have no investment at all in nuclear weapons or energy. It's best to check out what criteria are used, and make sure they are in agreement with your own. In unit trusts your money is spread across a number of companies to minimise risk. Because it is the nature of modern business to be mostly about large multi-nationals which have many subsidiary companies doing different things, it's very difficult to invest in the mainstream without including some investment in questionable areas, especially if your criteria are very tight. It can also be difficult to find out all the interests of a large company with many subsidiary companies.

If you decide to invest with a unit trust scheme, in addition to the sensible financial questions such as what degree of risk is involved, what charges are made and what the premium is, you can ask about what ethical criteria are used, how rigorously they are applied and whether the fund has an independent vetting committee and if so how it works. If the fund claims to be 'green', do they look only at the finished product, or do they take into account the processes of production, and even the company's general record on the environment?

Another way of researching your ethical investment is to apply to **EIRIS**, the Ethical Investment Research Service. They research companies' interests in several areas of concern, and cover all companies in the Financial Times All-Share index. Their address is *EIRIS, 401 Bondway Business Centre, 71 Bondway, London SW8 1SQ. (0171) 735 1351.* Send SAE with enquiries.

If you don't want to take your chances with the multi-nationals, then you can invest in small schemes which loan money for small projects. This has the advantage of being very ethical, though the premium may not be as good.

Among the unit trust schemes they offer is the TSB Environmental Investor Fund. The investments are vetted by an independent committee set up under the auspices of the Conservation Foundation.

Allchurch's Investment Management Service
19-21 Billiter Street, London EC3N 2RY.
(0171) 528 7364
Set up originally as the Ecclesiastical Insurance group to serve the church and clergy. Now run Amity fund for ethical investment.

Ecology Building Society
18 Station Road, Cross Hills, Keighley, West Yorkshire BD20 8TB.
(01535) 35933
Lends money for property or projects which are likley 'to lead to the saving of non-renewable resources, the promotion of self-sufficiency in individuals or communities, or the most ecologically efficient use of land'. Examples are: small-scale workshops, back-to-back houses, homes for people running ecological businesses, organic farms, houses with special energy saving or energy efficient features, properties which will help to promote the life of small communities etc.

Ethical Investment Fund
10 Queen Street, Mayfair, London W1X 7PF.
(0171) 491 0558
Unit Investment underwritten by Royal Heritage Life Assurance.

Ethical Investment Research Service
504 Bondway Business Centre, 71 Bondway, London SW8 1SQ.
(0171) 735 1351
Research into ethical behaviour of company groups on FTA All share index, to enable investors to make ethical decisions about potential investments. Independent research, not related to financial advice, specially for investors. Also publish a quarterly newsletter and a number of subject briefings for investors.

Friends Provident Unit Trust
Pixham End, Dorking, Surrey RH4 1QA.
(01306) 740123
Run the stewardship trust: includes unit trust, income trust, the North American stewardship trust and personal equity plan.

ICOF (Industrial Common Ownership Finance)
12-14 Gold Street, Northampton NN1 1RS.
Lend money to co-operatives.

Mercury Provident
3 Orlingbury House, Lewes Road, Forest Row, Sussex RH18 5AA.
(0134282) 3739
An ethical bank that makes loans to projects that are of benefit to the community. Allows investors to target their deposits to projects or activities of their choice. Avoids industries which damage the environment and are exploitative. Areas they like to invest in include organic agriculture, wind energy, recycling, natural health and community based education.

Merlin Jupiter Ecology Fund
Knightsbridge House, 197 Knightsbridge, London SW7 1RB.
(0171) 581 8015
Investment in companies with environmental concerns such as alternative energy, recycling, energy efficiency, pollution control, green consumer products, pollution detection cquipment. Avoids those who profit from defence, tobacco or nuclear industries. Support financial initiatives which promote community based investments. The type of investments are unit trust, investment trust and private client portfolio services.

Tilt Ltd
BIrdwood House, 44 High St, Totnes Devon.
A community company channelling local money to invest in local projects. Money is used to create ecologically and sociallly sustainable projects. Will not invest in anything that does not contribute to the environmental and social welfare of their region. Take investment from and loan money to people whose commitment is solely within the Dart Valley catchment area.

DATING AGENCIES

Friendship Register
29 Goldstone Way, Hove, Sussex BN3 7PA.

Friendships
51 Besbury Park, Minchinhampton, Stroud, Gloucestershire GL6 9EN.
(01453) 731196
Friendships is a nationwide friendship agency, established in 1978, for individuals who are interested in green issues, nature, conservation, rambling, holistic medicine, astrology, organic gardening, youth hostelling, yoga, New age understanding, amongst others. Pride themselves on their low-cost service, ranging from £26.00 to £40.00 per annum. Produce a monthly update magazine circulated to all members, with news on regional get togethers, UK holidays and abroad, and the 'market place' section where members themselves can advertise. Meetings are held every month in London, Kent, Bristol and Cheltenham.

Natural Friends
15 Benyon Gardens, Culford, Bury St Edmunds, Suffolk IP28 6EA.
(01284) 728315
Open to Everyone over 18, with a bias towards non-smokers, green-thinkers, new age non-materialists. About 2000 active members nationwide. Occasional 'get-togethers' organised by members and publicised without charge by Natural Friends. Annual membership fees range from £25.00 - £42.00. Offer personal, confidential service, with a high proportion of their members being recommended by friends. Natural Friends is a member of the Association of British Introduction Agencies (ABIA) which has a strict code of conduct and operates an independent arbitration scheme for any disputes, includes over 30 agencies.

Veggyfriends & Vegetarian Matchmakers
Century House, 100 Nelson Road, London N8 9RJ.
(0181) 348 5229
Covering all UK and some of Europe, Veggyfriends seeks to bring together vegetarians, vegans and aspiring vegetarians for romance, friendship and socialising with like minded people. They run approximately 2/3 social evenings per week nationwide, mainly in high population centres, and some weekends away. Fees range from £58.00 to £95.00 per year.

ROOMS FOR HIRE

Amadeus Centre
50 Shirland Road, Little Venice, London W9 2JA.
(0171) 286 1686

Association for Analystic and Bodymind Therapy and Training
8 Princes Avenue, Muswell Hill, London N10 3LR.
(0181) 883 5418
Sound-proofed, pleasant therapy rooms with garden.

Bodywise
119 Roman Road, Bethnal Green, London E2 0QN.
(0181) 981 6938
Small and large room for hire by groups or individuals. Large room £15/hr, £80/day, £140/weekend. Small group room £7.50/hr, £45/day, £80/weekend.

Community Health Foundation
188-194 Old Street, London EC1V 9BP.
(0171) 251 4076
Wide range of rooms to rent for workshops, courses and meetings. £25 for 18ft x 18ft room and £50 for 44ft x30 half day or evening. Good central location with restaurant downstairs and close to Old St tube station.

Gaunts House
Wimborne, Dorset BH21 4JQ.
(01202) 841522
Large conference, seminar, training and retreat centre available for hire (can accommodate up to 200 people) by community wishing to promote 'individual growth and fulfilment from a non-sectarian basis'. Facilities include gym and heated pool. Vegetarian food, with special diets available. Staff at Gaunts House are involved in learning how to live and work together with respect and to communicate with the inner essense in each other and all things. Interests lie in the realms of creative, cultural, ecological, environmental, philosophical, psychological and rural, particularly with a spiritual basis, reaching towards freedom. Refer to organisers for breakdown of costs.

Gestalt Centre London
60 Bunhill Row, London EC1Y 8QD.
(01727) 864806
Three group rooms and two consulting rooms for hire for small conferences (up to 40 people), team meetings, workshops and individual consultations. Recently refurbished suites are private, comfortable and informal. The rooms are light and airy being on the fifth floor. Layout can be varied to suit specific requirements from formal boardroom to informal circle of chairs or cushions. Cushions and chairs provided. Full range of business facilities (video camera, recorder, monitor, photocopier and fax). Lunch or supper can be provided.

Institute For Arts In Therapy & Education
70 Cranwich Rd, London N16 5JD.
(0171) 704 2534
Three very luxurious spacious group rooms for hire, 30ft x 30ft. 10 mins from Angel tube. Kitchen facilities.

Living Centre
32 Durham Road, Raynes Park, London SW20 OTW.
(0181) 946 2331
Large group room (up to about 40 sitting) available weekends and evenings. (£10 per hour). Carpeted. Kitchen.

Lower Shaw Farm
Old Shaw Lane, Shaw, Nr Swindon, Wilts SN5.
(01793) 771080

Monkton Wyld Court
Nr. Charmouth, Bridport, Dorset DT6 6DQ.
(01297) 60342
Provide venue groups of up to 34 people.

Neal's Yard Agency
14 Neal's Yard, Covent Garden, London WC2 9DP.
(0171) 379 0141
Two large rooms for hire at a central location. The rooms measure 22 x 27 feet and 14 feet square.

Portobello Green Fitness Centre
3-5 Thorpe Close, North Kensington, London W10 5XL.
(0181) 960 2221

RIGPA Fellowship
330 Caledonian Road, London N1 1BB.
(0171) 700 0185
Centre available for occasional hire.

Sound Health
261 Grove Street, London SE8 3PZ.
(0181) 691 7519
Consulting rooms and space for workshops. Victorian house with garden in Wandsworth.

Gerda Boysen Clinic
120 The Vale, London W3 7RQ.
(0181) 746 0499
Rooms for practitioners and space for workshops.

Violet Hill Studios
5-7 Violet Hill, St John's Wood, London NW8 9EB.
(0171) 624 0101 or (081) 458 5368
Spacious Consulting and Workshop Rooms beautifully converted from an 18th Century Barn.

West Usk Lighthouse
Lighthouse Road, St. Brides, Wendlooge, Nr. Newport, Gwent NP1 9SF.
(01633) 810126/815860

PRACTITIONERS SERVICES

Bates, Carrie
c/o Spectrum, 7 Endymion Road, London N4 1EE.
(0171) 263 5545
Established 1991. Aim to help holistic practitioners, small businesses and the self employed empower themselves and use radio to promote the benefits of their work. Runs workshops and one-to-one consultancy on helping prepare for, and make the most of radio interviews. Also offers individual advice on how to get on the radio. One day workshops costs £50, and one-to-one consultancy (which lasts one and quarter hours) for £40. Carrie is also an holistic massage practitioner.

Brainwave
226 Links Road, Tooting, London SW17 9ER.
(0181) 677 8000
Publishing and marketing specialist serving the holistic market. We

publish guidebooks to the field. We publish 'Holistic London', 'The Holistic Marketing Directory' and 'The Whole Person Catalogue'. We also publish free guides to the Mind Body Spirit field in London and the UK as well as providing mailing lists.

Breakthrough Centre
7 Poplar Mews, Uxbridge Road, Shepherds Bush, London W12 7JS.
(0181) 749 8525
An alternative business centre, providing support, training and networking for everyone seeking to combine work with personal growth and ethics. Introductory evenings twice monthly. Self-employed and career changes equally welcome.

Green Events
14 Curzon Road, Muswell Hill, London N10 2RA.
(0181) 365 2958
They mail out an 'event calendar' on a regular basis to people interested in therapy and the green movement. They can include your details in the listings. The event calandar is also on display in shops and other venues throughout London.

Greenshift
48 Beck Road, London E8 4RE.
(0171) 249 5584
Leaflet and poster distributor for London area. Greenshift offers an excellent, targeted network of venues with own exclusive racks to hold and display your leaflets. They specialise in the alternative field (i.e. health and green centres, new age

bookshops etc), but also link extensively to London's general public (i.e. libraries, AEI's, colleges, hospitals, cafes, cinemas etc.) Sample terms: minimum 1,000 leaflets £65, 10,000 for £175. Between these two amounts there is a sliding scale. For posters their is a flat rate of £20 for 50 posters. They also offer an effective targeted mailout service as well as very low printing.

Signalysis
Silver Birches, Private Road, Rodborough Common, Stroud, Gloucs GL5 5BT.
(0145387) 3446, 3668, 2618
Blood/urine analysis and remedies, service for medical doctors and natural medicine practitioners. £50, £99 and £185 depending on type of analysis. Remedies last for about 3 months.

Hyden House Ltd
Little Hyden Lane, Clanfield, Hants PO8 ORU.
(01705) 596500
Established 1990. Design, marketing, publishing, copy writing, practice management consultants, editors. Primary

activities are publishing and design. Their target market is the natural medicine student/practitioner. Serves the UK.

Latourelle, Maggie
58 Leverton St, London NW5 2NU.
(0171) 485 4215
Runs workshops for practitioners to help them market their business and get more clients.

Lisha Spar
49 Upcerne Road, London SW10 0SF.
(0171) 352 1540
Publicity and promotion service for clinics, centres, product suppliers and individuals.

London and South East Connection
Laurel Cottage, Watery Lane, Donhead St Mary, Shaftsbury, Dorset SP7 9DF.
(01747) 828913
They produce two guides to the holistic movement in London, 'London and South West Connection' and 'London and South East Connection. Three issues/yr. Size A5, 80pp. Given out free. Take classified and display advertising. Actively seeking submissions, especially on group experiences and new and diary dates. Preferred method of submissions by synopsis and whole article. Print reviews of books, audio tapes, video tapes and products. Main avenues of distribution is to centres, health shops and bookshops. 'Our guide/magazine is FREE and the 15,000 distributed are consumed very quickly and often by people on the edge of interested in the new age. Our

advertising is very cheap compared to most new age magazines.'

Natural Health Public Relations
188 Old St, London EC1V 9FR.
(0171) 336 7593
Offers media coverage for any organisation in the holistic field.

Neal's Yard Agency
14 Neal's Yard, Covent Garden, London WC2 9DP.
(0171) 379 0141
Are an agency which matches up the public with holistic businesses running courses, events, dance, art, psychotherapy, counselling, trainings, martial arts, men's and women's groups etc. If you have a course, training, event, holiday etc you wish to find clients for, Neal's Yard Agency do their best to find them for you. The public come into the shop and browse around and talk to somebody about further advice. Also large and small meeting rooms for hire (14 ft square and 22 ft x 27 ft).

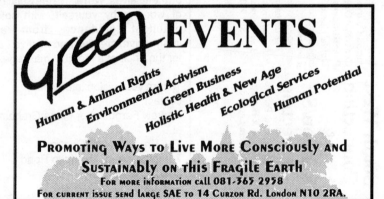

Practitioners Support Network
*25 Priory Court, Chipstead Road,
Barnstead, Surrey SM7 2HJ*
(01737) 370396
Once a month meeting to discuss all aspects of running a successful Practice and support for Practitioners'. Also workshops, newsletter, chance to give workshops and talks to others.

MACROBIOTICS

Macrobiotics is familiar to most people as a kind of diet. But it is also a whole theory of health and well-being based on the balancing of the opposite and complementary energies of Yin and Yang. Literally the word Macrobiotics means 'large life'.

Macrobiotic theory is based in the Oriental belief that good health is based on the balance of life energy. Yin energy is feminine, receptive, damp, cold and is symbolised by the moon. Yang energy is masculine, active, dry, hot and symbolised by the sun. Everything that exists partakes more or less of the qualities of these elemental energies. As in acupuncture, illness is seen as an imbalance of these forces in the body. Since food can be classified as Yin or Yang, a Macrobiotic diet is a way or restoring this balance through eating the right foods.

Cereals and brown rice form the basis of the Macrobiotic diet because they contain the best balance of Yin and Yang. Yin foods are those which contain a lot of water, grow above the ground and tend to be hot, sour or sweet in taste. They tend to be blue, green or purple. Yang foods tend to be hard, dense, dry, grow below ground and are often red or yellow in colour. Different methods of cooking can also increase the tendency towards Yin or Yang: quick cooking increases Yin, and slow cooking, Yang. Foods that will promote this balance depend on the temperament of the eater and his or her environment. It is better to eat local foods too, because there is a natural affinity between the food of a region and its people. But it is important to stress that each individual is unique and has his or her own requirements for healthy eating.

Although Macrobiotics is a good way of healing oneself, at first it is important to consult a trained macrobiotic dietitian, especially if you have a particular complaint. Diagnosis is carried out by observation of the colour and shape of the patient's body, an assessment of their temperament, and by taking the 'pulses' (see Acupuncture section for an explanation of the pulses). Emphasis is not only placed on eating healthily, but also on lifestyle. Disease can also be a result of not looking after the body properly, of having a negative attitude to life or of being in the wrong environment.

Though it can be hard to keep to a macrobiotic diet - if you like eating out then you may find it harder - many people have found it can help in treatment of very stubborn conditions, as well as promoting increased vitality and better digestion.

RESOURCES

Bumblebee Natural Foods
33 Brecknock Road, London N7 0AD.
(0171) 267 3884
Three neighbouring shops, each shop specialising in a different produce.
No. 30 sell a wide range of macrobiotic food, fruit and nuts, beans, jams, honeys, spreads, pastas, oils, teas, and soya milk.
No. 32 is the takeaway section with hot dishes prepared in their kitchen. Also breads, grains, juices, cereals and a large selection of O.G. wines.
No. 33 is the O.G. fruit and vegetable shop. It also stocks herbs and spice and herb teas. The dairy is sited towards the back of the shop.
No. 10 Caledonian Road (previously Peacemeal) does take aways and a large selection of wholefoods.

Bushwacker
59 Goldhawk Road, London W12.
(0181) 743 2359
Wholefood shop sells range of wholefood, organic fruit and vegetables, medicines, books and also macrobiotic specialities.

Community Health Foundation
188-194 Old Street, London EC1V 9BP.
(0171) 251 4076

VEGETARIANISM AND VEGANISM

A vegetarian diet is one which excludes all meat. A vegan diet excludes not only meat but also all animal products, such as milk, eggs and sometimes honey. Most vegans also prefer not to use or wear leather.

The past few years have seen an increasing number of people becoming vegetarian or vegan. A number of different factors have contributed to this change in eating habits. Recent publicity about the possible harmful effects of meat and dairy products has added to the argument that a vegetarian diet is healthier and has offset the popular and unfounded fear that unless your diet includes a lot of meat you will become undernourished in some way. The saturated fats present in animal products have been found to be contributory to the development of heart disease, and links appparently exist between high meat consumption and low fibre intake and breast and bowel cancer. Research shows that a high fibre, vegetable and fruit based diet is also less fattening and promotes healthy functioning of the digestive system.

However, most people who adopt a vegan or vegetarian diet do so for ethical reasons. Since the consumption of meat and dairy products is no longer necessary for our survival, it is argued that the suffering inflicted upon animals in the food creating process is also unnecessary. Factory farming and mass production of meat means that in the modern world animals are subjected to greater suffering that in the days of the smallholding. The publicity which has been given to the way in which meat is produced has left many people feeling that since they cannot condone the process, they cannot eat the product either.

Ecological awareness too has

played its part in the change in eating habits. Animal farming tends to use up more resources than plant farming and requires more acres of land for less food production. Forests throughout the world have been cleared for animal grazing and this has led to further ecological problems.

In the 1990s it is far easier to be a vegan or vegetarian than it was 20 years ago. Health food shops have sprung up all over the country, and vegetarian restaurants have become commonplace, at least in the big cities. Many restaurants offer special vegetarian dishes or a vegetarian menu. The growth of high quality vegetarian cuisine means that fewer people are cracking the old nut rissole and lentil jokes, and vegetarians are not seen as 'cranks' any more. Life can still be difficult for the vegan who wants to eat out though milk substitute products such as soya milk are available even in some local supermarkets in London.

Some people who would like to exclude meat from their diet still feel unsure about what they would eat instead, or still feel anxious about the prospect of a vegetarian coming for dinner. For further information on this and on other aspects of vegetarianism and veganism, contact the centres below.

Contact Centre
BCM Cuddle, London WC1V 6XX.
An international low fee friendship agency exclusively for vegetarians and vegans.

Vegetarian Society
Parkdale, Dunham Road, Altrincham, Cheshire WA14 4QG.
(0161) 928 0793
Campaigns to promote vegetarianism, gives information and advice, publishes books, leaflets and Vegetarian magazine, produces range of merchandise, supports non-animal research into the benefits of vegetarianism. Also runs cookery courses (see Vegetarian Society Cookery School in Residential Workshops section).

VEGETARIAN RESTAURANTS

Angel Gate
51 Queen Caroline Street, Hammersmith, London W6.
(0181) 748 8388
Vegan, wholefood and vegetarian.

Bunjie's Coffee House
27 Litchfield Street, London WC2.
(0171) 240 1796
12-11 every day. Sunday 5-11. Wholefood. Cheap, folk music some nights.

Cherry Orchard
241 Globe Road, Bethnal Green, London E2 0JD.
(0181) 980 6678
Tues-Fri 12-3 and 6.30-10.30, Sat 12-10.30, Sun & Mon closed. Vegan and vegetarian dishes at reasonable prices, canteen service at lunchtime changes to waitress service at night. Very pleasant garden in the Summer. Run by women members of the Buddhist centre next door.

RESOURCES

Cranks Health Foods
1 Central Avenue, Covent Garden Plaza, London WC2.
(0171) 379 6508
9.30-8.00, Sun 9.30-7. Covent Garden tube.

Cranks Health Foods
17-18 Great Newport Street, London W1.

Cranks Health Foods
8 Marshal Street, London W1.
(0171) 437 9431
Mon to Fri. 8-10.30 Vegan/ wholefood.

Cranks Health Foods
9-11 Tottenham Street, London W1.
(0171) 631 3912
8-8 Mon-Fri, 9-8pm Sat, closed Sun. Vegan/wholefood.

Dining Room
Winchester Walk, London Bridge, London SE1.
(0171) 407 0337
Tues-Fri 7-10. Vegan/wholefood.

Diwana Bhelpoori House
121 Drummond Street, Euston, London NW1.
(0171) 387 5556
12-11.45 daily. Indian. Cheap.

Diwana Bhelpoori House
50 Westbourne Grove, Bayswater, London W2.
(0171) 221 0721
12-3 and 6-10.30 daily. Indian. Cheap.

East West Restaurant
188 Old Street, London EC1.
(0171) 608 0300
Mon-Fri 11am-9.30pm. The only macrobiotic restaraunt in town.

Fallen Angel
65 Graham Street, Islington, London N1.
(0171) 253 3996
Mon-Sat 12-12, Sun 12-11.30. Wine bar/Cafe.

Food for Thought
31 Neal Street, Covent Garden, London WC2.
(0171) 836 0239
Covent Garden, Wholefood/ Vegan, 12-8, Sat 12-8 closed Sun.

Full of Beans
127 Rushey Green, Catford, London SE6.
(0181) 698 3283
9.30-5.30 Mon-Sat. Wholefood, hot meals, snacks, cakes. Vegan dishes sometimes avaialable.

Gate Vegetarian Restaurant
51 Queen Caroline Street, Hammersmith, London W6.
(0181) 748 6932
12 noon-11.30pm Mon-Fri, 12 noon-12 midnight Sats. Licensed (organic and non-organic wines). Private parties catered for. Linked to the Rudolph Steiner inspired Christian Community.

Govinda's
9 Soho Street, Soho, London W1.
(0171) 437 3662
Purely vegetarian restaurant

Greenhouse
16 Chenies Street, London WC1.
(0171) 637 8038
Goodge Street tube. Mon 10-6, Tues-Fri 10-10, Sat 1-8.30. Reasonable prices, vegan dishes available.

Hare Krishna Curry House
1 Hanway Street, London W1.
(0171) 636 5262
10.30-11pm all week. Has just re-opened and seats 50. Gujerati vegetarian dishes and wholefood. Licensed.

Rosanna's
17 Strutton Ground, London SW1.
(0171) 233 1701
Mon-Fri 9-9. Home made vegtarian food and organic wines and beers. Healthfood shop two doors up.

Hearth Cafe At Earthworks
132 Kings Street, Hammersmith, London W6 0QU.
(0181) 846 9357
Wholefood, Mon-Wed 11am-6pm. Fri & Sat 11am-10.30 pm.,

Hockney's
Croydon Buddist Centre, 98 High Street, Croydon, Surrey CR0 1ND.
(0181) 688 2899
Purely vegeterarian and vegan meals available. Mon - Sat 10.30am -5.30pm Friday evening 6pm - 10pm. Also adjacent health food shop.

London Ecology Centre
45 Shelton Street, Covent Garden, London WC2.
(0171) 379 4324
10.30am-10.30pm, closed 10. Covent Garden, Wholefood and vegan. Licensed.

Mandeer
21 Hanway Place, London W1.
(0171) 323 0660
10.30 Mon-Sat, closed Sun. Indian. Excellent food and cheap too. Well worth a visit.

Manna
4 Erskine Road, Chalk Farm, London NW3.
(0171) 722 8028
6.30-12 daily. Wholefood, sometimes vegan.)

Millwall
30 Stoke Newington Church St., Stoke Newington, London N16.
(0171) 254 1025
12-3 and 6-12 Mon-Thur, Fri 12-3 and 6-1, Sat 12-1am, Sun 12-12. Vegan/Wholefood.

Milward's
97 Stoke Newington Church St., Stoke Newington, London N16.
(0171) 254 1025
Mon-Fri 6-12, Sat and Sun 12-12. Vegan/Wholefood.)

Neal's Yard Bakery and Tea Room
6 Neal's Yard, Covent Garden, London WC2.
(0171) 836 5199
10.30-8 Mon Tue Thur Fr, Covent Garden, Wholefood, vegan dishes available and as many different types of tea as you could wish.

Nuthouse
26 Kingley Street, London W1.
(0171) 437 9471
10.30-7.00 Mon-Fri, 10.30-6 Sat, closed Sun. Vegan/wholefood. Cheap.

Ravi Shankar
133 Drummond Street, Euston, London NW1.
(0171) 388 6458
12-11 daily. Indian food.

Raw Deal
65 York Street, London W1.
(0171) 262 4841
10-10 Mon to Fri, Baker Street, Wholefood.

Rossana's Vegetarian Restaurant
17 Strutton Ground, Victoria, London SW1P 2UY.
(0171) 233 1701
Seats 34 people. A small intimate basement next door to health food shop. Serve vegetarian and vegan

food. Open12am-11pm Mon to Fri.
Wed, Thurs and Fri nights (not
days) women only. Licensed and air
conditioned.

Shan
*200 Shaftesbury Avenue, Soho, London
WC2.*
(0171) 240 3348
12-10 Mon-Sat, closed Sun.

Sunra
*26 Balham Hill, Clapham South, London
SW12 9EB.*
(0181) 675 9224
**A holistic health centre with a
vegetarian cafe on the premises.**

Well Bean
*10 Old Dover Road, Blackheath, London
SE3.*
(0181) 858 1319
Mon-Fri 9-6, Sat 9-5.30.
Wholefood: main dish and soup
every day, pies, pizzas, salads. Bring
your own bottle.

Wholemeal Cafe
*1 Shrubbery Road, Streatham, London
SW16.*
(0181) 769 2423
Midday to 10pm, 7 days a week.
Open Sat and Sun 9-11.30am for
breakfast. Wholemeal. Fully
licensed. No smoking.

Wilkins Natural Foods
*61 Marsham Street, Victoria, London
SW1.*
(0171) 222 4038
Mon-Fri 8-6. Wholefood cafe,
mainly lunctime trade. Some vegan
dishes.

Woodlands Restaurant
*37 Panton Street Off, Haymarket, London
W1.*
(0171) 839 7258
12-2.45 and 6-10.30 daily, Indian
food.

Woodlands Restaurant
77 Marylebone Lane, London W1.
(0171) 486 3862
12-2.45 and 6 - 10.30 daily, Indian
food.

Woodlands Restaurant
402 High Road, Wembley, Middlesex.
(0171) 930 8200
12-2.45 and 6-10.30 daily, Indian
food.

LONDON GETAWAY

RESIDENTIAL COMMUNITIES

A residential is a workshop which takes place over a weekend or longer, and in which the participants stay together in accommodation provided, usually because the venue is in the country. This builds up a more intensive atmosphere, and can enable people to enter more fully into the workshop. See also 'Residential Workshops' in this section.

Botton Camphill
Camphill Village Trust, Botton Village, Danby, Whitby, North Yorkshire YO21 2NJ.
(01287) 660871
Although basically Christian they try to follow the principles of philosophy as propounded by Rudolf Steiner.

Findhorn Foundation
The Park, Forres IV36 OTZ.
(01309) 690311

International Society for Krishna Consciousness
Bhaktivedanta Manor, Letchmore Health, Watford, Hertfordshire WD2 8EP.
(01923) 857244
Religious charity dedicated to practising and sharing the beliefs and lifestyle of Vaishnavisn (Krishna Consciousness) as has been known in Indian for hundreds of years. 'Our vision is to see respiritualisation of society by understanding we are not this body but are spirit souls, all individual eternal servants of the Supreme and can find true fulfilment in devotional service to Krishna'. Full list of local centres, meetings, festivals and publications available on request. Members do not necessarily live in community but practise the teachings at home. Food is lacto-vegetarian. Accommodation is double room or dormitory. Families participate in but live outside the community. Guests welcome for up to 3 days, initially, by prior arrangements. Refer to organisers for details of costs.

Loriestone Hall
Castle Douglas, Dumfriesshire DG7 2NB.
(016445) 275
Though no longer a 'commune', the 20 adults and 11 children on Lauriston Hall live together as individual members of a housing co-op, some in families, some by themselves, and others in small, non-family 'living groups' and share some aspects of their work. Hold visitors weeks when people can come and experience first hand what goes on. Run a number of residential workshops as well such as gay men's weeks, Reichian weeks, tai chi, music, alchemy and taoist weeks, and 'maximising our immunity' workshop. Sliding scale from £8.50 per day up to £15, depending on income, workshops may cost more.

Lower Shaw Farm
Old Shaw Lane, Shaw, Nr Swindon, Wilts SN5.
(01793) 771080
Community with no collectively stated religious or party political base other than environmental and permaculture. Workshops and

holidays, as well as working weekends etc. Prices are cheap starting at £55 per weekend which includes food and dormitory accommodation (few single and double rooms). Some of the weekend workshops they do are Shiatsu, fools weekend, yoga, massage, death exploration, pottery, women and crafts (such as photography), rug making etc. Offer concessions up to one third full price.

Monkton Wyld Court
Nr. Charmouth, Bridport, Dorset DT6 6DQ.
(01297) 60342
Monkton Wyld Court is an holistic education centre set in eleven acres of organic farm and gardens, three miles from the sea at Lyme Regis. They offer a wide range of workshops including: writing, pottery, batik, drumming, drum making, singing, dancing, massage, breathwork, shamanic studies, T'ai Chi, Shiatsu, personal development and a series of family weeks and visitor weeks, throughout the year. The centre is run by a resident community who live, work and celebrate the seasons together. Their rates are very competitive - from only £85 for a weekend course. They also offer a generous concession scheme.

Seekers Trust
The Close, Addington, West Malling, Kent ME19 5BL.
(01732) 843589
Prayer (Christian) and spiritual healing is offered at this residential community. Self catering flats

available for long or short stay. Centre situated at Addington Park in Kent within 37 acres of gardens and woodlands. The work entails constant prayer and very considerable clerical routine, most of which is carried out by voluntary helpers within the community. In some hundred half hour sessions each week, groups of dedicated resident members of the Trust meet in small chapels linking by concentrated prayer with the people who have asked for help and healing, who say the identical prayers at precisely the same times. No fees but donations accepted. Also conference hall. Accommodation starts at £60.00 per week, to £95.00 per week. Established for over 70 years, and aim to 'give help and encouragement in the form of spiritual healing to all who come to us in need, whatever their age, nationality, walk of life'.

RESIDENTIAL HEALTH CENTRES

Bethany Vegetarian and Vegan Nursing Homes
7/9 Oak Park Villas, Dawlish, Devon EX7 0DE.
(01626) 862794
Run on Christian principles, it offers care to all vegetarians and vegans, and is registered with the local health authority as a nursing home and rest home with 23 beds. Special diets such as diabetes, wholefood, Gerson type cancer therapy, gluten free are catered for.

Visiting chiropodist, hairdresser, masseuse, occupational therapist, homoeopath and acupuncturist. Aim to give residents holistic health care with a choice of naturopathic or allopathic therapy. Non smoking environment.Nursing bed £250 per week, rest home bed £175 per week. Also accept DHS patients.

Breakspear Hospital
1 High Street, Abbots Langley, Herts WD5 0PU.
(01442) 261333
Private Hospital opened March 1988 with in-patient, day-patient and out-patient facilities. Environmental control, filtered water and organic food. Patients seen by appointment only. Monthly seminars, lectures. Sale of books and vitamins. Prices £85 for initial consultation with doctor, thereafter prices individually ascertained. No concessions. Register of practitioners. Wheelchair access. Allergy desensitisation, sleep monitoring. Multi-gym, sauna and excercise programmes. Will perform home surveys for environmental contaminants.

Park Attwood Clinic
Trimpley, Bewdley, Worcestershire DY12 1RE.
(012997) 444
Nursing home run by qualified doctors using Anthroposophical Medicine - 'a therapeutic community in a clinical setting'. Have treated people for conditions both physical and mental. Also run in-service training for nurses, and are open to visits from interested health professionals.

Raphael Medical Centre
Coldharbour Lane, Hildenborough, Tonbridge, Kent TN11 9LE.
(01732) 833924
In- and out-patient facilities for Anthroposophical therapies.

Tyringham Naturopathic Clinic
Newport Pagnell, Milton Keynes, Bucks MK16 9ER.
(01908) 610450x204
Set in pleasantly secluded rural Buckinghamshire, the serene setting of Tyringham makes it an ideal location. 'This well appointed Georgian mansion house enjoys views over some 30 acres of gardens, woodlands and acres of surrounding farmland'. Osteopathy, acupuncture, massage, Balneotherapy, sitz bath, steam bath, Scottish douche, naturopathy, indoor pool with sauna and jacuzzi, gymnasium, hydrotherapy. Outdoor sports facilities. £228 - £465 per week depending on type of accommodation, treatments are included in the price.

RESIDENTIAL WORKSHOPS

Abshot Holistic Centre
Little Abshott Road, Titchfield Common, Fareham, Hants PO14 4LN.
(01489) 572451
'Maitri' means 'friend to oneself' and here they run self development courses including stress management, regression therapy, polarity therapy, synergetics, meditation and chanelling. Centre used to be the stables of the old Abshott Manor, which were converted 6 years ago. Swimming

pool, vegetarian food, special diets catered for with prior notice. Training centre for the International School of Polarity Therapy. £65 per weekend, £90 for a four day course.

Aura Soma
Dev Aura, Little London Telford, Nr Horncastle, Lincs LN9 6QL.
(01507) 533781
Teaching and sharing of all aspects of colour and light for healing and personal development particularly with reference to the soul. Workshops include a complete training in colour therapy, use of aura-soma, meditation and kinesology. Workshops are held at Dev Aura International, Telford and America, Australia and Europe. Accommodation comprises single, double or family rooms. Food is vegetarian or vegan. Booking through application forms. Tuition costs £40.00 per day and accommodation £20.00 per day.

Beacon Centre
Cutteridge Farm, Whitestone, Exeter, Devon EX4 2HE.
(01392) 811203
The centre is committed to personal, inter-personal and planetary healing and transformation. 'Our philosophy is based on an acknowledgement of the spiritual nature inherent in all people, and all of life'. Courses on self enlightenment and transformation, yoga, meditation, tai chi circle dancing, crystal healing and psychotherapy. Fully centrally heated with sauna and olympic size trampoline for those who are

feeling or want to feel 'bouncy'. Situated within 20 mins drive of Dartmoor, the sea and Exeter city centre. Working organic farm. Long weekend is approx £75.00 plus £4 (+ VAT) per night for shared accommodation - includes hire of self catering kitchen. Bed and breakfast also available. Write for programme. Available for hire for groups.

CAER (Centre For Alternative Education And Research)
Rosemerryn, Lamorna, Penzance, Cornwall TR19 6BN.
(01736) 810530
Wide range of workshops including Alexander technique, gestalt, massage, rebirthing, resonance therapy, stress management, yoga, Shamanism, women's and men's groups and body-oriented approaches, groupwork, RSA certified courses in groupwork and counselling etc. Introductory weekends in the above and two year part time Diploma in Human Development and Facilitation Skills. CAER's emphasis is broad based though growing focus on Shamanism and Buddhism. One of the longest established centres for residential workshops in personal and professional development in Europe. It is situated in seven acres of woods and gardens on the site of an Iron Age fort, near the sea in an area of Outstanding Natural Beauty. The house itself is an old Cornish manor house. Most diets are catered for. When there are no groups there, you can stay on a nightly basis. Wheelchair access.

Three tiered price structure for waged, low waged and unwaged from £30.00 to £60.00 per day including residential costs.

Centre of Light
Tighnabruaich, Stuy, by Beauly, Inverness-shire IV4 7JU.
(0146) 376 254
Residential healing and therapy centre in the peace and beauty of the Scottish highlands. The centre is comfortable and remote, but not isolated. Practise healing, channelling, kinesiology, massage, healing, with colour and light. Week long courses and individual sessions.

Eden Centre
Eden House, 38 Lee Road, Lynton, Devon EX35 6BS.
(01598) 53440
A centre for holistic approach to health and creative development. Holiday retreats £56 per week, accommodation only. £112 including food. Week workshops all-in £170. Weekend workshops £75. Minimum booking is for one week. Offer a wide range of therapies - massage, aromatherapy, relaxation, meditation, colour therapy, writing/poetry, Alexander technique and stress management. The house is available for small groups in August.

Findhorn Foundation
The Park, Forres IV36 OTZ.
(01309) 690311
Courses include Learning to Love, Letting Go - Unfolding Your Inner Self, Massage, Deep Ecology, Primal Painting, Towards Sexual Wholeness, Myths we Live By, Gestalt to name but a few. Participants live and work in the Findhorn Community in the 'Experience Week', completion of which is a requirement for participation in most courses longer than a weekend. For prices see under List of Centres section. For details of the philosophy of Findhorn see Other Groups in Spirit section.

Flight of the Phoenix
3-4 Moor View, Torpoint, Cornwall PL11 2LH.
(01752) 813438
A spiritual community of people from many walks of life who have

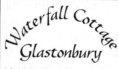

been living, meditating and working together for up to six years. Hold workshops on personal healing, esoteric yoga, song, meditation, and dance. £35 per day which includes lunch, £5 reduction per day for people on low income.

Gablecroft College of Natural Therapy
Church Street, Whittington, Shropshire SY11 4DT.
(01691) 659631
Residential training in massage, reflexology, aromatherapy, sports injury treatment, healing and dowsing. ITEC recognised. Finnish sauna and vegetarian, organic meals.

Grimstone Manor
Yelverton, Devon PL20 7QY.
(01822) 854358
Residential group training centre run by Grimstone Community. The Community runs several workshops each year and hosts many more. Courses on rebirthing, yoga, reflexology, massage, shiatsu, gestalt, psychodrama, tai chi. Also retreats, holiday breaks and season celebrations. The manor is situated in 27 acres on the edge of Dartmoor and has an indoor swimming pool, jacuzzi and sauna. Prices vary according to nature of the workshop. Short stays, bed and breakfast sometimes possible.

Hawkwood College
Painswick Old Road, Stroud, Glocs GL6 8QW.
(01453) 764607
Provides an exceptionally peaceful and beautiful setting for weekend or week long residential workshops.

It can accomodate 54 people in single and twin bedded rooms. It does not serve alcohol, but visitors are welcome to bring their own if they wish. It caters for vegetarians and meat eaters, and vegetables are grown biodynamically in the gardens for the kitchen. Typical course on offer include: dreams, stress, family, Alexander technique, dowsing, death, painting. Approx £90 for a weekend.

Hazelwood House
Loddiswell, Nr Kingsbridge, S Devon TQ7 4EB.
(01548) 821232 / (0171) 538 5633
Workshops on voice work, and music weekends with classical performers in concert. Also offer painting as art courses.

Holwell Centre for Psychodrama and Sociodrama
East Down, Barnstaple, Devon EX31 3NZ.
(01271) 850 267/597
Training and experience in psychodrama from beginners to advanced, with varying themes all year round. Some weekend course, mostly week long courses and one 5 week course. Accommodation is in shared rooms in a farmhouse, with food provided and vegetarian diets catered for. Costs are £395.00 per week, £165.00 per weekend. Workshops are for professional therapists and non-professionals with an interest in psychodrama. Holwell is an ancient farm in the Devonshire hills situated on ley lines.

Hourne Farm
Steel Cross, Crowborough, Sussex.
(01892) 661093
Set in the Sussex countryside, they offer a programme of weekend workshops, courses, open weekends and summer schools. Study of leylines, divination, yoga, holistic therapies, crystals. Approx £60 per weekend workshop.

Okido Natural Health Education Trust
Basement Flat, 45 Elgin Crescent, London W11.
(0171) 727 1575
Yoga holidays in Holland, Belgium, Italy and Suffolk as well as regular classes and seminars in London at various venues. Activities include breathing, purification, corrective, spine, balancing, hara-strengthening exercises and Yoga asanas, Do-in, Shiatsu, relaxation and meditation. Okido Yoga is a synthesis of elements from Indian Yoga, Chinese Taoism, Oriental Medicine and especially the Japanese Zen tradition. It was developed by Master Masahire Okis personal experience of many disciplines.

Pegasus Foundation
Runnings Park, Croft Bank, West Malvern, Worcs WR14 8BR.
(01684) 565253
Weekends about aspects of healing such as counselling skills, developing healing potential, healing relationships. Residential fees £95-£110.

Pellin Training Courses
15 Killyon Road, London SW8 2XS.
(0171) 720 4499
Intestive residential personal and professional growth programme in southern Italy. Described by the organisers as 'arduous and challenging' in a safe and nourishing environment. Morning and evening group for individual Gestalt work. £275 per programme week, including full board, excluding air fares.

Portman Lodge
Durweston, Blandford, Dorset DT11 0QA.
(01258) 452168
Portman Lodge is a centre for workshops and therapies. It is set in beautiful countryside and provides a peaceful atmosphere for inner leaning. Accomodation in spacious en suite bedrooms provided with bed and breakfast. We produce regular updated mailings available on request which outline what is coming up from season to season.

Songbear Creations
95 Devonport Road, Shepherds Bush, London W12 8PB.
(0181) 740 4991
Workshops on native American Indian practices. They are held in Suffolk and Dorset. Weekend retreats in different locations. £120 per weekend. Concs. Offer massage, medicine wheel therapy, past life healing, sweat lodge ceremonies, vision questing, shamanic drumming, crystal and colour therapy. Men and women only groups available.

Studio 8

10 Wycliffe Row, Totterdown, Bristol BS3 4RU.

(0117) 9713488

Open arts workshops, tutorial groups, Art Synthesis course exploring creativity, imagination and adventure through drawing, painting and other visual arts - 'awareness through art'. Venues are London, Somerset and France. Details of costs provided on application to Studio 8. Also run a 'Living Creatively' course at the above venues: bringing together meditation, and gentle healing with practical outlets for one's creativity using paint clay and sound. Offer day, weekend and week courses.

Sunra

26 Balham Hill, Clapham South, London SW12 9EB.

(0181) 675 9224

Taraloka

Cornhill Farm, Bettisfield, Nr Whitchurch, N. Shropshire SY13 2LV.

(0194875) 646

Buddhist residential workshop centre for women. Part of 'Friends of the Western Buddhist Order'. State they are the only women-only Buddhist retreat centre in Europe, and aim to teach as many women as are interested about meditation and Buddhism. Weekends £60.00 (£33.00 concs.), week £147.00 (£84.00 concs.), 10 days £210.00 (£120.00 concs.). Dormitory accommodation and vegetarian and vegan food are included in these prices.

The Beacon Centre

Cutteridge Farm, Whitestone, Exeter, Devon EX4 2HE.

The Beacon Centre offers a variety of workshops and weekly activities in areas such as counselling, Gestalt and meditation, and is situated three miles from Exeter.

Tighnabruaich

Tighnabruaich, Struy, by Beauly, Inverness-shire IV4 7JU.

(01463) 761254

Healing centre in Scotland. Run 'The Watershed', a course exploring the self through nature. Can take up to 4 people to stay combining holiday with daily two-three hour therapy session. Vegetarian organic food. Watershed £350, stay £305 per week.

Vegetarian Society Cookery School

Co-ordinator Parkdale, Dunham Road, Altrincham, Cheshire WA14 4QG.

(0161) 928 0793

Courses at various levels on how to cook vegetarian food for vegetarians and non-vegetarian participants. Weekends, weeks and the 'Cordon Vert' Diploma course.

Waterfall Cottage

20 Old Wells Road, Glastonbury, Somerset BA6 8ED.

(01458) 831707

Workshops on crystals, colour therapy, inner growth and transformation. They provide bed and breakfast and have a library on site. Also do tours of the local sacred sites.

West Usk Lighthouse

Lighthouse Road, St. Brides, Wendlooge, Nr. Newport, Gwent NP1 9SF.
(01633) 810126/815860
West Usk Lighthouse offer a wide range of workshops in astrology, palmistry, Tarot, aura soma colour healing, relaxation, meditation, ufology, dream interpretation, healing, past life regression and many more! Workshops take place on weekends. Accommodation comprises of 2 single and 4 double rooms, plus 1 meeting room. Average cost per weekend is £85.00 inclusive. All types of food are provided including vegetarian and vegan. The Centre also offers floatation tank, orgone accumulator and pyramid sessions.

RETREATS

A retreat is an intensive period of meditation, study or other religious practices which is residential. They almost always take place in the country. All retreats have a programme of activities. There are usually set times for meditation or prayer, and this structure provides a framework within which the retreatant can let go of having to organise his or her life and concentrate on inner spiritual experience.

Retreats can vary enormously in terms of what the programme is and whether the organisers expect you to participate fully in all activities, or whether you can just be there and join in as you wish. It is as well to decide beforehand what you do want and to check with the organisers about the programme.

Some retreats have an intensive programme with a great deal of meditation or prayer, and others may be silent some, or all, of the time. Others have a looser programme. There may be an early start, as early as 4am on certain retreats, and accommodation may be in dormitories or occasionally in smaller rooms. You may be asked to bring a sleeping bag. Sometimes participants are expected to work on the retreat, sometimes all the work is done for them. Food is usually vegetarian.

A good publication for finding a place for a retreat, even in central London, is **The Vision**, the Journal of the National Retreat Association *(24 South Audley Street, London W1 (0171) 493 3534)*, which costs £1 plus post and packing. This lists all the Christian retreat houses in Britain and group and individual retreat facilities.

All Hallows House
Idol Lane, London EC3R 5DD.
(0171) 283 8908

Creative and Healing Arts
222 Westbourne Park Road, London W11 1EP.
(0171) 229 9400
Mainly weekend retreats in the country with yoga, shiatus, dance and music.

Dartington Centre
Dartington Hall, Totnes, Devon TQ9 6EL.
(01803) 862271

Findhorn Foundation
The Park, Forres IV36 OTZ.
(01309) 690311

Gaia House
Woodland Road, Denbury, Nr. Newton Abbot, Devon TQ12 6DY.
(01803) 813188
Provide a facility for the practice of insight meditation both group and personal retreats (solitary). Insight meditation is known as Vispassana in Buddhist tradition. Vegetarian food provided, with special dietary requirements catered for where possible. Anyone is welcome on retreats. There is a variable daily structure, although it is not compulsory to participate in all of this. In fact, retreaters can make up their own structures. 'Aim is to free the mind from distortions of self-centredness, negativity and confusion. Balanced awareness grounded in the present moment leads to wisdom and compassion'. Costs cover board and lodging only. Teachings and meditation instruction given freely. Voluntary donations to teachers and staff according to means welcome. £14.00 daily. £40.00 weekends.

Gaunts House
Wimborne, Dorset BH21 4JQ.
(01202) 841522

Grimstone Manor
Yelverton, Devon PL20 7QY.
(01822) 854358

Insight
Lighthouse Road, St. Brides, Wentlooge, Nr. Newport, Gwent NP1 9SF.
(01633) 815582 (0633) 810126
New Age centre retreat in a lighthouse. Situated on ley lines, near the sea. Wedge Runs regular Yoga classes for members and friends, hold seminars weekly and weekend retreats inviting expert speakers. Monthly Satsang (discussion group). Membership is open to anyone and enquiries are dealt with by telephone and in writing. Accommodation on retreats comprises of separate compartments in caravans, or single rooms when retreats are held externally. A weekend (Friday to Sunday) costs about £70.00, costs vary. Week long and longer retreats available. Patanjali aim to help people 'become useful and responsible members of society by knowing themselves and bring Peace to the whole universe'.

SamyeLing Tibetan Centre
Eskdalemuir, Langholm DG13 0QL.
(013873) 73232

Taraloka
Cornhill Farm, Bettisfield, Nr Whitchurch, N. Shropshire SY13 2LV.
(0194875) 646
Provide residential retreats for women interested in meditation and Buddhism. Part of the new Western Buddhist movement, called Friends of the Western

Buddhist Order. Retreat programmes vary, full details given on application to the centre. Shortest retreat is a weekend, most people staying a week to 10 days. Weekends £60.00 (£40.00 concs.), week £154.00 (£119.00 concs.), 10 days £220.00 (£170.00 concs.). Accommodation and vegetarian/vegan food are included in these prices.

West Usk Lighthouse
Lighthouse Road, St. Brides, Wendlooge, Nr. Newport, Gwent NP1 9SF.
(01633) 810126/815860
Healing/New Age centre housed in a real lighthouse picturesquely set on the coast between Newport and Cardiff, with easy access from the M4. Stands impressively in its own grounds, with panoramic views of the surrounding countryside. Wide range of activities availalbe, including astrology, palmistry, tarot, auro soma colour healing, relaxation, meditation, ufology, dream interpretation, healing, past life regression. Also available are floatation tanks, orgone accumulators and pyramids.

Accommodation is 2 single and 4 double rooms with one large meeting room. All types of food available. Average cost £85.00 per weekend.

HOLIDAYS

The centres listed below provide the opportunity for residential workshops or healthy activities coupled with a holiday location. For more information about wholesome breaks, try **The Complete Healthy Holiday Guide** by *Catherine Mooney, Headway Books £6.95* which lists over 300 places to stay where healthy food is served and healthy activities are on offer.

Campus
Fletcherscombe, Diptford, Totnes TQ9 7NQ.
(01548) 821388
Camping holidays include festival, music, theatre, therapies, workshops. Welcome families.

RESOURCES

Churchill Centre
22 Montagu Street, Marble Arch, London W1H 1TB.
(0171) 402 9475
Massage learning holidays in Lanzarote.

Cortijo Romero UK
24 Grange Avenue, Chapletown, Leeds LS7 4EJ.
(0113) 2374015
A comprehensive programme of holiday courses available to anybody, and some specifically aimed at development for people in the helping professions. The courses are run in small groups, in a beautiful, unspoilt environment, with gardens and a pool, set in an eight hundred-year-old olive grove. The premises are also availble for others to hire to run their own events. Guided trips to the 'real' Spain. A week in the south of Spain, including travel is generally no more expensive than a training course in the UK. This is not a standard package holiday.

Educo of the Sea
Mickleton House, Mickleton, Gloucestershire GL55 6RY.
(01386) 438251
Not so much a holiday, but provide specialist events, courses or seminars at sea with a specific orientation and purpose.

Hatha
33 Percy Road, Pocklington, York YO4 2LZ.
(01759) 304140
With their aim being to introduce people to yoga and provide an opportunity for relaxation and an introduction to complementary therapies, Hatha organise yoga

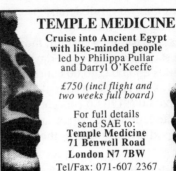
holidays in peaceful places in UK and France. Most holidays are full board, vegetarian food, and prices are inclusive of everything except individual yoga therapy, other complementary therapies and transport. Other activities include walking, the Edinburgh festival, events and a lot of fun.

Holidays For Health
20 Southeby Road, London N5 2UR.
(0171) 359 6690
Relaxation holidays in Spain.

La Val Dieu
11 Meadow Green, Welwyn Garden City, Herts.
(01707) 324631
Workshop holidays in southern France. Typically: yoga, meditation, art, medicine wheel, circle dancing. Workshops are held on a farm. Vegatable garden, horse riding, cows, good food. The address is 11190 Rennes-le-Chateau, (from UK phone 010-33-6874-2321).

Living Planet Travel Ltd
PO Box 922, London N10 3UZ.
(01582) 429365
Adventure holidays to Peru, India, Mexico and Nepal. Will arrange

individual iteneries - for instance will introduce you to the Buddhist kingdom of Zanskar and Ladakh and their tradition Tibeten culture (£1600 for a 34 day holiday).

Neal's Yard Agency
14 Neal's Yard, Covent Garden, London WC2 9DP.
(0171) 379 0141
Are not a holiday company, but act as agents for alternative holiday companies. Either drop in or phone and they will let you have leaflets and talk with you about the different kinds of holidays that are on offer.

CORTIJO ROMERO
Alternative Holidays in Spain

---

* A stunningly beautiful, unspoilt environment - mountains, rivers, sea, ancient villages and the fabled city of Granada

* Workshops by some of the finest people in the Human Potential movement worldwide

* Delightful buildings, gardens and pool, set in an 800 year old olive grove

* 325 sunshine days per year

* See the real Spain, with a devoted Anglo-Spanish staff

* Refreshment and renewal for Body, Mind and Spirit

For our 1994 colour brochure phone 01494-782720

New Day Dawning
71 Benwell Road, London N7 7BW.
(0171) 607 2367
Offer cruises into ancient Egypt with like-minded people. £750 including flight and two weeks full board.

Oak Dragon Camps
PO Box 5, Castle Cary, Somerset BA7 7YQ.
(01269) 870959/550225
Run a yearly series of outdoor, educational camps centred around various subjects such as spirituality, myth, creative arts, healing and green issues for both adults and children. Camp facilities include vegetarian food, children's funspace, hot showers, etc. Each day there is a camp pow-wow, workshops in marquees, ongoing practical projects, celebrations and spontaneously arising events. Numbers limited to 70-100 people. £70 - £95 for 8 days adults, small charge for children. Half price for low incomes.

Skyros Centre
92 Prince of Wales Road, London NW5 2NE.
(0171) 267 4424 / 431 0867
Situated on the beautiful Greek island of Skyros, Skyros holidays provide a unique adventure for the mind, the body and the spirit. There are two centres on the island of Skyros - Atsitsa and the Skyros Centre. Atsitsa, situated right by the sea in the pine forested Atsitsa bay aims at relaxing and revitalising the whole person. Activities include yoga, massage, tai chi, windsurfing, dance, meditation, and much more at approximately £490 (depending

on season) which includes courses, accommodation and full board, flight not included. Skyros Centre is situated in the heart of Skyros village and offers a more intensive programme, focusing on personal development courses such as psychodrama, gestalt, bioenergectics at approximately £450, includes courses accommodation and half board, flight not included. Skros now offers writers workshops led by distinguished and respected authors such as D. M. Thomas, Hugo Williams and Bernice Rubens. All the courses and workshops are run by some of the world's most experienced facilitators. Prices given are for two weeks.

Sunra
26 Balham Hill, Clapham South, London SW12 9EB.
(0181) 675 9224
Health holidays in the sun. £520 including flight for two week holiday. Yoga and meditation and massage. Also yoga holidays in the UK.

Synthesis of Light Holidays (SOL)
112 Wood Vue, Spennymoor, Co Durham DL16 6RZ.
(01388) 818151
Yoga holidays in India and USA. Spiritual tours of India. Also Greek and South American holistic holidays. £125-£290 per week. Bursaries available at short notice.

Vinyasa Yoga
17 De Montfort, Merley, Wimborne, Dorset BH21 1TG.
(01202) 842853
Two week yoga vacations in Southern Greece. £395-£450.

Whole Life Holidays
Fox Hole, Dartington, Totnes, Devon TQ9 6EB.
(01803) 867075

LECTURES

Alternatives
St James's Church, 197 Piccadilly, London W1V 9LF.
(0171) 287 6711
This is a project dedicated to providing a platform for New Age ideas - creative and spiritual alternatives to currently accepted Western thought. It does this through a regular lecture series incorporating topics such as new age, new science, psychology, green issues, workshops, meditations, sacred dance and celebration. It also provides a counselling service for other New Age groups, advising them how to start their own projects or helping them with any group dynamics problems. A healing centre is also located at St. James's.

Centre for Creation Spirituality
St James's Church, 197 Piccadilly, London W1V 9LF.
(0171) 734 4511 (2-5pm)
The centre has a programme of workshops, talks and courses on green issues, sexuality, spirituality, creativity etc. £4, concs £2. Workshops £20 per day.

Hahnemann College of Homoeopathy

243 The Broadway, Southhall, Middlesex UB1 1NF.
(0181) 574 4281
Lectures on homoeopathy are held at the Polytechnic of Central London, 35 Marylebone Road, London, on alternative Sundays.

Rainbow Ark

PO Box 486, London SW1P 1AZ.
(0171) 738 4296
They operate 'Vision Network', organising lectures, workshops, discussions groups and social events covering ecology, new age, alternative medicine, animal welfare issues.

Turning Points

Office: 21a Goldhurst Terrace, London NW6 3HB.
(0171) 625 8804
Tuesdays 7-10pm. Established in 1982, originally at St James's, Piccadilly, then branching out to include other venues in central London, Wales and Greece. Topics include personal and planetary change, healing, creativity, men and women, etc. Light refreshments are served and there is time for socialising. Workshops and conferences. Sell tapes and books. Wheelchair access sometimes. £3 per evening, £25-£30 per day. Concessions.

FESTIVALS

Animal Aid

The Old Chapel, Bradford St, Tonbridge, Kent TN9 1AW.
(01732) 364546
Aim to promote lifestyle free of cruelty to animals and in connection to this which does not exploit humans/environment. Primary activities are education and raising public awareness. Organise a 3 day 'Living Without Cruelty' exhibition held at Kensington Town Hall, London in June each year.

Dimensions Promotions

2 Stag Cottage, Chapel St, Milborne St Andrew, Nr Blandford, Dorset DT11 0JP.
(01258) 837720
Established 1991. Aim to education the general public primarily to spread the word of 'the New Age'; to provide a platform for traditional crafts, new age therapies etc. All lectures and workshops are free to attend. Craft, new age and ecology festivals, incorporating traditional handmade crafts, new age practitioners, new age and ecological goods for sale and various readers. Areas served are Dorset and Avon. Held March, May, October, November. Regular events lasting 2 days.

Vision Associates

134 Leicester Road, Groby, Leics LE6.
(0116) 2870780

New Life Promotions

170 Campden Hill Road, London W8 7AS.
(0171) 938 3788
Organise 1) Festival for Mind, Body, Spirit (May bank holiday

weekend)- the original 'New Age' festival which has been going for 13 years. Covers natural health, personal growth, spiritual/ philosophical organisations, psychic arts, ecology, crafts and products. As well as the stalls, there's an ongoing programme of lectures, demonstrations and workshops. 2) The Healing Arts (usually held in November). Alternative medicine and complementary therapies exhibition - therapies, products, training bodies etc. Lectures and workshops, and a physical therapy room where a team of bodyworkers will give you a taste of the technique of your choice.

Sirius Fairs
Golsoncott Cottage, Golsoncott, Rodhuish, Minehead, Somerset TA24 6QZ.
(01984) 40005
Run the Bath and West of England Body, Mind and Soul fair in July. Alternative medicine, green issues, divination.

P&O Events
Earls Court Exhibition Centre, Warwick Road, London SW5 9TA.
(0171) 370 8185
Organise The Natural Health Show usually held in June at the National Hall at Olympia (NOT at Earls Court, even though the address of the organisers is there) . Covers green living, fitness, beauty and healthy eating as well as natural remedies and therapies.

GALLERIES

Freud Museum
20 Maresfield Gardens, Hampstead, London NW3.
(0171) 435 2002
The museum was the home of Sigmun Freud, the founder of psychoanalysis, who lived, worked and died here after he and his family left Nazi-occupied Vienna as refugees in 1938. On view are rooms containing original furniture, paintings, photographs, letters, and personal effects of Freud and his daughter Anna. Of particular interest is Freud's study and library with his famous couch and his large collection of Egyptian, Roman and Oriental antiquities. Exhibitions and archive film programmes are also on view. There is also a bookshop. Admission is £2.50 for adults, £1.50 for students, free for children under 12. Open Wednesday - Sunday, noon till 5pm. Finchley Road tube.

CLUBS AND DANCES

Woodie's
1 Parke Road, London SW13 9NF.
(0171) 603 4594
Weekly boogie in London. Held at 416 Holloway Road, London N7

Whirl-y-gig
(0181) 864 6760
Weekly dance every Saturday night at 8pm-12pm. for people of all ages. Light show, cafe, face painting

and world music. Prices £7, £5 concs.

HELP

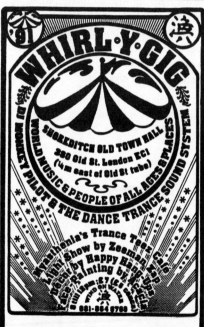
ORGANISATIONS FOR SPECIFIC PROBLEMS

Alternative Centre
The White House, Roxby Place, Fulham, London SW6 1RS.
(0171) 381 2298
Specialise in the treatment of psoriasis and eczema.

Cancer Help Centre
Grove House, Cornwallis Grove, Clifton, Bristol BS8 4PG.
(0117) 9743216
Provides a complementary/holistic approach to cancer, which can be used alongside orthodox medical treatment. Programme includes counselling, dietry advice, relaxation and meditation, healing by touch. Patients can make day visits or stay over a longer period and participate in both one-to-one and groups sessions, and are put in touch with local support group. Fees are £100 for patient plus one relative for initial day, £25 for subsequent days. £605 for one week patient, £165 for one week relative. Two bursaries available, one for day and one for residential patients.

CHI Centre
Riverbank House, Putney Bridge Approach, Fulham, London SW6 3JD.
(0171) 371 9717
Clinic specialising in the treatment of eczema, acne, psoriasis, dermatitis and other skin conditions through Chinese herbal medicine. Consultants are two Professors from China.

Fellowship of Sports Masseurs and Therapists

B M Soigneur, London WC1N 3XX.
(0181) 886 3120
Run training courses for those wishing to become masseurs for sportspeople.

New Approaches To Cancer

5 Larksfield, Egham, Surrey TW20 0RB.
(01784) 433610
A registered charity which promotes the benefits of holistic and self-help methods of healing to cancer patients.

St James Centre for Health and Healing

197 Piccadilly, London W1V 9LF.
(0171) 734 4511
As well as offering a range of therapies and counselling, St James centre also runs free cancer support groups.

Traditional Chinese Medicine Clinic

10 Sandown Way, Northolt, Middx UB5 4HY.
(0181) 743 0706
Specialise in treating gynaecological problems and cancer patients that cannot be treated by othodox medicine. Appointment only. Patients are seen by Dr Hsu who also trys to prevent the side effects of western drugs on cancer patients. Children's problems also treated. First visit £55, subsequent visits £35. Unemployed and low waged get up to 25% discount.

Wandsworth Cancer Support Centre

PO Box 17, 20-22 York Rd, London SW11 3QE.
(0171) 924 3924
A cancer support centre offering one-to-one counselling and massage courses. Newsletter and resource library. Drop in support group for people under 40 with cancer. Offer a holistic approach to those with cancer utilising a wide range of complementary therapies which can be used alongside orthodox medicine. Run courses in relaxation and visualisation, workshops, on-going groups, counselling service, offer healing and massage, also workshops for health professionals. There are also books, tapes, periodicals and videos about cancer available on loan to members. Established 1983.

PRODUCTS

There are a whole range of holistic products on the market. Below we list places or businesses where you can buy them. The list includes either shops or businesses that offer a mail order service.

AIR PURIFIERS

Air Improvement Centre
23 Denbigh Street
London SW1V 2HF. (0171) 834 2834.
Mon-Fri 9.30-5.30. Sat10-1. Showroom stocking and supplying a wide range of air improvement products by different manufacturers. As well as air purifiers and ionisers, also stock humidifiers, dehumidifiers and mobile air conditioners. Also have stands in the electrical departments of Harrods and Selfidges.

AROMATHERAPY OILS

Aromatherapy oils or 'essential' oils are extracted from plants, flowers or trees and used in aromatherapy (see relevant entry in 'Body' section). Aromatherapy has recently become extremely popular and essential oils have even started appearing in some high street chain stores, often accompanied by leaflets on self-help use. However, while food and herbal medicine are regulated to a certain extent in terms of contents, standards and quality, at present there is no official standard by which the purity of essential oils can be measured, though some reputable essential oils manufucturers are now looking at this problem. The quality of the plants used and the conditions they have been grown in also affect the therapeutic potency of the oils. For instance, if artificial fertilizers or pesticides have been used, the oils could be adulterated with toxins. The best means of extracting the oils is through distillation, but adulteration can also take place in this process of extraction. Furthermore, the oils are suspended in vegetable oils and some manufacturers may dilute their oils much more than others, so it is difficult to tell which oils are good value for money. Some products called aromatherapy oils may not even contain the plant essence they are named after, because synthetic oils can be produced which contain the same active substances and smell the same as the original oil.

Perhaps the best way to ensure the quality of oils is to buy from a supplier with a background in aromatherapy, or those who work closely with consultant trained aromatherapists. Get information from them about their oils, how they ensure quality and ask about dilution ratios.

Aromatique
Sarnett House, Repton Drive
Gidea Park, Essex RM2 5LP. (01708) 720289.
Mail order. Cosmetics and toiletries containing essential oils for different skin and hair conditions.

Cosmos Herbs
329 Chiswick High Road
London W4 4HS. (0181) 995 7239.
11am-6pm Mon-Sat. Medicinal herbs and remedies sold, as well as occult ritual supplies and an intriguing range of incense and oils (from Luv Luv Luv oil to Graveyard dust). Member of British Herbal Medicine Association. Mail order available.

Baldwin and Co
173 Walworth Road, Camberwell
London SE17 1RW. (0171) 703 5550.

Institute of Clinical Aromatherapy
22 Bromley Road , Catford
London SE6 2TP. (0181) 690 2149.
Mail order essential oils and vegetable oils.

Hermitage Oils
East Morton
Keighley BD20 5UQ. (01274) 565957.
Retail and wholesale. Extensive range of oils of different qualities. Rapid turn round on orders. Telephone above number or send SAE for list and order form.

Fleur
Pembroke Studios
Pembroke Road
Muswell Hill
London N10 2JE. (0181) 444 7424.
Can visit by appointment. They supply new age shops, health food shops and they do mail order.

Ionisers (UK)
3 Gordon Cresent, Broad Meddows
South Normanton DE55 3AJ. (01773) 863034.
Ionisers range between £39-£495. They also sell a range of about 20 of differnt Aromatherapy oils which are infused with Homoeopathic remedies.

Quinessence
3a Birch Avenue , Whitwick
Leicestershire LE6 3GB. (01530) 838358/180779.
Affiliated to the International Federation of Aromatherapists, mail order essential oils and essential oil remedies, ready mixed lotions and massage oils, vaporisers and mood enhancers - from 'wild passion' to 'celestial dream' ! Free advice service from qualified aromatherapist.

Neal's Yard Apothecary
2 Neal's Yard, off Shorts Gardens
London WC2H 9DP. (0171) 379 7222.
Mon, Tues, Thurs 10-6, Wed, Sat 10-5.30. Also at Chelsea Farmers Market, Sydney Street, London SW3 (which is also open Sun 11-4) and 68 Chalk Farm Road, London NW1. (0171) 284 2039. Cosmetics and toiletries, nutritional supplements, essential oils, herbal tinctures (including Chinese), medicinal herbs and powders, gifts. Nice line in naturally scented vegetable oil soaps, and toiletries and preprations packed in cute blue bottled.

Micheline Arcier Aromatherapy
7 William Street, Knightsbridge
London SW1X 9HL. (0171) 235 3545 .
The shop sells face oils, body oils and bath oils made from essential oils.

Shirley Price Aromatherapy Ltd.
Essentia House, Upper Bond Street, Hinckley
Leicestershire LE10 1RS. (01455) 615466.
Comprehensive range of essential oils and aromatherapy skin care. Mail order.

Falcons
25 Kite House, Grant Road
London SW11 2NJ. (0171) 585 3445.
Can supply essential oils, not only to students on their courses, but any others interested.

Holistic Aromatherapy Practice
10 Bamborough Gardens
London W12 8QN. (0181) 743 9485.
Organic Essential oils, organic Aromatherapy blended oils, Carrier oils. All oils are organic, gas liquid chromatography tested, each oil has details of origin, nature, laboratory reports etc. Also available are relaxation tapes etc. Mail order only - send for free catalogue.

Verde
75 Northcote Road
London SW11 6PL. (0171) 924 4379.
This little known shop sell only their own brand of essential oils which are of excellent quality. Worth a visit.

Frames and Fragrance
83 Kingsgate Road
London NW6 4JY. (0171) 372 6621.
A shop selling picture frames, candles and essential oils.

Id Aromatics
12 New Station Street, Leeds
West Yorkshire LS1 5DL. (0113) 2424983.
Over 90 essential oils and over 90 perfume oils in stock, pot pourris, candles.

Kobashi
50 High St, Ide, Exeter
Devon EX2 9RW. (01392) 217628.
Supply pure essential oils, massage oils, bases to be used with oils. Burners, light bulb rings, gift pack, books and posters. Organic liquid soaps and shampoos.

Talimantra Aromatherapy Supplies
19 Allwood Road, Cheshunt
Herts EN7 6UA. (01992) 640665.
Mail order service as well as being a wholesaler. Supply pure essential oils, massage oils, bases to be used with oils. Burners, light bulb rings, gift pack, books and posters. Organic liquid soaps and shampoos.

Visionaries
97 Caledonian Road, Kings Cross
London N1 9BT. (0171) 278 8481.
All their products have a fantasy, mystic and new age theme. Trade catalogue available on request. Showroom/Cash and Carry open Mon-Fri 10am to 6pm.

ASTROLOGY PRODUCTS

Equinox
The Astrology Shop, 78 Neal St
London WC2.
Specialise in astrological and heavenly goods. This is also the base for Equinox, computer generated star charts. They aim to provide goods and services connected with astrology and celebrating the glory of the heavens.

BACK PRODUCTS

Alternative Sitting
PO Box 19, Chipping Norton
Oxford OX7 6NY. (01608) 658875.
Specialists in work and domestic ergonomic problems. Sell ergonomic furniture.

Back Store Ltd
330 King Street, Hammersmith
London W6. (0181) 741 5022.
Mon-Fri 10-6, Sats 10-4. Everything for the back is here. Allow yourself some time to choose.

Back Shop
24 New Cavendish Street
London W1M 7LH. (0171) 935 9120.
10am-6pm Mon-Sat. All manner of things for the back are here including chairs, pillows, beds, shoes, exercise equipment and meditation stools which give correct support to the back, and even a 'massage pillow' — a cushion which vibrates to give you your own portable massage. Also books, videos, mail order

Pelvic Support Chairs
New Mill Lane, Eversley
Hants RG27 0RA. (01734) 732365.
Pelvic support chairs, car accessories and the Nada chair - not really a chair but a portable back support sling.

Banana Chair Company
Barton Road, Long Eaton
Nottingham NG10 2FN. (0115) 9464799.
Sell the 'banana chair'. A revolutionary version of a rocking chair, but designed to be easy on the back.

Wholistic Research Company
Bright Haven, Robin's Lane, Lolworth
Cambridge CB3 8HH. (01954) 781074.

BIOFEEDBACK MACHINES

Biofeedback machines are electrical equipment which give information about mood and state of mind through either measuring brain wave patterns or muscle tension. The machine has to be in contact in some way with the body and measures physical changes which reflect emotional or mental changes. The so-called lie detector is an example of the biofeedback machine, as is equipment used to measure the brain wave frequency of, for instance, people meditating.

Biomonitors
26-28 Wendell Road
London W12. (0181) 749 3983.
Several machines designed to measure brainwave frequencies and monitor states of mind. Also manufacture the therapeutic strobe to alter mood.

John Bell and Croyden
Medical Dept., 54 Wigmore Street
London W1. (0171) 935 5555.
Biofeedback machines that also have instruction tapes attached to them. They also have a wide range of aids for disabled people.

Life Tools
Sunrise House, Hulley Road
Macclesfield SK10 2LP. (01625) 502602.
'Mind' machines for relaxation and accelerated learning are all available at excellent trade prices. Also supply a range of relaxing music tapes.

BIRTHING POOLS

These are (usually circular or oval) pools filled with water in which women can give birth. Giving birth in water is said to ease the pain of contractions and provide an enviroment in which women can relax in the favoured position for active birth, crouching or kneeling. The agencies listed below provide pools for hire or sale.

Active Birth Centre
55 Dartmouth Park Road, Kentish Town
London NW5 1SL. (0171) 267 5368.
Hire out portable water birth pools. Ring for catalogue.

Jaya's Company
Unit 4E, Brent Mill Trading Estate
South Brent
Devon TQ10 9YT. (01364) 73909
Available for sale or hire at £35 per week. Two types available: circular one which can be dismantled, and fixed rectangular one for hospitals.

Splashdown Birth Pools
17 Wellington Terrace
Harrow-on-the-Hill
Middlesex HA1 3EP. (0181) 904 0202.
Water birth pools for hire or sale, with a choice of round and oval. Pools measure 5ft in diameter by 26 ins deep. £125 plus £20 for sterilised liner for four weeks standby hire. Door -to-door delivery anywhere in the UK. Free advice and information packs on water birth to enquirers, free water birth workshops. Sell and loan books and cassettes.

Birthing Tub Company
Pakyns Lodge, Albourne Road, Hurstpierpoint
W Sussex BN6 9ET. (01273) 835245.
Manufacturers and suppliers of portable, collapsable, wooden water pools for use in labour and childbirth. The cost including delivery and return to anywhere in the U.K. is £150 for a period of two weeks before the birth until a suitable time afterwards.

CANDLES

Id Aromatics
12 New Station Street, Leeds
West Yorkshire LS1 5DL. (0113) 2424983.
Over 90 essential oils and over 90 perfume oils in stock, pot pourris, candles.

Visionaries
97 Caledonian Road, Kings Cross
London N1 9BT. (0171) 278 8481.
All their products have a fantasy, mystic and new age theme. Trade catalogue available on request. Showroom/Cash and Carry open Mon-Fri 10am to 6pm.

CARDS

Oakapple
Lanhams Buildings
High St, St. Ives
Cornwall TR26 1RS. (01736) 798493.
Provide greetings cards, mainly wholesale, but also through mail order. 'Oakapple is a concept providing Keith English with a vehicle to bring spiritual truths, teachings, love and light to fellow travellers on their paths to ultimate enlightenment.

Little Gem
8 High Street, Glastonbury
Somerset BA6 9DU. (01458) 831116.
New Age greeting Cards

Moon Garden
5 Tunnel Terrace, Newport
Gwent NP9 4BT. (01633) 267164.
Alternative greeting cards with green/pagan/mythic themes. Mail order as well as wholesale.

Agency (The)
2D Jerrard Drive, Sutton Coldfield
West Midlands B75 7TR. (0121) 311 1440.
Market the now famous 'astro-cards'.

CEREMONIAL PRODUCTS

Windhorse Imports
PO Box 7, Hay-on-Wye
Hereford HR3 5TU. (01497) 821116 .
Aim to provide Buddhist objects for meditation practise and shrine objects, plus Tibetan ethnic jewellery, incense etc. This includes crystals, wool shawls, Buddha images, healing incense, cymbals, brocades, etc.

Zam Trading
330 Caledonian Road
London N1 1BB. (0171) 700 0334.
Buddhist books and images. Tibetan singing bowls, ritual objects, jewellery and textiles.

CRYSTALS

Crystal 2000
37 Bromley Road, St Annes-on-Sea
Lancs FY8 1PQ. (01253) 723735.
Also crystal light torches for colour crystal healing and crystal light boxes.

Kernowcraft
Bolingey, Perranporth
Cornwall TR6 0DH. (01872) 573888.
Mail order supplier, retail and wholesale. Precious and semi-precious stones, crystals, available also in bead form. Mounts, chains and fastenings for jewellery making, as well as silversmithing equipment. Pyramids, spheres, obelisks, wands, standing points etc. - ask for the crystal list when applying for information.

Rainbow Gems
6 Rookwood Court, Castlewood Road
London N16 6DR. (0181) 802 9196.
Rainbow gems trades on Saturday and Sunday from 9.30-6 at Camden Lock market, and as well as a selection of crystals and minerals both polished and natural sells pyramids, spheres, eggs and wands. Also do gem elixiers.

Aurora
16A Neal's Yard, Covent Garden
London WC2. (0171) 379 5972.
Open Mon-Sat 10-6. This shop is open to the public and stocks a wide range of natural quartz crystals, dowsing pendulums, rainbow crystal jewellery and balls, cards and posters and 'New Age' music and videos. Also mail order.

Snapdragon
12 South Park, Sevenoaks
Kent TN13 1AN. (01732) 740252.
mystical cards, tarot cards, crystal balls, special incense, healing pendants, pendulums. Keep a list of alternative medicine practitioners in the area. Tapes for healing.

RESOURCES

Wessex Impex Ltd

Stonebridge Farmhouse
Breadsell Lane, Crowhurst
St Leonards on Sea
East Sussex TN38 8EB. (01424) 830 659.
Visitors by appointment only please.
Importers of rough crystals,
manufacturers of crystal jewellery,
gemmologists, lapidaries, wholesale and
retail.

Charlie's Rock Shop

Merton Abbey Mills, Wimbledon
London SW19 2RD. (0181) 544 1207.
This shop is set within a large craft market
in South London and sells a large selection
of crystals as well as music tapes, video tapes,
native American products, ceremonial
products and figurines.

Paradise Farm

182A Kings Road
London SW3. (0171) 376 5264.
This shop is open to the public and stocks a
wide range of natural quartz crystals,
dowsing pendulums, rainbow crystal
jewellery and balls, cards and posters and
new age music and videos. Also mail order.

Latitude

Peel House, Peel Road, Skelmersdale
Lancs WN8 9PT. (01695) 23207.
Large and constantly changing range of
silver jewellery from various parts of the
world. Also specialise in crystals and semi-
precious stones. Free catalogue available
upon request.

Everlasting Gems

46 Lower Green Road, Esher
Surrey KT10 8HD. (0181) 398 7252.
Large and constantly changing range of
silver jewellery from various parts of the
world. Also specialise in crystals and semi-
precious stones. Free catalogue available
upon request.

DAYLIGHT BULBS

Otherwise known as full spectrum lighting,
this is used to treat seasonal affective disorder
(shortened to 'SAD') which is a form of
depression caused by lack of sunlight, and
which some people get in the winter. The
lack of sunlight affects the pineal gland,
which starts to secrete too much of a hormone
called melatonin, which causes depression.

Full Spectrum Lighting

Unit 1, Riverside Business Centre
Victoria St, High Wycombe
Bucks HP11 2LT. (01494) 526051.
Bulbs fitted with full spectrum light,
particularly for the alleviation of Seasonal
Affective Disorder (SAD) or 'Winter
Depression', now a recognised medical
condition that can be helped by expsoure to
a light level of 2500 lux which accurately
simulates the spectrum of natural day light.

Hygeia College of Colour Therapy

Brook House
Avening
Tetbury
Gloucestershire GL8 8NS. (0145383) 2150.
Health-oriented illumination: lamps, true-
lite tubes. Also colour therapy instruments.

EAR CANDLES

Biosun

Sheepcoates Lane, Great Totham
Maldon, Essex CM9 8NT. (01621) 788411.
Sell Hopi ear candles.

FLOAT TANKS

South London Natural Health Centre
7A Clapham Common South Side
Clapham Common
London SW4 7AA. (0171) 720 9506/8817
Phone 720 9506 for Gracemill Ltd who are manufacturers and installers of the 'ocean float room'.

Float Centre
20 Blenheim Terrace
St Johns Wood
London NW8 OEB. (0171) 328 7276.
Sell the 'Open Float Room' ™, which is 8ft high x 8ft long x 4ft wide. They can be custom built to suit your premises. Provide staff training and back up consultancy to those interested in starting up their own commercial centre. Staff training on how to run a float centre - £225 per day incl VAT.

FOOD/FOOD SUPPLEMENTS

3HO Kundalini Yoga Foundation
55 Sunny Gardens Road
London NW4 1SJ. (0181) 203 7302.
Sell their famous 'Yogi Tea'.

Chlorella Health
4th Floor, Russell Chambers
Covent Garden, WC2E 8AA. (0171) 240 4775.
Sell algae tablets for detoxifiction purposes.

Nutri
Buxton Road
New Mills
Stockport
Cheshire SK12 3JU. (01663) 746559.
Nutritional supplements.

GAMES

Trading Centre
Findhorn Foundation
The Park
Forres IV36 0TZ. (01309) 691074.
Produce the Transformation Game: "a playful yet substantial way of understanding and transforming the way you play your life. Just as life is filled with insights, setbacks, pain and miracles, so is the Transformation Game. It mirrors players lives, highlighting strenghts, identifying blind spots and bringing fresh perspectives to current challenges". Also sell Angel cards, nature and tree calendar, tree diary.

HEALTH AIDS

Dove Healthcare Ltd.
2 West Road, Weaverham
Cheshire CW8 3HQ. (01606) 854684.
No needle acupuncture kits.

Earthdust Products
46 Wainfleet Road, Skegness
Lincolnshire PE25 3QT. (01754) 768336.

HERBS AND HERBAL REMEDIES

Culpeper Herbalists
8 The Market
Covent Garden Piazza
London WC2. (0171) 379 6698.
Mon-Sat 10-8, Sun 11.30-7. Range of herbs, also cruelty free toiletries.

Cosmos Herbs
329 Chiswick High Road
London W4 4HS. (0181) 995 7239.
11am-6pm Mon-Sat. Medicinal herbs and remedies sold, as well as occult ritual supplies and an intruiging range of incense and oils (from Luv Luv Luv oil to Graveyard dust). Member of British Herbal Medicine Association. Mail order available.

RESOURCES

Herbalists
74 Lee High Road
London SE13. (0181) 852 9792.
They have been established since 1926.
Open between 8.30 am-5.15pm for
consultations.

East Asia Company
101 - 103 Camden High Street, Camden
London. (0171) 388 5783 or 388 6704.
Wide range of books on Alternative Medicine
as well as books on general health,symptom
alleviation, natural living, oriental
philosophy and lifestyle. They do charts
(such as reflexology charts) on health for
practitioners as well as for the public. Sell
herbal and homoeopathic remedies.

Neal's Yard Apothecary
2 Neal's Yard, off Shorts Gardens
London WC2H 9DP. (0171) 379 7222.
Mon, Tues, Thurs 10-6, Wed, Sat 10-5.30.
Also at Chelsea Farmers Market, Sydney
Street, London SW3 (which is also open Sun
11-4) and 68 Chalk Farm Road, London
NW1. (071) 284 2039. Cosmetics and toiletries, nutritional supplements, essential oils,
herbal tinctures (including Chinese), medicinal herbs and powders, gifts. Nice line in
naturally scented vegetable oil soaps, and
toiletries and preprations packed in cute
blue bottled.

Bach Flower Remedies Ltd
Dr Bach Centre, Mount Vernon
Sotwell, Wallingford,
Oxon OX10 0PZ. (01491) 833712.
Sell a range of Bach flower remedies. If you
wish to place an order then send to Bach
Flower Remedies, Unit 6, Suffolk Way,
Drayton Road, Abingdon, Oxon OX14 5JX.

CHI Centre
Riverbank House, Putney Bridge Approach
Fulham, London SW6 3JD. (0171) 371 9717.
Manufacturers (and suppliers) of a range of
skin care products, especially helpful for
sensitive skins, and balms for aches, strains,
insect bites etc. Everthing handmade in the
UK from Chinese Herbs. Further information and price list available on request.

Earth Force
The Beeches, 20 Ballygraffan Road
Comber, Co. Down
Northern Ireland BT23 5SU. (01247) 873797.
Sell 'Planetary Formulaes'. High quality vitamin/herbal products.

HOMOEOPATHIC PHARMACIES

Ainsworths Homoeopathic Pharmacy
38 New Cavendish Street
London W1M 7LH. (0171) 935 5330/(018833)
40332.
Same day postal supply of all traditional
homoeopathic medicines including many
novel remedies. Veterinary remedies as well.

E Gould and Son
14 Crowndale Road
London NW1 1TT. (0171) 388 4752.
Mon-Fri 9-5.45. Closed Sats. Open Sun am.

East Asia Company
101 - 103 Camden High Street
Camden, London
(0171) 388 5783 or 388 6704.
Wide range of books on Alternative Medicine as well as books on general
health,symptom alleviation, natural living,
oriental philosophy and lifestyle. They do
charts (such as reflexology charts) on health
for practitioners as well as for the public.
Sell herbal and homoeopathic remedies.

Noma (Complex Homoepathy) Ltd
Unit 3, 1-16 Hollybrook Road, Upper Shirley
Southampton SO16 6RB. (01703) 770513.
Acupuncture and homoeopathy equipment.

INCENSE

Moksha
7 Hillview, Churchill
Oxon OX7 6NQ. (01608) 658937.
Quality Tibetan incense.

Tutankamen
Tasburgh Hall, Low Road
Tasburgh, Norfolk NR15 1LT. (01508) 471405.
Incense.

Visionaries
97 Caledonian Road, Kings Cross
London N1 9BT. (0171) 278 8481.
All their products have a fantasy, mystic and new age theme. Trade catalogue available on request. Showroom/Cash and Carry open Mon-Fri 10am to 6pm.

JEWELLERY

Kernowcraft
Bolingey, Perranporth
Cornwall TR6 0DH. (01872) 573888.
Mail order supplier, retail and wholesale. Precious and semi-precious stones, crystals, available also in bead form. Mounts, chains and fastenings for jewellery making, as well as silversmithing equipment. Pyramids, spheres, obelisks, wands, standing points etc. - ask for the crystal list when applying for information.

Rainbow Gems
6 Rookwood Court, Castlewood Road
London N16 6DR. (0181) 802 9196.
Rainbow gems trades on Saturday and Sunday from 9.30-6 at Camden Lock market, and as well as a selection of crystals and minerals both polished and natural sells pyramids, spheres, eggs and wands. Also do gem elixiers.

Aurora
16A Neal's Yard, Covent Garden
London WC2. (0171) 379 5972.
Open Mon-Sat 10-6. This shop is open to the public and stocks a wide range of natural quartz crystals, dowsing pendulums, rainbow crystal jewellery and balls, cards and posters and 'New Age' music and videos. Also mail order.

Wessex Impex Ltd
Stonebridge Farmhouse
Breadsell Lane, Crowhurst
St Leonards on Sea
East Sussex TN38 8EB. (01424) 830 659.
Visitors by appointment only please. Importers of rough crystals, manufacturers of crystal jewellery, gemmologists, lapidaries, wholesale and retail.

Latitude
Peel House, Peel Road
Skelmersdale
Lancs WN8 9PT. (01695) 23207.
Large and constantly changing range of silver jewellery from various parts of the world. Also specialise in crystals and semi-precious stones. Free catalogue available upon request.

Hames Enterprises
Woodbine Cottage
Old Mill Lane
Oldbury, Bridgnorth
Shropshire WV16 5EQ. (01746) 763056.
Supply a Dutch silver magnet pendant that equalises out your excess negative and positive body tensions.

Wild Goose Studio
66 Lower O'Connell St
Kinsale, County Cork .
Cast iron, bronze sculptures and wall plaques of celtic crosses, animals and birds, celtic myths and symbols of transformation.

JUICERS

Juicers extract the juices of fruit, vegetables and sometimes of herbs and plants. Consuming fresh juice is a way of ingesting high doses of nurtrients for therapeutic purposes - for instance in the Gerson cancer therapy diet which features fresh juice as part of the detoxification process. Many healthy people also like to drink juice, because they feel it helps to maintain good health.

There are different types of juicer. Centrifugal juicers grate the fruit or vegetable and then spin the pulp, forcing the juice out by centrifugal force. These are the cheapest juicers, but they tend not to extract such a high level of nutrients as other models. Nose cone pressure juicers break down the material with a cutter or masticator. This is then forced into a cone under high pressure, and the juice is forced out. This method produces juice which is rich in nutrients, but it is more expensive than the centrifugal juicer. With juice presses the material is first pulped, then put into a strong nylon cloth which retains the pulp when the juice is squeezed out by a press.

Wholistic Research Company
Bright Haven
Robin's Lane
Lolworth
Cambridge CB3 8HH. (01954) 781074.

MARTIAL ARTS SUPPLIERS

Dragon Martial Arts
128 Myddleton Road
London N22 4NQ. (0181) 889 0965.
Weds, Thurs, Sats 9.30-5.30. Books, equipment, suits and martial arts weaponry.

Shaolin Way
10 Little Newport Street
London WC2. (0171) 734 6391.
A shop which sells martial arts supplies of different designs. 11-7pm seven days a week.

MASSAGE AIDS

Back Shop
24 New Cavendish Street
London W1M 7LH. (0171) 935 9120.
10am-6pm Mon-Sat. All manner of things for the back are here including chairs, pillows, beds, shoes, exercise equipment and meditation stools which give correct support to the back, and even a 'massage pillow' — a cushion which vibrates to give you your own portable massage. Also books, videos, mail order

NATIVE AMERICAN PRODUCTS

Latitude
Peel House, Peel Road, Skelmersdale
Lancs WN8 9PT. (01695) 23207.
Large and constantly changing range of silver jewellery from various parts of the world. Also specialise in crystals and semi-precious stones. Free catalogue available upon request.

NUTRITIONAL SUPPLEMENTS

Emerald Life
5 Cheyne Place, Suite 4
London SW3 4HH. (0171) 352 5665.
Sell 'Chlorella' which is a natural medicinal algae. It is a rich source of protein, chlorophyll, vitamins, minerals and is claimed to stregthen the immune system and aid in detoxification. Mail order only.

ORGANIC WINE

Organic wine is made from grapes grown without chemical fertilisers or weedkillers, and which have not been sprayed with insecticide. To earn the name of organic, no synthetic additives should be used to preserve or flavour the wine. Farmers and producers of organic wine should use only ecologically sound techniques. Wine-producing countries have their own bodies which lay down guidelines for organic wine and monitor its production. Bottles of organic wine will display the symbol of approval by such a body as proof of their integrity.

Available now in addition to wine, are organic beers and spirits. Enthusiasts claim that drinks grown organically are less likely to cause hangovers because they don't contain harmful additives. However, this is a claim which hasn't as yet been put to clinical trials!

Organics
290 Fulham Palace Road
London SW6 6HP. (0171) 381 9924.

Vinceremos Wines
Unit 10, Ashley Industrial Estate
Wakefield Road, Ossett
West Yorkshire WF5 9JD.
Range of organic wines, beers and spirits from around the world including rum from Cuba, Armenian brandy and sparkling white wine from India. Prices start from £2.85 per bottle.

Vintage Roots
Sheeplands Farm, Wargrave Road
Wargrave
Berkshire RG10 8DT. (01734) 401222
Range of organic wines mostly from France and include the French 'classics'. They are planning to stock organic beer and vinegar in the near future. Also able to provide wines that are suitable for vegtarians, and some wines that are also bio-dynamic.

TAPES - PERSONAL DEVELOPMENT

Dharmachakra Tapes
PO Box 50
Cambridge CB5 8EG. (01223) 460 252.
Taped lectures by Ven. Sangharakshita, founder of Friends of the Western Buddhist Order, on many aspects of Buddhism.

New World Cassettes
Paradise Farm, Westhall,
Halesworth
Suffolk IP19 8RH. (01986) 781682, (0986) 781642 wholesale.
Music for relaxation, inspiration and pure listening pleasure. 'Audio and video recordings to create positive changes in your life'.

Aurora
16A Neal's Yard, Covent Garden
London WC2. (0171) 379 5972.
Open Mon-Sat 10-6. This shop is open to the public and stocks a wide range of natural quartz crystals, dowsing pendulums, rainbow crystal jewellery and balls, cards and posters and 'New Age' music and videos. Also mail order.

SCWL
55 Kellner Road
London SE28 0AX. (0171) 630 7732 or (0181) 855 8575.

Triangle Truth Ltd
PO Box 89
London SE3 7JN. (0181) 305 2317.
Series of tapes on on subjects such as forgiveness, weight loss, confidence, prosperity, relationships etc. £8.95 per tape.

TSA Publishing
23 New Road
Brighton BN1 1WZ. (01273) 693311.
Tapes on the problems of teenage life for worried parents, produced by the Trust for the Study of Adolescence.

New Day Dawning
71 Benwell Road
London N7 7BW. (0171) 607 2367.

RESOURCES

TAPES (MUSIC)

Cloud Nine Music
123 Francis Avenue
Ilford
Essex IT1 1TS. (0181) 478 9992.

Free Flow Music
The Cabin
Donstone
Hereford HR3 6BL. (01981) 550786.
Distribute tapes from Voices of Silence group.

Earthsounds Music
Old Mill
Skeeby
Richmond
North Yorks DL10 5EB. (01748) 825959.
Series include 'Fire of Ritual', 'Seed Thoughts' and 'World Musics'.

Inner Harmonies
Rose Cottage
Draycott
Moreton in the Marsh
Glos. GL56 9LB. (01386) 701252.
Relaxing music from four composers, including "Living Earth' by Annie Locke, copies of which has been presented by a US peace delegation to the Soviet Union.

Elfington Cassettes
The Old Forge Studio, Back Road
Wenhaston, Halesworth
Suffolk IP19 9EP. (01502) 478 678 No answer
The music of Mike Rowland composer of The Fairy Ring, gentle music for relaxation and meditation.

Aurora
16A Neal's Yard, Covent Garden
London WC2. (0171) 379 5972.
Open Mon-Sat 10-6. This shop is open to the public and stocks a wide range of natural quartz crystals, dowsing pendulums, rainbow crystal jewellery and balls, cards and posters and 'New Age' music and videos. Also mail order.

Music Suite Ltd
Cenarth, Newcastle-Emlyn
Dyfed SA38 9JN. (01239) 710594 .
Original compositions by Adrian Wagner, Francis Monkman (ex of 'Curved Air' - remember them?), Prana, and various story tapes. Also offer bulk cassette and video duplicating service, CD and record manufacturing and electronic music studio.

Snapdragon
12 South Park,
Sevenoaks
Kent TN13 1AN. (01732) 740252.
Mystical cards, tarot cards, crystal balls, special incense, healing pendants, pendulums. Keep a list of alternative medicine practitioners in the area. Tapes for healing.

Seventh Wave Music
Vogwell Cottage, Manaton
Devon TQ13 9XD. (01647) 22437.
Uplifting atmospheric music, creating landscapes using sound and rhythm composed by Nigel Shaw. Four albums available.

Labyrinth Distribution
2 Hargrave Place
London N7 0BP. (0171) 267 6154.
Distribute and sell, both wholesale and through mail order, ambient, new age music for relaxation, meditation or for just plain enjoyment. Also authentic indigenous (not ethnic!) music, thus infusing interest and hopefully understanding of the worlds diverse nations and styles.

Paradise Farm
182A Kings Road
London SW3. (0171) 376 5264.
This shop is open to the public and stocks a wide range of natural quartz crystals, dowsing pendulums, rainbow crystal jewellery and balls, cards and posters and new age music and videos. Also mail order.

Eventide Music
P O Box 720, Hemel Hempstead
Herts HP3 9BF. (01442) 217787.
Produce, distribute and promote new instrumental, restful, atmospheric albums.

Monolith Records
119 Swindon Road, Wroughton
Wilts SN4 9AD. (01793) 814946.
Publishers and suppliers of Shamanic music and relaxation tapes.

Dawn Awakening Music
Foxhole, Dartington, Totnes
Devon TQ9 6ED. (01803) 864866.
They aim to supply an ever increasing market with their carefully selected music titles. Aim to supply quality music across the wide spectrum of what is described as 'New Age Music'. Instrumental music.

New World Cassettes
Paradise Farm, Westhall, Halesworth
Suffolk IP19 8RH. (01986) 781682, (01986) 781642 wholesale.
Music for relaxation, inspiration and pure listening pleasure. 'Audio and video recordings to create positive changes in your life'.

Select Music and Video Distribution Ltd
34a Holmethorpe Avenue
Redhill
Surrey RH1 2NN. (01737) 760020.
Distributors of classical music to record retailers. They are setting out to do for music related 'New Age' products.

New Day Dawning
71 Benwell Road
London N7 7BW. (0171) 607 2367.

TAPES (RELAXATION)

New Day Dawning
71 Benwell Road
London N7 7BW. (0171) 607 2367.

VIDEOS

Aurora
16A Neal's Yard
Covent Garden
London WC2. (0171) 379 5972.
Open Mon-Sat 10-6. This shop is open to the public and stocks a wide range of natural quartz crystals, dowsing pendulums, rainbow crystal jewellery and balls, cards and posters and 'New Age' music and videos. Also mail order.

Yoga Dham
67 Pinner Park Ave
North Harrow
Middlesex HA2 6JY. (0181) 428 6691/9402.
Yoga video.

WATER PURIFIERS

If you want to find out what your water contains, apply to your local water authority for a report on its chemical and bacterial composition and compare these levels of metals and chemicals with permitted EC levels. Information on these levels can be obtained from your local water authority or by sending an SAE to **Friends of the Earth**, 26-28 Underwood Street, London N1 7JQ (0171 490 1555). If there are greater levels of impurity than the EC recommendations, then complain to the EC.

Water filters come in jug form, or can be fitted to the tap, or can be plumbed into the water supply pipe. They vary enormously in cost and effectiveness. The cheapest are jug filters which use charcoal to remove unpleasant tastes and smells, especially chlorine. The charcoal must be replaced regularly - usually at least once a month. Tests show that they are not as effective in removing a whole range of toxic pollutants as plumbed-in filters.

Plumbed-in filters can use a variety of methods to extract pollutants and bacteria from the water. Granular silver activated carbon filters remove some chemicals, including chlorine. The silver in this type of filter helps to remove bacteria, though only after the water has been left from 2 to 24 hours. Ultraviolet radiation is used in some filters to kill bacteria, though this is less effective if there is a lot of iron in the water. Microstraining purifiers are the most effective in cleaning water, and only they can really be called 'purifiers' rather than just 'filters'. They work using highly refined filtration and absorption to remove bacteria and chemicals. These systems also use electrokinetic attraction which draws the dissolved impurities to it. Since this then becomes clogged, the filtration unit must be replaced every 1 to 2 years with cartridges available from the supplier.

Aquapure
Suite 9, Richmond Mansions, Denton Road, East Twickenham, Middlesex TW1 2HH
(0181) 829 9010

Alphabetical List of Centres

We have included when possible, information on what each organisation offers and a breakdown of costs, including concessionary rates

3HO Kundalini Yoga Foundation
55 Sunny Gardens Road London NW4 1SJ. (0181) 203 7302.
Spiritual teacher is Yogi Bhajan who is resident in USA and teaches around the world. Many members of 3HO are practising Sikhs. Run evening, weekend courses, seminars, residentials and retreats in France and the USA. Have residential communities and some people involved are natural healing practitioners. They also run a health food business and sell 'Yogi Tea' a healthy tea drink. They offer Yoga.

5 to Midnight
Nappers Crossing, Staverton, South Devon TQ9 6PD. (01803) 762 655.
Ritual theatre, photo therapy. Residential workshops at various locations, some in London. They offer Dance therapy.

Abraxas
27 Bathhurst Mews London W2 2SB. (0171) 402 0290.
Run seminars and workshops on dreams. On-going evening and weekend workshops. Broadly Jungian but gestalt, art therapy and music is embraced. They offer Dream, Jungian Psychotherapy.

Abshott Holistic Centre
Little Abshott Road Titchfield Common, Fareham Hants PO14 4LN. (01489) 572451.
Run a variety of residential growth workshops in Hants. They offer Bioenergetics, Massage, Polarity Therapy, Resonance Therapy, Shiatsu, Meditation.

Academy of Systematic Kinesiology
39 Browns Rd, Surbiton Surrey KT5 8ST. (0181) 399 3215.
A natural health centre. Run workshop on balanced health. They run a training in Touch For Health. They offer Touch For Health, Acupuncture.

Acca and Adda
BCM Akademia London WC1N 3XX. (0181) 677 5837.
Workshops, tuition in esoteric subjects, magic and Wicca. Consultations in tarot, runes, palmistry, geomancy, I-Ching etc. Also publish O Fortuna, journal of spiritual, magical and ecological progress. Esoteric subjects, beliefs and philosophies (of all kinds). Challenging (and impossible) big prize crossword every time. Quarterly. Sample issue £1.50 plus stamp, or £6 subscription. They offer Paganism.

Action Against Allergy
24-26 High St, Hampton Hill Middx TW12.
A self help for people with allergic illness. Newsletter. £5 subs. SAE to above address. Provide information only; leaflets, booklets, advice etc. They offer Allergy Therapy.

Active Birth Centre
55 Dartmouth Park Road Kentish Town London NW5 1SL. (0171) 267 5368.
Provides an educational service for expectant parents which centres around yoga in pregnancy and preparation for an active birth. Full programme of workshops and seminars. Programme for mums and babies such as baby gymnastics and baby massage. Free national information and networking service by post or telephone. Sell books, pregnancy clothes, natural pregnancy and babycare products. Catalogues on request. They run a training in Active Birth. They offer Active Birth.

Acumedic Centre
101-105 Camden High Street Camden, London NW1 7JN. (0171) 388 5783/(0171) 388 6704.
Specialist supplies and health products sold in shop on the premises. Bookshop. Chinese acupuncture and Chinese herbs. Professional supply showroom for equipment and products. See East Asia Company in this book. £20 per

session typical. They offer Biofeedback, Stress Management, Acupuncture, Herbalism, Shiatsu.

Acupuncture and Osteopathy Clinic
34 Alderney Street, Pimlico London SW1V 4EU. (0171) 834 6229/1012.
They offer Hypnotherapy, Acupuncture, Osteopathy, Shiatsu, Aromatherapy, Reflexology, Homoeopathy, Alexander Technique.

Acupuncture Clinic of North London
Winchester Court 237 Green Lanes London N13. (0181) 886 9494.
They offer Acupuncture.

Adlerian Society for Individual Psychology
55 Mayhill Road London SE7 7JG. (0181) 858 7299 / 445 7879.
Counselling and psychotherapy based on principles of individual psychology. They are a UK association of practitioners and associate members interested in Alfred Adler and the movement based upon his work called 'individual psychology'. Aim to advance public knowledge of the work of Alfred Adler and train counsellors and psychotherapists' to practice in this tradition. They hold a programme of public lectures, a conference in Oxford and one day sessions in various parts of the country. The counselling centre is based in Swiss Cottage, London is open Monday evenings 7-9. Low cost counselling by diploma trainees. Wheelchair access to public meetings and counselling centre. They run a train-

ing in Adlerian Psychotherapy. They offer Adlerian Psychotherapy.

Adlerian Society
Boltisham Village College Cambridge . (01223) 314827.
They offer a training in Adlerian Psychotherapy.

Aetherius Society
757 Fulham Road, London SW6 5UU. (0171) 736 4187.
Open to public Mon-Sat 9am-10pm. Centre where lectures/ healing services and personal instructional courses are held, with a health food shop nearby. Also have a northern headquarters and groups throughout the country. Sell books and have a mail order service. Manufacture and sell radionic pendulums and holy stone shapes. Give spiritual counselling. Run a 'UFO hotline' on (0171) 731 1094. Hold conferences and seminars. Wheelchair access. They offer Homoeopathy, Flower Essence Remedies, Hand Healing, Colour Therapy.

African Herbs Ltd
104 Kingsley Road, Hounslow East Middlesex TW3 4AH. (0181) 570 5795.
Astrology, spiritualism. They also offer Herbalism.

Alexander Teaching Centre
188 Old Street London EC1V 9BP. (0171) 250 3038.
Established since 1983. Register of practitioners. Concs. Bookshop in the main building. They offer Alexander Technique.

All Hallows House
Idol Lane London EC3R 5DD. (0171) 283 8908.
Holistic health centre in the Wren Tower in the City of London. Open Mon-Fri 9-7pm. They offer Allergy Therapy, Stress Management, Acupuncture, Biodynamic Massage, Autogenic Training, Hellerwork, Counselling, Aromatherapy, Herbalism, Reflexology, Polarity Therapy, Yoga, Diet Therapy.

Alternative Medicine Clinic
56 Harley House, Marylebone Road, London NW15 HW. (0171) 486 7490.
Complimentary health centre. Five therapists. One level apartment with lift facility. Appointments necessary. The client is seen at consultation as a whole person and problem is assessed and advice given on an ongoing programme. Deal with weight problems, scars, and skin problems. Specialising in allergies and ethnic skin conditions. They try to assist the client with their expertise and teamwork. Fees on request. They run a training in Relaxation Training. They offer Allergy Therapy, Iridology, Kineosotherapy, Hypnotherapy, Stress Management, Acupuncture, Anti-smoking Therapy, Aromatherapy, Ayurevedic Medicine, Diet Therapy, Eating Problem, Gestalt Therapy, Herbalism, Homoeopathy, Massage, Neuro-linguistic Programming, Reflexology, Regression, Relaxation Training, Touch for Health (Kinesiology), Co-counselling, Counselling, Couple Therapy, Family Therapy.

Alternative Therapies Centre
52 & 52a Church St
Stoke Newington
London N16 0NB. (0171)
241 5033.
Appointments necessary. £30 per one hour session. They offer Hypnotherapy, Homoeopathy, Acupuncture, Antismoking Therapy, Aromatherapy, Astrological Psychotherapy, Bereavement Counselling, Eating Problem, Chiropody, Hand Healing, Massage, Meditation, Osteopathy, Reflexology, Regression, Reiki, Relaxation Training, Sex Therapy, Spiritualism, Stress Management, Yoga.

Andrew Still College of Osteopathy
30 Rosebank Road
London W7 2EN.
They offer a training in Osteopathy

Anna Freud Centre
21 Maresfield Gdns,
Hampstead, London NW3
5SH. (0171) 794 2313.
They run a training in Child psychotherapy. They offer Child psychotherapy.

Anthroposophical Association
Rudolph Steiner House
35 Park RoadRegents Park
London NW1. (0171) 723
4400.
Centre for the furthering and development of the work of Rudolf Steiner. Office open 10-6 Mon to Fri, 10-5 Sat. Lectures, performances, classes in eurhythmy (£10 per session), painting, drawing, creative speech, groups, workshops and courses exploring Rudolf Steiner's anthroposophy and its implications. Opened in 1926, bookshop, library open to public. Information about Steiner schools, homes and other activities. Teacher Training weekend seminars for Teachers in Steiner schools. Also offered is a two year part time Waldorf Kindergarten training course. Wheelchair access via lift. Lectures and evening workshops £3.00 (£1.50 concs). Day workshops

Arbours Association
6 Church Lane
London N8. (0181) 340
7646.
They offer a training in Psychoanalytic Therapy

Arbours Consultation Service
6 Church Lane
London N8. (0181) 340
8125.
They offer Psychoanalytic Therapy.

Arcadia Creative Therapy Centre
130 Wellmeadow Road
London SE6 1HP. (0181)
698 6312.
Radical psychoanalysis and advocacy. They offer Psychoanalysis, Gestalt Therapy.

Aromatherapy Associates
68 Maltings Place
Bagleys Lane, Fulham
London SW6 2BY. (0171)
371 9878/(0171) 731
8129.
The three partners have been practising for over 20 years: they and four other therapists work in the centre. All associates are fully qualified, insured members of the International Federation of Aromatherapists. The aim of the centre is to offer a haven of tranquility where clients can enjoy this most relaxing of treatments in the care of highly qualified and experienced therapists. Aromatherapy approx. 1hr 20mins £35. Osteopathy £28.They run a training in Aromatherapy. They offer Aromatherapy, Osteopathy.

Art from Within
119 Grosvenor Avenue,
Highbury
London N5 2NL. (0171)
354 1603.
Groups held at the Highbury Centre. Booking necessary. Groups are maximum of 12 people and are not drop-in. Individual sessions are usually six initial sessions after which it is open ended. Short term and long term in-depth work. They offer Art Therapy, Psychosynthesis.

Art of Dream Fulfilment
28 Woodlea Road, London
N16 0TH. (0171) 241
6415.
Creative visualisation and life improvement. Workshops and courses and metaphysical counselling and healing. Counselling with the Tarot. They offer Dream Therapy.

Arts Psychology Consultants
29 Argyll Mansions, London
W14 8QQ. (0171) 602
2707.
A psychology practice for people in the arts and media, specialising in typical problems like stage-fright, creativity, motivation, burnout, creative blocks, and problems of self confidence. Appointments only. No wheelchair access. Established 1987. Also offer career counselling. Counselling £20-£25. Career analysis £125. Some grants available. They offer Clientcentred Therapy, Counselling, Creativity.

LIST OF CENTRES

Asatru Folk Runic Workshop
43 St Georges Avenue London N7. (0171) 607 9695.
Northern mysteries study group. Courses in runecraft, lectures, consultations. They offer Paganism.

Association for Analystic and Bodymind Therapy and Training
8 Princes Avenue, Muswell Hill, London N10 3LR. (0181) 883 5418.
The centre is small, personal, friendly and supportive. An association of caring men and women, each with a distinctive style and expertise, together with. It has been established for 20 years. There are also talks on the principles and methods therapists use. They run a training in Integrative Psychotherapy. They offer Couple Therapy, Hypnotherapy, Primal Therapy, Gestalt Therapy, Group Oriented Therapy.

Association for Group and Individual Psychotherapy
1 Fairbridge Road Upper Holloway London N19 3EW. (0171) 272 7013.
They run a training in Psychoanalytic Therapy. They offer Group Oriented Therapy, Psychoanalytic Therapy.

Association for Marriage Enrichment
c/o Westminster Pastoral Foundation 23 Kensington Square London W8 5HN. (0171) 937 6956.
Hold residentials through the UK for couples in 'marriage enrichment'. Non-residential activities can be arranged for suitable groups. Small selection of books from USA available. Offer a three weekend training course in marriage enrichment. They offer Couple Therapy.

Association for Neuro-Linguistic Programming
27 Maury Road London N16 7BP. (01384) 443935.
Umbrella organisation. Register of practitioners of NLP. Contact and information point for general public and practitioners. Introductory and applications seminars on NLP. Two conferences a year. They run a training in Neuro-linguistic Programming. They offer Neuro-linguistic Programming.

Association of Biodynamic Psychotherapists
153 Goldhurst Terrace London NW6 3EU. (0171) 401 3582.
Referral list only for biodynamic psychotherapy. Professional newsletter, discussion with other psychotherapists. They offer Biodynamic Massage.

Association of General Practitioners of Natural Medicine
The Hon Secretary 38 Nigel House, Portpool Lane London EC1N 7UR. (0171) 405 2781.
They offer a training in Complementary Medicine

Association of Independent Psychotherapists
PO Box 1194 London N6 5PW. (0171)
700 1911 or (071) 281 6219.
Established 1988. 22 members. Reduced fee scheme for therapy with trainees. Members in London, Essex, Oxfordshire, Hertfordshire and Surrey. Assessment consultation £35. Psychotherapy £10-£30.They run a training in Psychoanalytic Therapy. They offer Couple Therapy, Jungian Psychotherapy, Men's Therapy, Psychoanalytic Therapy, Transpersonal therapy.

Association of Jungian Analysts
3-7 Eton Avenue, South Hampstead, London NW3. (0171) 794 8711.
They run a training in Jungian Psychotherapy. They offer Art Therapy.

Association of Natural Medicines
27 Braintree Road, Witham Essex CM8 2DD. (01376) 511069 / 502762
Natural healing centre. They run a training in Complementary Medicine. They offer Acupuncture, Allergy Therapy, Hypnotherapy, Homoeopathy, Reflexology.

Association of Reflexologists
27 Old Gloucester Street London WC1N 3XX. (0181) 445 0154.
Professional association for reflexologists. Gives information to general public, and on schools for those wishing to train. Instructional meetings on other therapies and quarterly newsletter to members. Meetings arranged at various venues. Register. They run a training in Reflexology. They offer Reflexology.

Astro-Psychotherapeutic Practice
23 Whitehall Gardens London W3 9RD. (0181) 992 9514.
Established 1986. Three practitioners in all. Work on a referral network. Also offer "Sandplay therapy". Clients must make an appointment. Wheelchair access. Also available for talks and lectures. Their vision is "soul searching on a journey to make sense personally and collectively". Psychotherapy session £30. Horoscope readings £45. They offer Astrological Psychotherapy, Men's Therapy, Art Therapy, Couple Therapy, Dream, Feminist Therapy, Integrative Psychotherapy, Jungian Psychotherapy.

Augenblick Centre
39b Bonnington Square London SW8. (0171) 735 4513.
Friendly centre run in a communal setting. Individual and group work. They offer Massage, Voice Therapy, Biodynamic Psychotherapy, Alexander Technique, Flower Essence Remedies.

Aura Vision
199 Mortlake Road, Kew Surrey TW9 4EW. (0181) 878 6693.
They offer Kirlian Diagnosis.

Awakened Mind
9 Chatsworth Road London NW2 4BJ. (0181) 451 0083.
Individual training using biofeedback techniques. Aimed at people who wish to reduce their stress levels and improve their ability to relax. They offer Biofeedback, Stress Management.

Baha'i Faith
27 Rutland Gate, Knightsbridge London SW7 1PD. (0171) 584 2566.
Contact for details of local meetings.

Bach Flower Remedies Ltd
Dr Bach Centre, Mount Vernon, Sotwell, Wallingford, Oxon OX10 0PZ. (01491) 833712.
They offer a training in Flower Essence Remedies

Barnes Physiotherapy Clinic
2a Elm Bank Gardens, Barnes London SW13 0NT. (0181) 876 5690.
Established 1983. Physiotherapy, psychotherapy. They offer Counselling.

Barry Long Foundation
BCM Box 876 London WC1N 3XX. (01984) 623426.
Mail order books and tapes of Barry Long. No callers or activities on site. They offer Meditation.

Bates Association of Great Britain
11 Tarmount Lane Shoreham-by-Sea, West Sussex BN43 6RQ. (01273) 452623.
Professional body for teachers of the Bates method. They can put you in touch with practitioners (send SAE) - there are six practising in London at the time of going to press - and can give general information on the method and supply a booklist. Visiting lectures and workshops can be arranged. £15-25 per session. Workshops vary. Most teachers work with children at reduced fees. Low cost training clinics. They run a training in Bates Eyesight Training. They offer Bates Eyesight Training.

Bates, Carrie
c/o Spectrum, 7 Endymion Road, London N4 1EE. (0171) 263 5545.
Offers holistic massage - helping people reconnect and get back in touch with their bodies. Carrie is a qualified massage practitioner, who aims to create a sense of well-being that can have far reaching physical, mental and emotional benefits. She believes in the importance of on-going personal growth and professional development.

Bayly School of Reflexology
Monks Orchard, Whitbourne Worcs WR6 5RB. (01886) 821207.
They are the official teaching body of the British Reflexology Association. Will provide a register of members for £1.50. Newsletter, books and charts. Details of Introductory and Advanced Reflexology trainings and courses on related subjects. They run a training in Reflexology. They offer Reflexology.

Bayswater Clinic
25B Clanricarde Gardens Bayswater, London W2 4JL. (0171) 229 9078.
Natural holistic treatment for environmentally induced illnesses, such as food and chemical allergy. Biochemical testing for food and chemical allergies, nutrition and treatment of candidosis. Correction of diet and dietary counselling. They offer Allergy Therapy, Diet Therapy, Homoeopathy.

LIST OF CENTRES

Belgravia Beauty
11 West Halkin St
London SW1X 8JL. (0171)
259 6033.
Beauty salon specialising in holistic therapy. They offer Aromatherapy, Massage, Relaxation Training, Biofeedback.

Bennett & Luck
54 Islington Park Street
Islington, London N1 1PX.
(0171) 226 3422.
Established for 3 years, this centre is also a health food shop selling books and a range of organic produce. Can refer if necessary. Wheelchair access to building but not to toilets. Range between £16-25 per session. They offer Counselling, Acupuncture, Aromatherapy, Flower Essence Remedies, Diet Therapy, Massage, Naturopathy, Osteopathy, Reflexology, Shiatsu.

Bereavement and Loss Workshops
107 Antill Road, London
N15 4AR. (0181) 801
2296.
They offer Bereavement Counselling.

Beshara Trust
Frilford Grange, Frilford
Near Abingdon
Oxon OX13 5NX. (01865)
391344.
Runs seminars with visiting leaders.

Bexleyheath Natural Health Clinic
6 Sandford Road,
Bexleyheath
Kent DA7 4AX. (0181) 303
9571.
Established for 4 years, there are four practice rooms and waiting area. Consultations are by appointment only, but they are open to visitors. Sell books, tapes, cosmetics, dietary supplements and a selection of health foods. They offer Hypnotherapy, Regression, Acupuncture, Aromatherapy, Cranial Osteopathy, Homoeopathy.

Bhratiya Vidya Bhavan (Institute of Indian Culture)
4a Castletown Road
West Kensington
London W14 9HQ. (0171)
381 3086/4608.
The philosophy of the Bharatiya Vidya Bhavan is summed up in their mottos: "Let noble thoughts come to us from all sides", and "The world is one family". Spiritual director is Mathoor Krishnamurti. Celebrate with music, prayer and sacred dance. Every weekend, hold gatherings of people to sing bhajans (religious songs). Also discourses and seminars by well-known scholars and swamis. Hindu religious festivals are observed with prayers and offerings. Meditation hall for those of all religions, bookshop with sections on various religions and philosophy. Sell tapes, records and CDs of religious songs. Concs to students and the elderly. Bookshop on premises. They offer Yoga, Hinduism, Meditation.

Biodynamic Psychotherapy and Teaching
13 Mansell Road
London W3 7QH. (0181)
749 4388.
Two psychotherapists with 10 and 15 years of clinical experience offering Jungian psychotherapy which includes the body-dimension. Work with individuals, couples and groups; supervision available, especially for body therapists who want more analytical input: hypnotic trance work (past-life regression) available. Foreign languages available: German, some French and Spanish spoken. Sale of publications/ video by A B and G Heuer. They offer Jungian Psychotherapy, Biodynamic Massage.

Bioenergetic Partnership
22 Fitzjohn's Avenue
Swiss Cottage
London NW3. (0171) 435
1079.
Bioenergetic Analysis as developed by Dr Alexander Lowen and his trainers with an analytic orientation. They offer an on-going evening group, weekly, subject to initial interview. Open to all. Individual on-going bioenergetic therapy offered. Advanced monthly group to therapists and trainees. They offer Bioenergetics.

Biomonitors
26-28 Wendell Road
London W12. (0181) 749
3983.
Day and evening courses. Also individual biofeedback training, massage. They offer Biofeedback, Relaxation Training, Meditation.

Bloomsbury Alexander Centre
Bristol House
80a Southampton Row
Bloomsbury
London WC1B 4BA. (0171)
404 5348.
Lessons are on a one to one basis, so appointments have to be made. A course of lessons can be from 10 to infinity! People are welcome to drop in for information or to book appointments, and teachers are at the centre from 8am-8pm. There are five rooms, with about fifteen teachers using the centre, which has been established

since 1987. The longest qualified teacher has been teaching for 13 years, and the centre provides a home for two senior teachers who have been teaching since the 1930s. Occasional introductory courses, courses for those with some experience, and for qualified teachers. Speakers on request. Books. Training starting in 1993 approximately. Access: ground floor, 2 steps to manage, slightly awkward door. Also run workshops and evening classes. They offer Alexander Technique.

Bluestone Clinic
Flat 20 Harmont House
20 Harley Street
London W1N 1AL. (0171)
637 4533.
Pulsed electro-magnetic energy (PEME) which it is claimed speeds up healing in the body by 50%. Cold beam laser treatment and remedial beauty treatments. Visiting spiritual healers. They offer Aromatherapy, Massage, Complementary Medicine, Osteopathy.

Body Balance
14 Golders Rise
London NW4 2HR.

Body Clinic
32 The Market Place
Falloden Way
Hampstead Garden Suburbs
London NW11 6JJ. (0181)
458 9412.
Electrolysis, neuro-muscular massage, feradic therapy, G5 massage, facials, leg waxing, paraffin wax therapy, manicures, steam cabinet, sunbed, specialists in sports injuries and back problems. Has been established since January 1987. It is open 7 days a week and has late evenings Tues, Weds and Thurs till 9pm. There are 5 therapy rooms and 8 practitioners. Clients

can usually pop in without an appointment, but this is not so on the late evenings or Sunday as these tend to get booked up in advance. Sell range of vitamins, essential oils, sports aids, therapeutic bath salts and books. Wheelchair access. They offer Hypnotherapy, Acupuncture, Aromatherapy, Chiropody, Laser Therapy, Massage, Naturopathy, Osteopathy.

Bodyspace
Guy Gladstone
The Open Centre
188 Old St. London EC1.
(0181) 549 9583.
They offer Bioenergetics, Psychodrama and Pulsing.

Bodywise
119 Roman Road
Bethnal Green
London E2 0QN. (0181)
981 6938.
Established 1983. Alternative health centre with five practice rooms, 25 practitioners, two group rooms. Reception cover from 9am-7pm and Sat mornings. Quiet friendly atmosphere. No wheelchair access. Appointments necessary except for 'open' Yoga classes. Their aim is to provide a high standard of complementary medicine at affordable prices in a conducive environment. The centre was set up and is run by a team of Buddhist women on the Buddhist principles of honesty, co-operation and friendliness. Yoga class £2-£4 (1 hour). Average costs of therapies on offer is £20-£30 per hour. Concessions available. They run a training in Massage. They offer Counselling, Acupuncture, Alexander Technique, Feldenkrais, Homoeopathy, Tai Chi, Massage, Naturopathy, Osteopathy, Reflexology, Shiatsu, Yoga, Aromatherapy, Art Therapy,

Bereavement Counselling, Cranial Osteopathy, Dance therapy, Herbalism, Hypnotherapy, Men's Therapy, Polarity Therapy, Psychosynthesis.

Brackenbury Natural Health Centre
30 Brackenbury Road
Hammersmith
London W6 0BA. (0181)
741 9264.
9am-9pm Mon-Fri, 9am-1pm Sat. Established in 1983, this is a large centre with over 25 qualified therapists and seven treatment rooms with cane furniture and indoor plants. Offer free advice to anyone unsure about treatment. Friendly, welcoming atmosphere. Some natural products sold, give talks and Qi Gong sessions in local church hall, hold workshops and occasional open days. Baby massage taught to two mums at a time. Register. Creche. No access. They offer Counselling, Acupuncture, Alexander Technique, Allergy Therapy, Aromatherapy, Flower Essence Remedies, Biodynamic Massage, Colonic Irrigation, Colour Therapy, Diet Therapy, Herbalism, Homoeopathy, Massage, Naturopathy, Osteopathy, Polarity Therapy, Reflexology, Shiatsu, Couple Therapy, Feldenkrais, Hypnotherapy, Stress Management, Hand Healing.

Brahma Kumaris World Spiritual University
Global Co-operation House
65 Pound Lane
London NW10 2HH.
(0181) 459 1400.
Courses in positive thinking, meditation and interpersonal skills. Non-governmental organisation affiliated to the U.N. Centres in sixty coun-

tries. Working for peace based on change in human values. They offer Meditation.

Breakspear Hospital
1 High Street, Abbots Langley
Herts WD5 0PU. (01442) 261333.
They offer Allergy Therapy.

Bretforton Hall Clinic
Bretforton, Vale of Evesham Worcestershire WR11 5JH. (01386) 830537.
Cymatics (acoustic treatment/ treatment by sound). They offer Aromatherapy, Colour Therapy, Massage.

British Acupuncture Association and Register
Stoneleigh, 218 Washway Road
Sale, Cheshire M33 4RA. (0161) 973 2309.
Controlling body for acupuncture. They have an handbook with the list of the practitioners in London, £1.50 They offer Acupuncture.

British and European Osteopathic Association
6 Adelaide Road, Teddington Middlesex
0181) 977 8532.
They keep a register of members. They offer Osteopathy.

British Association for Counselling
1 Regent Place
Rugby CV21 2PJ. (01788) 578328.
They are a national membership organisation providing information on a wide range of counselling topics and training. They keep a nationwide register of counsellors and offer a referral service for people looking for a counsellor or psychotherapist in their area. Please send an A4 SAE.

Produce journal 'Counselling' (£15 subs, £4 individual copies), and two national directories: 1) Training in Counselling and Psychotherapy and 2) Inhouse and tailor-made training in Counselling skills as well as many other leaflets and publications. They sell cassettes and videos (also for hire) on counselling. They do a useful resource pack for those involved in AIDS counselling (£100). In London there is the North London Branch and the South London Branch (listed in this book). You can become a member, phone or write for details. Prices are determined by the counsellor who is recommended to you, but the fees are usually very reasonable. They offer Counselling.

British Association for Social Psychiatry
112A Harley Street
London W1. (0171) 555 2603.
They offer Art Therapy, Bereavement Counselling, Family Therapy.

British Association of Analytical Body Psychotherapists.
47 Dean Court Road, Rottingdean, Brighton BN2 7DL. (01273) 303382.
Bioenergetic Analysis as developed by Dr Alexander Lowen and his trainers. They offer an on-going evening group, weekly, subject to initial interview. Open to all. Individual on-going bioenergetic therapy offered. Workshops £15 evening, £30 day. Individual therapy £25 - £35 by negotiation. They run a training in Bioenergetics. They offer Bioenergetics.

British Association of Psychotherapists
37 Mapesbury Road
London NW2 4HJ. (0181) 346 1747.
Individual psychoanalytic psychotherapy for adults and children. The BAP was founded in 1951 and in 1981 became a charity. They have been in their centre for two years, which was purpose designed to fit their needs with seminar rooms, a lecture room and clinical rooms. The Clinical Service offers advice and information through consultation to anyone suffering from emotional and psychological problems. Those seeking help can discuss with an experienced psychotherapist, whether psychotherapy would be an appropriate form of help and treatment. Fees vary for each therapist but approx. £25 per session. Also run a reduced fee scheme for £10 per session, for a limited number of clients. They run a training in Jungian Psychotherapy. They offer Child psychotherapy, Psychoanalytic Therapy, Eating Problem, Family Therapy, Jungian Psychotherapy.

British Buddhist Association
11 Biddulph Road, Maida Vale, London W9 1JA. (0171) 286 5575.
Non-sectarian Buddhist group under direction of A Haviland-Nye Dhammacariya. Teach meditation and run part-time study courses for various levels of experience and knowledge. Shrine room for meditation, bookshop. Open by appointment. They offer Buddhism, Meditation.

British College of Acupuncture
8 Hunter Street
London WC1N 1BN.
(0171) 833 8164.
Have clinic where students work. Register of practitioners. They run a training in Acupuncture. They offer Acupuncture.

British College of Naturopathy and Osteopathy
Frazer House
6 Netherhall Gardens
Hampstead, London NW3
5RR. (0171) 435 7830
(clinic), 435 6464 (college).
Founded in 1935, this is a private training college with clinic open to general public. Wheelchair access. They have available a register of practitioner members: send large SAE for 24p and £1.50 for list plus leaflets. They run a training in Naturopathy. They offer Naturopathy, Osteopathy.

British Homoeopathic Association
27A Devonshire Street
London W1N 1RJ. (0171)
935 2163.
Register of qualified medical doctors trained in homoeopathy, and homoeopathic vet and chemists. Send SAE for list. They offer Homoeopathy.

British Hypnosis Research
St. Matthews House
Brick Row, Darley Abbey
Derby DE22 1DQ. (01332)
541030.
Centre at St Ann's Hospital, London (appointments through Brighton centre). Training videos and books available. Training in Eriksonian hypnosis, psychotherapy and NLP. Register. No access. They run a training in Neuro-linguistic Programming. They offer Hypnotherapy, Neuro-linguistic Programming.

British Ki Aikido Association
c/o The Secretary, 48
Oakshott Court, Polygon
Road
London NW1 1ST. (0171)
281 0877.
Classes mainly in north London. They offer Aikido.

British Osteopathic Association
8-10 Boston Place,
Marylebone
London NW1 6QH. (0171)
262 5250.
Run clinic (see London College of Osteopathic Medicine) which specialises in offering low-cost treatment to those with low income. Register. They offer Osteopathy.

British Psycho-Analytical Society and The Institute of Psycho-analysis
63 New Cavendish Street
London W1. (0171) 580
4952 or (0171) 636 2322.
This establishment was founded by Ernest Jones, the biographer of Freud. They run a training in Psychoanalysis. They offer Psychoanalysis, Psychoanalytic Therapy.

British Reflexology Association
Monks Orchard, Whitbourne
Worcs WR6 5RB. (01886)
21207.
They offer a training in Reflexology.

British School - Reflex Zone Therapy of the Feet (Ann Lett Ltd)
87 Oakington Avenue
Wembley Park
London HA9 8HY. (0181)
908 2201.
Established in 1980 to train nurses, physiotherapists, midwives and doctors in reflex zone therapy. Affiliated to European schools in Holland, Scandinavia, Belgium, Spain, France, Italy, Israel, Switzerland and Germany with the same training programme. 20,000 practising therapists most of whom use their training in hospitals, clinics, and some in private practice. Register. Wheelchair access. They run a training in Reflexology. They offer Reflexology.

British School of Oriental Therapy and Movement
61a Rosendale Road
West Dulwich SE21 8DY.
(0181) 761 3526.
Drop in classes in Kitaiso, Tues (advanced) and Thurs (beginners). Training in Shiatsu. They use a large hall five minutes from Richmond tube station. Register of practitioners. No access. They run a training in Shiatsu. They offer Complementary Medicine, Shiatsu, Acupuncture, Meditation, Herbalism.

British School of Osteopathy
1-4 Suffolk Street
London SW1Y 4HG. (0171)
930 9254.
The British School of Osteopathy is a registered charity. Open Mon-Fri 9-6pm, also Sat 10-1. They run a training in Osteopathy. They offer Osteopathy.

LIST OF CENTRES

British School of Reflexology
92 Sheering Road, Old Harlow Essex CM17 0JW. (01279) 429060.
Register. Clinic and training school for 18 students, established 15 years. Wheelchair access. They run a training in Reflexology. They offer Reflexology.

British School of Shiatsu-Do
6 Erskine Road, London NW3 3AJ. (0171) 483 3776.
Treatments by appointment. Send SAE to their office for full details of courses. Established 1983, they have 6-10 practitioners and 180 students. Their aim is to make Shiatsu-do available to as many people as possible, and in treatment, to help improve people's attitude towards life and towards one-another. Shiatsu-Do treatment £30/£20 concessions. Introduction weekend £50.They run a training in Shiatsu. They offer Shiatsu, Meditation, Yoga.

British School of Yoga
The Old Vicarage, Clauton Nr. Holsworthy Devon EX22 6PS. (01409) 27432.
They offer a training in Yoga

British Society of Hypnotherapists
37 Orbane Road, Fulham, London, SW6 7JZ. (0171) 385 1166.
Established 1950. Register of practitioners. Training for treatment of neurotic behavioural problems, traumas and psychosomatic illness. They offer Hypnotherapy.

British Wheel of Yoga
1 Hamilton Place, Boston Road Sleaford, Lincs NG34 7ES. (01529) 306851.
They offer a training in Yoga.

Brothers
207 Waller Road London SE14 5LX. (0171) 639 9732.
Growth programme for men using psychosynthesis, education and analytic techniques. Established for 5 years, Brothers runs introductory and on-going workshops. Admission is based on written application. Also offer individual sessions for men. Annual conference 'Embodying the Masculine'. They offer Men's Therapy, Psychosynthesis.

Brunel Management Programme
Brunel University, Uxbridge Middlesex UB8 3PH. (01895) 256461 or 812058.
Courses on self knowledge and self development for managers. Stress at work. Courses on interpersonal effectiveness in management and on organisational design and development. Plus other short courses. They offer Management, Stress Management.

Buddhapadipa Temple
14 Calonne Road, Wimbledon London SW19. (0181) 946 1357.
It is a Tai Buddhist Temple they offer free Vipassana Meditation. It is also a retreat for people to stay. They offer Meditation, Retreats.

Buddhist Society
58 Eccleston Square, Victoria London SW1V 1PH. (0171) 834 5858.
Introducing Buddhism course open to public - a series of 8 lectures running continuously throughout the year. Library open to public to browse, but not to borrow. Members may attend courses on Zen, Theravadin and Tibetan Buddhism. Residential summer school. Correspondence course in basic Buddhism, cassettes and bookstall. Seminars, lectures. Quarterly journal, 'The Middle Way', free to members . They offer Buddhism, Retreats.

Bumblebees Natural Remedies
35 Brecknock Road London N7 0AD. (0171) 267 3884 0171 607 1936.
Offer a wide range of treatments and have a shop on the premises. The shop sells natural medicines including: herbal, homoeopathic medicine, nutritional items, cruelty free products, skin care and aromatherapy oils. Near Kentish Town tube station. Opening hours are 9.30-6.30 Monday to Saturday. The clinic is open in the evening. They offer Acupuncture, Alexander Technique, Cranial Osteopathy, Chiropractice, Homoeopathy, Massage, Naturopathy, Osteopathy, Reflexology, Shiatsu.

C.H.I Clinic
River Bank House Putney Bridge Approach London SW6 3JD. (0171) 371 9590.
They deal with skin complaints like Psoriasis and Eczema the treatment includes consultation, herbs. The clinic has 3 practitioners from

China. Psychotherapy is also available along side the herbs treatment. They offer Stress Management, Herbalism.

Cabot Centre
41 Battle Bridge Road
London NW1 2TJ. (0171)
833 0570.
Established 1993 with currently eleven practitioners. Appointments essential. Cabot is a charity aiming to offer the widest range of body and mind trainings and therapies to the widest range of clients. They run a range of groups for special needs clients and groups, some of these are free. £30-£35 per hour, some low cost available. They offer Aikido, Anti-smoking Therapy, Art Therapy, Assertion Therapy, Astrological Psychotherapy, Biodynamic Massage, Biodynamic Psychotherapy, Client-centred Therapy, Co-counselling, Counselling, Couple Therapy, Dance therapy, Drama Therapy, Dream, Eating Problem, Existential Psychotherapy, Family Therapy, Integrative Psychotherapy, Massage, Meditation, Psychodrama.

CAER (Centre For Alternative Education And Research)
Rosemerryn, Lamorna
Penzance, Cornwall TR19
6BN. (01736) 810530.
They offer a training in Counselling

Camden Osteopathic and Natural Health Practice
96 Malden Rd. Camden
Town
London NW5 4DA. (0171)
482 1248.
They offer Acupuncture, Naturopathy, Osteopathy.

Capital Hypnotherapy Centre
Temple Lodge
51 Queen Caroline Street
Hammersmith
London W6 9QL. (0171)
737 1929.
Counselling, hypnotherapy, primary cause analysis. They offer Anti-smoking Therapy, Hypnotherapy.

Care-Healing Centre
3 Bristol Gardens
Little Venice
London W9 2JG. (0171)
286 2003.
Sell audio tapes on these subjects. Run a training in hands-on spiritual healing which can be adjusted to a persons requirements. They offer Hand Healing, Hypnotherapy, Neuro-linguistic Programming, Crystal Therapy.

Central London School of Reflexology
15 King St, Covent Garden
London WC2. (0171) 240
1438 / 284 1817.
This centre is situated at the heart of Covent Garden and overlooks the peaceful garden of St. Paul's Churchyard. Established 10 years, appointment required. They are constantly seeking to advance their knowledge of reflexology in the therapeutic context with the aim of improving the efficiency of treatments. Prices range from £20 for reflexology to £20+ for chiropody and podiatry. They run a training in Reflexology. They offer Reflexology, Chiropody.

Central School of Counselling and Therapy
56b Hale Lane, London

NW7 3PR. (0181) 906
4833.
A teaching resource centre which trains, supports and publishes in the field of counselling for statuary, voluntary and commercial organisations. They run a number of trainings and courses all based on counselling. Send for their free information pack. They offer Counselling.

Central School of Speech and Drama
Sesame Course, Embassy
Theatre, Eton Avenue
London NW3 3HY. (0171)
722 8183.
They offer a training in Drama Therapy

Centre for Counselling and Psychotherapy Education
21 Lancaster Road, Notting
Hill, London W11 1QL.
(0171) 221 3215.
Professional training. Individual, couple and group therapy. Centre established 1983; comprising two houses (130 students). Holistic approach which includes the spiritual dimension. Weekend workshops (£50 and short-term groups). They run a training in Counselling. They offer Counselling, Couple Therapy, Transpersonal therapy.

Centre for Creation Spirituality
St James's Church
197 Piccadilly
London W1V 9LF. (0171)
734 4511 (2-5pm).

LIST OF CENTRES

Centre for Health and Healing
St James's Church
197 Piccadilly
London W1V 9LF. (0171)
437 7118.
This centre is attached to St James's Church Piccadilly and offers holistic therapies. Includes cancer care and women's group. Drop-in in the caravan. They offer Counselling, Music therapy, Diet Therapy, Massage, Homoeopathy, Osteopathy, Aromatherapy.

Centre for Nutritional Studies
The Garden House, Rufford Abbey, Newark, Notts NG22 9DE. (01623) 822004.
They offer a training in Diet Therapy

Centre for Pagan Studies
Flat b, 5 Trinity Rise
Tulse Hill, London SW2
2QP. (0181) 671 6372.
Healing, pathworking and meditation. Established for educational, therapeutic and spiritual purposes to provide academic classes and experiential workshops in north European shamanism, wicca and ritual mythic drama. Also aims to act as a guide to seekers through the labyrinth of competing wares in the esoteric marketplace. Classes, workshops, apprenticeship training. Practice through ritual drama, mythic re-enactment, ecstatic dance, pathworking, chanting, making music etc. Consultation and advice available for seekers trying to find their way through the confused labyrinth of the New Age marketplace. Offers free information on different current strands in the esoteric field, particularly in London. They offer Paganism.

Centre for Past Life Healing
118a Regent's Park Road
London NW1 8XL. (0181)
586 0690.
Offer practitioner trainings in Past Life Healing. One weekend a month for five months. £90 per weekend. Small groups only. Nine day residential trainings also available in Devon. They offer Regression.

Centre for Personal & Professional Development
Lancaster House
583 High Road
London N17 6SB. (0181)
444 9217/(0181) 342
9956.
Established 1988, large centre in N17. Garden, reception area, carpeted and cushioned throughout. Massage suite, group rooms and private interview rooms. Six practitioners plus faculty. No wheelchair access, initial telephone contact. Specialise in sexual issues, including counselling for survivors and perpetrators of sexual abuse, bisexuality, male rape etc. Their aim is to educate and train competent psychotherapists, counsellors and sex therapists; to support male and female survivors of sexual abuse and to confront male and female sex offenders. They are equally supportive and accessible to both women and men, and have great expertise in the field of physical, emotional and sexual abuse and their prevention. On a sliding scale of £20-£45 per session. They run a training in Integrative Psychotherapy. They offer Adlerian, Assertion Therapy, Bereavement Counselling, Biodynamic Massage, Biodynamic Psychotherapy, Bioenergetics, Child psychotherapy, Client-centred Therapy, Counselling, Couple Therapy, Dream, Eating Problem, Encounter, Family Therapy, Feminist Therapy, Gestalt Therapy, Group Oriented Therapy, Hand Healing, Integrative Psychotherapy, Jungian Psychotherapy, Massage, Meditation, Men's Therapy, Reflexology, Regression, Reichian Therapy, Relaxation Training, Sex Therapy, Spiritualism, Stress Management, Transactional Analysis, Transpersonal therapy.

Centre for Psychoanalytical Psychotherapy
20 Renters Avenue
London NW4 3RB. (0181)
202 8351.
Individual work at £35 per session. Fees negotiable. They run a training in Psychoanalytic Therapy. They offer Psychoanalytic Therapy.

Centre for Psychological Astrology
PO Box 890
London NW3 2JZ. (0181)
749 2330.
They offer Astrological Psychotherapy.

Centre for Release and Integration
5 Norfolk Lodge
114 Richmond Hill
Richmond TW10 6RJ.
(0181) 332 6979.
The office is in Teddington but they can refer you to practitioners in London and through the UK. They run a training in Postural Integration. They offer Postural Integration.

Centre for Stress Management
156 Westcombe Hill
Blackheath, London SE3
7DH. (0181) 293 4114.
Cognitive/behavioural therapy, anxiety management, psychodynamic counselling. Established 1987, included training room and two counselling rooms. Training in cognitive/behavioural approaches to psychotherapy, and counselling and stress management. Mail order, books, relaxation tapes, hypnosis tapes, videos on health, daily logs, biofeedback machines, biodots. In house workshops for organisations. Free leaflets on health (send SAE). Lectures, workshops. Management consultancy for industrial stress. No access. They run a training in Stress Management. They offer Assertion Therapy, Biofeedback, Counselling, Hypnotherapy, Stress Management.

Centre for the Expressive Arts
22a Topsfield Parade
London N8 8PP. (0181)
340 4988.
They offer Art Therapy, Dance therapy.

Centre for Transpersonal Psychology
7 Pembridge Place
Bayswater
London W2 4XB.
The centre is a co-operative of like-minded psychologists, counsellors, psychotherapists and members of related professions that have a commitment to the path of self realisation. They run a training in Transpersonal therapy. They offer Transpersonal therapy.

Centre of Integral Psychoanalysis
6 Colville Road
London W11 2BP. (0171)
727 4404.
The centre was established in London in 1986, and is affiliated to the International Society of Analytical Trilogy, which was started in Brazil and now has centres around the world. It is a society of a scientific and cultural nature, dedicated to research into Keppe's discoveries. They also publish and distribute 30 books, in six different languages. They run a training in Integrative Psychotherapy. They offer Psychoanalytic Therapy.

Changes
5 Romney Court
Haverstock Hill
London NW3 4RX. (0171)
722 9353.
The North West London stress management consultancy. Established 1992. Five therapists, by appointment only. Ground Floor with ample parking or 3 mins from Belsize Park station. Also offer self-hypnosis courses. Their aim is to offer a holistic approach to dealing with the stress of living in an uncaring modern metropolis. They offer Anti-smoking Therapy, Aromatherapy, Assertion Therapy, Autogenic Training, Bereavement Counselling, Counselling, Creativity, Diet Therapy, Eating Problem, Hand Healing, Hypnotherapy, Massage, Meditation, Mind Clearing, Neurolinguistic Programming, Relaxation Training, Shiatsu, Stress Management.

Chantraine School of Dance
47 Compayne Gardens
West Hampstead
London NW6 3DB. (0171)
624 5881.
They teach the dance of contemporary expression, an approach to dance and movement created by Francoise and Alain Chantraine. Established in France in 1958 and in England in 1977. Emphasis is on the development of the person as the dancer and towards a unity of mind, body and spirit. There is no one building; classes are held at Adult Education institutes mostly in North London, but also in South Kensington. Not so much dance therapy, more dance as a way of expression.

Cheirological Society
16 Bridge St, Osney
Oxford OX2 0BA. (01865)
241086.
The Society is a national network of qualified Cheirological consultants and tutors (hand analysis). It was founded in 1889, to promote Cheirology as a serious diagnostic and aid to self understanding. The society is the only one of its kind in the world, and is dedicated to the study of the hand in all its aspects. One and a quarter hour consultation: £25, Two and a half hours: £45. They run a training in Hand Healing.

Chelsea Complementary Natural Health Centre
172 Ifield Road
London SW10 9AF. (0171)
373 8575.
This centre in Chelsea has been established since 1991 and has continued to grow, now accommodating 12 practitioners. It is housed in a lovely old building with large

and peaceful therapy rooms and lots of flowers. There is wheelchair access for some of the therapies, but if pre-warned they will do their best to accommodate. Appointments are necessary, but not for the Homoeopathic drop-in clinic. Apart from the therapies listed below they also have a sports injuries clinic. Their aim is to create a peaceful, healing friendly environment, with excellent curing practitioners who are committed to their therapy. Massage £30, Homoeopathy £20-40, Chiropody £15, Shiatsu £25, Yoga £5. They offer Aromatherapy, Acupuncture, Chiropody, Counselling, Herbalism, Homoeopathy, Massage, Osteopathy, Reflexology, Shiatsu, Yoga, Cranial Osteopathy.

Chessington Hypnotherapy Clinic
130 Guilders Road
Chessington, Surrey
(0181) 397 3146.
Psychologist. Wheelchair access, one step on entry. They offer Hypnotherapy, Aromatherapy, Diet Therapy.

CHI Centre
Victoria House
98 Victoria St
Victoria
London SW1E 5JL. (0171) 828 9292
They offer Traditional Chinese Medicine and can treat many chronic conditions including Eczema, Psoriasis and Acne, women's problems etc. Resident Dermatologists and Physicians from China. Psychotherapy available alongside herbal treatment if needed. They also offer a Helpline offering information and advice on TCM and a free information pack. They

offer Herbalism, Traditional Chinese Medicine, Psychoanalytic Therapy.

Children's Hours Trust
28 Wallace House
410 Caledonian Road
London N7 8TL. (0171) 609 5568.
They listen to children and their play. Client-centred approach based on Rachel Pinney's theories of 'creative listening'. Full attention and no interpretation. Small centre. Registered charity formed in 1983. You can visit by appointment. Workshops twice a month in London and by arrangement elsewhere, children welcome. Creche. Wheelchair access. Register of practitioners. Mail order. Library. Volunteers welcomed. They offer Child psychotherapy.

Chinese Clinic
12 Bateman Street
London W1V 5TD. (0171) 494 3593.
Chinese herbalism and western orthodox medicine practised by two fully qualified doctors. The clinic has been established for five years. Their aim is to spread traditional Chinese Medicine to England. They offer Acupuncture, Herbalism, Sex Therapy.

Chiron Centre for Holistic Psychotherapy
26 Eaton Rise, Ealing
London W5 2ER. (0181) 997 5219.
Offers body psychotherapy drawing on the work of Lowen (bioenergetics), biodynamic psychology (Boyesen), gestalt body therapy (Rosenberg) and core energetics (Pierrakas). On going evening psychotherapy groups. Weekend workshops. Member of UK standing conference for

psychotherapy. They run a training in Integrative Psychotherapy. They offer Bioenergetics, Couple Therapy, Gestalt Therapy, Biodynamic Massage, Massage.

Chiropractic Clinic
141 Golders Green Road
London NW11 8HG.
(0181) 201 8992.
Established 7 years. By appointment only. Two treatment rooms. Concs. Wheelchair access. They aim to help people with mechanical joint disorders. Manipulation £28. Massage £35/hr. X-rays £45 They offer Chiropractice, Massage.

Christian Community
Temple Lodge
51 Queen Caroline Street
London W6 9QL. (0181) 748 8388.
Set up by Rudolph Steiner in 1922 to practice the spirit of Christianity rather than merely to uphold the traditional forms. Celebrate the sacraments, Christian festivals, hold study groups, services, workshops. Counselling is available, and a homoeopathic doctor visits on Thursday (phone 458 4304 for appointment). Bookshop and vegetarian restaurant. They offer Christianity.

Chung San Acupuncture School
15 Porchester Gardens
Maida Vale
London W2 4DB. (0171) 727 6778.
Clinic on Sunday with students of school. Treatment also available from qualified practitioners. They run a training in Acupuncture. They offer Acupuncture.

LIST OF CENTRES

Churchill Centre
22 Montagu Street
Marble Arch, London W1H
1TB. (0171) 402 9475.
Mainly part-time courses in
health care and relaxation
with massage for Churchill
and ITEC certificate. Individual treatments by appointment. The centre was
founded in 1973 by Ken
Holme. Design and make
treatment couches to order,
including backrests, cover and
cushions. Sell books, tapes and
oils. They run a training in
Massage. They offer Massage,
Reflexology.

Circle of Creative Arts
Therapy
1 Ravenstone Road
London N8 0JT. (01273)
884256.
Spiritual counselling. Workshop on various themes to do
with self-development and
spirituality, inspiring new
ideas from creative art images. Group and individual
work. They offer Art Therapy,
Creativity.

City Health Centre
36-37 Featherstone Street
London EC1Y 8QX. (0171)
251 4429.
Western and Chinese herbal
pharmacy, iris photography
and consultation service, vega
diagnosis. Established 1982,
6 treatment rooms, consultations by appointment. Practitioners available for short free
consultations to help people
decide the best form of treatment or therapy. Mail order
herbal pharmacy. They offer
Counselling, Neuro-linguistic
Programming, Acupuncture,
Alexander Technique,
Herbalism, Homoeopathy,
Iridology, Massage, Osteopathy, Shiatsu.

Clapham Common Clinic
1st Floor
151/153 Clapham High
Street
Clapham Common
London SW4 7SS. (0171)
627 8890 or 622 4382.
Also offer Well Woman Clinic,
Chinese Herbalism, Sports
injury clinic, Family Planning.
They have 25 practitioners
and have been operating since
1986. They offer free consultation with most practitioners. Open 9am - 9pm, with
appointments not always necessary. They integrate medical, complimentary and alternative therapies in one centre. £18-£35 per session with
concessions and sliding scales.
They offer Counselling, Acupuncture, Alexander Tech-
nique, Aromatherapy, Mas-
sage, Osteopathy, Allergy
Therapy, Anti-smoking
Therapy, Assertion Therapy,
Bereavement Counselling,
Biodynamic Massage, Chi-
ropody, Client-centred
Therapy, Couple Therapy,
Cranial Osteopathy, Diet
Therapy, Eating Problem, Ex-
istential Psychotherapy, Fam-
ily Therapy, Feminist
Therapy, Flower Essence
Remedies, Herbalism, Ho-
moeopathy, Hypnotherapy,
Integrative Psychotherapy,
Kineosotherapy, Natural
Birth Control, Naturopathy,
Personal Construct Therapy,
Psychoanalytic Therapy,
Reflexology, Relaxation
Training, Sex Therapy,
Shiatsu, Stress Management,
Touch For Health, Tradi-
tional Chinese Medicine,
Transactional Analysis.

Clare Maxwell Hudson
NW2 4ER. (0181) 450
6494.
All forms of massage. Clinic
for members of the public.
Home visiting service for
those living in London. They
run a training in Massage.
They offer Massage, Shiatsu.

Clinic of Alternative
Therapies
18 The Drive, South
Woodford
London E18 2BL. (0181)
989 2216.
Vegatesting. Treatment for
arthritis, rheumatism, migraine. They offer Acupuncture.

Clinic of Herbal Medicine
8 Whitgift Street, Croydon
Surrey CR0 1DH. (0181)
681 0924.
Herbal medicine. Member of
National Institute of Medical
Herbalists.

Clinic of Herbal Medicine
61 Fernside Road, Balham
London SW12. (0181) 675
6405.
Established since 1983, the
Centre is close to Balham tube
station and has easy parking.
Open Tues-Sat inclusive, have
six practitioners and a variable number of students in
attendance. The training
clinic is manned by senior students under the supervision
of a qualified medical herbalist. Appointment only for sessions but you are welcome to
drop-in to get the feel of the
place. Creche. Wheelchair
access. They have very reduced fees. First consultation
waged £12, unwaged £6. Subsequent consultations waged
£8, unwaged £4. Plus the cost
of medicines. They run a
training in Herbalism. They
offer Herbalism, Diet
Therapy.

283

Clissold Park Natural Health Centre

154 Stoke Newington Church Street, Stoke Newington
London N16 0JU. (0171) 249 2990.

Have been established since 1984 and have 5 treatment rooms where patients may be seen by appointment. Offer an acute 'homoeopathic drop-in' 3 evenings a week on Monday, Wednesday and Friday at 5pm where patients can be seen without an appointment. Also offer various evening and weekend courses on different aspects of health. Sell homoeopathic first aid kits and books. They offer Counselling, Acupuncture, Aromatherapy, Herbalism, Osteopathy, Alexander Technique, Homoeopathy, Reflexology, Shiatsu.

Co-Counselling International

17 Lisburne Road
London NW3 2NS. (0171) 485 0005.

Part of a network, Co-counselling Community International. Co-counselling is a two-way process enabling both parties to act as a client/counsellor. About £70-£100. They run a training in Co-counselling. They offer Co-counselling.

College of Cranio-Sacral Therapy

160 Upper Fant Road
Maidstone
Kent ME16 8DJ. (01622) 729231.

They offer Cranial Osteopathy.

College of Healing

Runnings Park, Croft Bank West Malvern, Worcs WR14 4DU. (01684) 566450.

The college is an educational charity, and the longest established organisation of its kind in Britain. They offer a three year part-time diploma course in the art of healing. They run a training in Hand Healing. They offer Hand Healing, Stress Management, Relaxation Training, Meditation.

College of Homoeopathy

Regents College, Inner Circle Regents Park, London NW1 4NS. (0171) 487 7416.

College and clinic of homoeopathy. They run a training in Homoeopathy. They offer Homoeopathy.

College of Homoeopathy Clinic

26 Claredon Rise
London SE13 5EY. (0181) 852 0573.

Teaching clinic for students. Four practise rooms. Open six days a week. They offer Homoeopathy, Acupuncture, Alexander Technique, Aromatherapy, Cranial Osteopathy, Massage, Osteopathy, Reflexology.

College of Opthalmic Somatology

24 Chapel Market, Islington London N1 9E2. (0171) 278 1212.

A lecture takes place in central London at Regent's College, one Sunday per month. They run a training in Iridology. They offer Iridology.

College of Osteopaths Education Trust

Administrative Services
110 Thorkill Road
Thames Ditton
Surrey KT7 0UW. (0181) 398 3308.

NB Teaching Clinic is at Neals Yard Therapy Rooms. The above address is the admin office only. They run a training in Osteopathy. They offer Osteopathy.

College of Practical Homoeopathy

Oakwood House
422 Hackney Road
London E2 7SY. (0171) 613 5468.

They offer Homoeopathy.

College of Psychic Studies

16 Queensberry Place
London SW7 2EB. (0171) 589 3292/3.

An educational charity seeking to promote spiritual values and a greater understanding of the wider areas of human consciousness. Lectures, workshops and courses on spiritual, psychic and personal development. Lending library with over 10,000 books on all areas of spiritual growth. Send an SAE for complete programme of events. Also publish 'Light' three times a year, £1.75 each. Membership of the CPS, which includes use of library and discounts on events, is £14 per year. They offer Hand Healing, Bereavement Counselling, Counselling, Eating Problem, Meditation.

College of Traditional Chinese Acupuncture

Tao House, Queensway Leamington Spa Warks CV31 3LZ. (01926) 422121.

They offer a training in Acupuncture

Colon Health
27 Warwick Avenue
London W9 2PS. (0171)
289 7000.
Uses colonic irrigation to help with many disorders such as skin and heavy toxic conditions. Free implants and free charts. They offer Allergy Therapy, Colonic Irrigation, Diet Therapy.

Communication and Counselling Foundation
Haflodas, Tregoran
Dyfed, Wales SY25 6UG.
(01686) 630439
Programme of workshops, some residential: The Psychology of Transition and Envisioning the Future retreat. Also run the Women, Earth and Spirit programme a series of workshops and retreats for women. Wheelchair access. They run a training in Psychosynthesis. They offer Feminist Therapy, Psychosynthesis.

Community Health Foundation
188-194 Old Street
London EC1V 9BP. (0171)
251 4076.
Established in 1976 is one of the largest natural health centres. They aim to provide health education by concentrating on cooking, exercise and massage. They run a wide range of courses dedicated to natural health care. There is a 'popular clinic for individual advice on macrobiotics, shiatsu and massage'. Also have rooms to rent for workshops/courses. There is a macrobiotic/vegan restaurant on the premises as well as a book and food shop. They hold open days and free introductory evenings. They run a training in Macrobiotics. They offer Macrobiotics, Tai Chi, Massage, Shiatsu, Yoga, Iridology, Hypnotherapy, Neuro-linguistic Programming.

Confederation of Healing Organisations
The Red and White House
113 High St
Berkhamsted, Herts
HP4 2DJ. (01442) 870667.
Head office of a confederation of 16 associations deploying about 8,500 healers in the UK and others abroad. Their aim is to make healing available on the NHS and in private medicine. They offer Hand Healing.

Constructive Teaching Centre
18 Landsdowne Road
Holland Park
London W11. (0171) 727 7222.
The centre was established in 1960 to teach the Alexander Technique. They run a training in Alexander Technique. They offer Alexander Technique.

Core Trust (The)
1-12 Lisson Cottages
Lisson Grove
London NW1 6UD. (0171) 258 3031.
An holistic treatment centre for people with problems with addiction. .

Cortijo Romero UK
24 Grange Avenue
Chapletown, Leeds LS7 4EJ.
(0113) 2374015.
One to two week residential courses in the foothills of the Sierra Nevada, Spain. £260-£300 per week depending on the time of year. Occasional bursary. They offer Creativity, Psychosynthesis, Meditation, Dance therapy, Massage.

Cranial Osteopathic Association
478 Baker Street, Enfield
Middlesex EN1 3QS. (0181) 367 5561.
Aim to undo cranial lesions i.e. damage to the head. Register of members. They run a training in Cranial Osteopathy. They offer Cranial Osteopathy.

Craniosacral Therapy Education Trust
29 Dollis Park, Finchley
London N3 1HJ. (0181) 349 0297.
They run a training in Complementary Medicine. They offer Complementary Medicine.

Creative and Healing Arts
222 Westbourne Park Road
London W11 1EP. (0171) 229 9400.
This small practice was established in 1989, and consists of two rooms in a private house, with one therapist working at a time. The initial approach is to give therapy and treatment, tailored to the patient's needs and provide a self-help. They also act as a referral network to put people in touch with affiliated therapists. There is no wheelchair access. Consultations are by appointment only. £25-£35 per hour, with concessions available. They offer Osteopathy, Shiatsu, Yoga, Massage.

Creative Arts and Therapy Consultants
Terpsichore
70 Cranwich Road
London N16 5JD. (0181) 809 5866.
They run a training in Integrative Psychotherapy. They offer Dance therapy.

Croydon Buddhist Centre
98 High St
Croydon CR0 1ND. (0181)
688 8624
A centre of the Friends of the Western Buddhist Order (see London Buddhist centre for details). The Centre was established in 1981, primarily as a Buddhist centre, but Meditation and Yoga classes are suitable for all faiths. Drop-in classes are available. Phone for a full programme. Evening courses in meditation £42 for 7 weeks, Yoga £36 for 8 weeks. They offer Yoga, Buddhism, Meditation, Tai Chi.

Crystal 2000
37 Bromley Road
St Annes-on-Sea
Lancs FY8 1PQ. (01253)
723735.
Run crystal healing training, also correspondence courses. Publish Crystal News (£1.25). They offer Crystal Therapy.

Dancing Dragon Massage
50 Burma Road
London N16 9BJ. (0171)
275 8002.
Psychic development. Massage is based on a combination of Swedish and intuitive massage and energy balancing. It is taught as a dance-like form. They run a training in Massage. They offer Counselling, Hand Healing, Massage.

Dancing on the Path
Flat 1
39A Glengarry Road
London SE22. (0181) 693
6953.
Individual sessions and shamanic dance workshops by psychotherapist trained in the Dancing Path by Gabrielle Roth. They offer Counselling,
Dance therapy, Transpersonal therapy, Hand Healing.

Demigod
2 Berenger Towers
off Kings Road, Chelsea
London SW10 0EF. (0171)
351 2220.
Dream analysis and therapy. Also clairvoyance, crystal ball and psychometry. They offer Counselling.

Dick Read School for Natural Birth
14 Pitt Street
London W8. (0171) 937
4140.
Established 1976. Natural childbirth procedures according to the Dick-Read approach. Individual tuition given. Visiting speakers to groups. Book and teaching cassette also available. They offer Active Birth.

Dr Edward Bach Centre
Mount Vernon, Sotwell
Wallingford, Oxon OX10
0PZ. (01491) 834678.
Bach Flower Remedies available by post, books, free advice service, consultations by appointment. Are planning seminars which are scheduled to start 1990. They offer Flower Essence Remedies.

Drakefield Homoeopathic Centre
122a Drakefield Road
London SW17 8RR. (0181)
672 5253.
They offer Homoeopathy.

Druid Order
161 Auckland Road
London SE19 2RH. (0181)
771 0684.
Public meetings at London Ecology centre fortnightly on Fridays at 7.15. Public ceremonies on Tower Hill at Spring equinox (12 noon GMT), at Stonehenge at Summer solstice, on Primrose Hill at Autumn equinox (12 noon GMT). Teaching and training given to companions in Groves and classes, available to those who wish to be initiated into the Druid order.

Eagle's Wing Centre for Contemporary Shamanism
58 Westbere Road
West Hampstead
London NW2 3RU. (0171)
435 8174.
Established 1983 as Playworld and 1987 as the Centre for Contemporary Shamanism. They offer a comprehensive programme of courses and events on Shamanism which is issued twice a year. Individual sessions by appointment. Offer a one year part-time residential course in elements of Shamanism, based on the medicine wheel teachings of the American Indian. One day and weekend Workshops and dance evenings also available. The centre aims to bring the gifts of the ancient way of Shamanism to the people of today in a way that is appropriate to 20th Century circumstances. As far as they are aware 'Eagles Wing' is the only centre that bridges Shamanism and trans-personal psychotherapy. Day workshop £30 (concessions £15). Dance evenings £10-15. Residential weekends £85. One year course (part-time residential -26 days in total) £875 (concessions available). They run a training in Shamanism. They offer Paganism, Shamanism.

Eagle's Wing Centre for Contemporary Shamanism
58 Westbere Road
West Hampstead
London NW2 3RU. (0171)
435 8174.
Established in 1986. One year course 'Elements of Shamanism', weekends and residentials on teachings of native American Indians. Native American smudge sticks for sale £4 each. Typical weekend £45/50, residential £65. One year course (mainly residential) £625. They run a training in Shamanism. They offer Paganism, Shamanism.

Ealing Psychotherapy Centre
St Martin's Rooms
Hale Gardens Acton
London W3 9SQ. (0181)
993 5185.
Individual and group analytic psychotherapy. Established for ten years with around twenty psychotherapists. Appointments need to be made in advance by letter or telephone to the general administrator. Therapists at the centre are available for teaching, lecturing, staff group consultancy etc. Wheelchair access. They offer Psychoanalytic Therapy, Couple Therapy.

Eckankar
8 Godolphin Road
Shepherds Bush
London W12 8JE. (0181)
746 0131.
Contact only for local group.

Edgware Centre for Natural Health
128 High Street
Edgware, Middx HA8 7EL.
(0181) 952 9566.
They have been in Edgware since the 1970's and comprise a Natural health clinic of 10-15 practitioners and a dispensary for herbal and homoeo-pathic medicines both located at the rear of their Health food shop. Also offer Accupressure. Wheelchair access. Appointments necessary. Average £12 per half hour session, £30 per one hour session. They offer Acupuncture, Alexander Technique, Herbalism, Massage, Counselling, Diet Therapy, Homoeopathy, Hypnotherapy, Reflexology, Anti-smoking Therapy, Astrological Psychotherapy, Chiropody, Chiropractice, Eating Problem, Polarity Therapy, Shiatsu, Touch For Health, Yoga.

Edinburgh School of Chiropody
Queen Margaret College
Clerwood Terrace
Edinburgh EH12 8TS.
(0131) 317 3482.
They offer a training in Chiropody

Edmonton Acupuncture Clinic
322 Fore Street, Edmonton
London N9 OPN. (0181)
803 8102.
Established 8 years. They offer Acupuncture.

Eigenwelt London
12 Howitt Rd
London NW3 3LL. (0171)
586 3254 Anna and Alice
Weekend courses in London run by nationwide organisation based in Newcastle. Run courses in Edinburgh, Cumbria, Ilkeston, Worcester etc. Also offer in-service training. They offer Client-centred Therapy, Counselling, Existential Psychotherapy, Psychodrama.

Equilibrium Therapy Centre
117 Granville Road,
Southfields,
London SW18 5SF. (0181)
870 8761.
The centre has eight core team members who all meet regularly to support one another and ensure their own health. There are no waiting lists and they adopt a very holistic approach. All the therapists are fully qualified and have been through counselling themselves. They also offer Traditional Chinese Medicine and run a Basic Counselling course at their venue in Greenwich SE10. £10-35. They run a training in Counselling. They offer Counselling, Couple Therapy, Eating Problem, Relaxation Training, Acupuncture, Osteopathy, Hypnotherapy, Reflexology, Shiatsu, Diet Therapy, Anti-smoking Therapy, Aromatherapy, Bereavement Counselling, Chiropody, Client-centred Therapy, Homoeopathy, Kineosotherapy, Massage, Naturopathy, Neuro-linguistic Programming, Regression, Sex Therapy, Stress Management.

Essentials for Health
PO Box 2216
London E11 3TA. (0181)
556 8155.
They offer a training in Massage and Aromatherapy.

European Hellerwork Association
c/o 23 The Grove, Parkfield
Latimer, Buckinghamshire
HP5 1UE. (01494)
765481.
Hellerwork is a combination of deep tissue bodywork, for releasing chronic tension and to align the body better in the field of gravity, movement

education, and dialogue to relate the mind and the body. The programme was formulated by Joseph Heller in the USA in 1978. The Association is a member network of Hellerwork practitioners who work at different locations and can do home visits. The aim of the E.H.A. is to promote the practice of Hellerwork and to support further professional training. They offer a two week intensive and full scale practitioner training in Hellerwork. £35-£60 per session of 1-1 1/2 hours. A full course is 11 sessions. They run a training in Hellerwork. They offer Hellerwork.

European School of Osteopathy
104 Tonbridge Road, Maidstone, Kent ME16 8SL. (01622) 671558
They offer a training in Osteopathy

European Shiatsu School
222 Westbourne Park Road London W11. (0171) 229 9400.
They offer Osteopathy, Shiatsu.

European Shiatsu School
ESS Workshop Venue Neal's Yard, Covent Garden London WC2. (01672) 861362.
They offer Shiatsu.

European Shiatsu School
High Banks, Lockeridge Nr Marlborough, Wilts SN8 4EQ. (01672) 861362.
They offer a training in Shiatsu

Faculty of Astrological Studies
The Registrar, Urania Trust 396 Caledonian Road London N1 1DN. (0171) 700 3556 (0962) 713 134.
They run a training in Astrological Psychotherapy. .

Faculty of Homoeopathy
2 Powis Place, Great Ormond Street, Bloomsbury London WC1N 2HR. (0171) 837 2495.
Must be referred by your GP because it is a national health hospital. They run a training in Homoeopathy. They offer Homoeopathy.

Faculty of Traditional Chinese Medicine of the UK
13 Gunnesbury Avenue London W5. (0181) 993 2549.
They run a training in Acupuncture. They offer Acupuncture.

Falcons
25 Kite House, Grant Road London SW11 2NJ. (0171) 585 3445.
Consultation and facilities for small groups. Use of leisure complex: swimming, jacuzzi, sauna by arrangement. They offer Stress Management, Aromatherapy, Diet Therapy, Reflexology.

Family Planning Association
27-35 Mortimer Street London W1N 7RJ. (0171) 636 7866.
They can put you in touch with your local family planning clinic. Will answer all queries about contraception, sexuality and health over the phone. Leaflets. They offer Natural Birth Control.

Feldenkrais Guild UK
PO Box 370 London N10 3XA.
Write above address for a directory of qualified teacher/practitioners (include SAE). They offer Feldenkrais.
Feldenkrais Professional Training Programme
PO Box 1207, Hove East Sussex BN3 2GG. (0181) 549 9583.
They offer a training in Feldenkrais

Finchley Alternative Medicine Centre
253 Ballards Lane, Finchley London N3 1NG. (0181) 445 2631.
Practice Bioresonance which is a combination of homoeopathy and acupuncture. .

Findhorn Foundation
The Park, Forres IV36 OTZ. (01309) 690311.
Very large community in northeast Scotland, situated in and around the seaside village of Findhorn. Courses attract up to 4,000 visitors per year. Residents of the 200 strong 'open' community run various businesses, including solar panel making, a computer consultancy, a Steiner school and Meadowlark nursing home. Experience Week £180-240, Weekend workshop £50-£110, week course £200-290, retreat weeks from £80-210. .

Float Centre
20 Blenheim Terrace St Johns Wood London NW8 OEB. (0171) 328 7276.
The Centre has been established for four years. The Tanks have underwater lighting to avoid claustrophobia. They aim to provide create tranquil, meditative condi-

tions, tailored towards each person. A new design of float spas were introduced in 1993 and are unique to the Float Centre, which completely changes the idea that you have to be enclosed. One week introductory course (3 x 1 hour sessions) £48.
Each one hour session costs £24. They offer Flotation Tank Therapy.

Food and Chemical Allergy Clinic
149 Primrose Lane
Shirley Oaks, Croydon
Surrey CR0 8YP. (0181)
654 1700.
Established 8 years. Testing for allergies, desensitisation. Also treat asthma, eczema, ME, candida, multiple sclerosis, hayfever. Ring for appointment. Wheelchair access. They offer Allergy Therapy, Massage, Reflexology.

Fook Sang Acupuncture and Chinese Herbal Practitioners Training College UK
1037B Finchley Road
Golders Green
London NW11 7ES. (0181)
455 5508.
Chinese osteopathy. Traditional Chinese diagnosis. Acupuncture treatments last from 1-3 hours, depending on the severity of the condition. Associated clinic in Reading, and affiliated training college. They run a training in Acupuncture. They offer Acupuncture, Herbalism, Osteopathy.

Forty Hill Natural Therapy Centre
478 Baker Street, Enfield
Middlesex . (0181) 367
5561.
Relaxation and bee venom therapy (in which the patient is stung by a bee - used to relieve arthritis). Also supervised fasts. Wheelchair access. They offer Acupuncture, Cranial Osteopathy, Naturopathy, Reflexology.

Foundation for International Spiritual Unfoldment
71 Trumpington Road
Forest Gate
London E7 9EH. (0181)
555 4643.
Established for 13 years, they offer a 'unique form of mediation'. They also offer a course in spiritual unfoldment. Courses by appointment only. They run a training in Meditation. They offer Meditation.

Fountain London
PO 1383
London N14 6LF.
They offer Meditation.

Gaia House
Woodland Road
Denbury
Nr. Newton Abbot
Devon TQ12 6DY. (01803)
813188.
Founded by Christopher Titmuss and Christina Feldman, Buddhist Vipassana (insight) meditation is taught here on retreat. Zen and Reiki energy balancing. There is a residential community here too, and facilities for solitary retreats They offer Buddhism, Meditation, Retreats.

General Council and Register of Osteopaths
56 London Street
Reading
Professional association linked with British College of Naturopathy and Osteopathy. Register. They offer Naturopathy, Osteopathy.

Gerda Boyesen Centre
Acacia House
Centre Avenue, Acton Park
London W3 7JX. (0181)
743 2437.
Established 1975. Appointments necessary for all 25 practitioners. Car parking available. 24 hour phone. They are dedicated to spreading the word about Gerda Boyesen's method of Biodynamic Psychotherapy. This is the only London centre personally supervised by Gerda Boyesen. £22-£30 per hour. Low cost massage given by trainees. Concessions. They run a training in Biodynamic Massage. They offer Biodynamic Massage, Massage, Aromatherapy, Biodynamic Psychotherapy, Homoeopathy, Osteopathy, Psychoanalytic Therapy, Radionics.

Gerda Boysen Clinic
120 The Vale
London W3 7RQ. (0181)
746 0499.
Centre for complementary medicine. Currently have 37 therapists working at the centre. They offer Biodynamic Psychotherapy, Aromatherapy, Acupuncture, Osteopathy, Naturopathy, Reflexology.

Gestalt Centre London
60 Bunhill Row
London EC1Y 8QD.
(01727) 864806.
Established in 1983 the centre's initial focus was on gestalt therapy and training. They have 7 Gestalt practitioner, 1 Homoeopathist, and 3 Alexander Technique practitioners. The centre is an association of accredited therapists working throughout London and the home counties with an administrative base at St. Albans. Appointment is by phone, with a drop in clinic held on the last Friday of each month. Full cost £25 per hour. Low cost therapy for £14-18 per hour. They run a training in Counselling. They offer Gestalt Therapy, Alexander Technique, Counselling, Eating Problem, Homoeopathy.

Gestalt Consortium (The)
49 Croftdown Road
London NW5. (0171) 624 4322/ (081) 559 3568.
This is a new organisation created to provide premises for Gestalt and other practitioners - there are 8 Gestalt therapists currently running the consortium. Also in the process of creating a referral system for clients. Run individual and group sessions, days for parents and specialised weekends for teams at work. They are looking to attract other practitioners to work at the consortium in order to further expand the range of services on offer. Their aim is to 'provide safe, attractive premises at reasonable prices for practitioners and their clients. All the consortium members are qualified and experienced, and seeking to use their knowledge in new and creative ways for practitioners and clients,

producing an environment that is beautiful in which to grow.' £18-£30 according to therapy per individual session. They offer Gestalt Therapy, Group Oriented Therapy.

Gestalt Studio
Basement Flat
49 Croftdown Road
London NW5 1EL. (0171) 485 2316.
Offer weekly beginners and advanced mixed groups, and beginners and advanced women's groups. Individual therapy, advanced events, including training and supervision events. Women's weekends, mixed weekends. Contact for brochure. They run a training in Gestalt Therapy. They offer Feminist Therapy, Gestalt Therapy.

Gestalt Therapy & Contribution Training
18 Granville Park
London SE13 7EA. (0181) 852 4647.
They offer Contribution training and Gestalt Therapy.

Gestalt Therapy in West London
36 Newburgh Road, Acton
London W3 6DQ. (0181) 993 0868.
Established 1987. Three practitioners, appointments necessary. Good parking, the nearest tube is Acton Town, BR is Acton Central. Wheelchair access by arrangement. They offer counselling and therapy for individuals and couples, and supervision for practising counsellors and therapists. Individual sessions £20-£30 per hour. Concessions negotiable. They offer Couple Therapy, Gestalt Therapy, Counselling.

Goldsmiths' College
Art Psychotherapy Unit
23 St James New Cross
London SE14 6AD. (0181) 692 1424.
They offer a training in Art Therapy

Graigian Community
10 Lady Somerset Road
Kentish Town
London NW5 1UP. (0171) 485 1646 (after 12 noon and before 6pm).
The centre is small Graigian Green Monastery, a spiritual 'focal point' where New Age Monks meditate, pray, work, eat, live, give talks, hold meetings every morning for worship (Matins), paint, draw, sculpt, photograph, write books & design leaflets, collate and publish booklets etc.etc. Established as a monastery for ten years and as a centre for 33 years. Beautiful house open to visitors on Sundays. Activities include 'Being in a Group' group (Sundays 4-6pm), art therapy, tarot and pottery tuition. Telephone or write before visiting between 8-10am and 2-8pm. Members get four newsletters per year, access to regular Sunday group, access to art and pottery tuition, discounts on booklets and pottery, and are entitled to attend communal holidays in Wales after a year's membership. Members are expected to help support the society's environmental campaigning. For general information about the Graigian Community and it's work please write enclosing an SAE (no letters answered without one). Their aim is to "enable all serious, sensible, sincere 'one-pointed' people to get rid of blocks which prevent them from self-development and harmonisation of conflicting arche-

types. To spread the extraordinary discoveries of natural psychology" For groups: first visit a contribution (e.g. milk, fruit juice or vegetarian biscuits); on second visit people are expected to become members for a year. Membership: £3 per annum (concessions), £5 per annum (waged). Couples (of any kind) £7 per annum. Communities, companies and societies £12 per annum. They offer Art Therapy, Dance therapy, Jungian Psychotherapy, Meditation.

Greater World Christian Spiritual Association
3 Conway Street
Fitzrovia
London W1P 5HA. (0171) 436 7555.
Religious charity, seeking to spread the truths of Christian spiritualism and encourage the individual to develop his/her full potential as a spiritual being, achieving a true balance of mind/body/spirit. Give private consultations with recommended mediums. Lectures, bookshop, workshop and postal courses. They offer Hand Healing.

Green Wood College
'Parkside', Ravenscourt Park
W6 0UU. (0181) 741 5668
(and Fax).
They offer Aromatherapy, Massage, Reflexology, Relaxation Training, Stress Management, Shiatsu.

Group Relations Training Association
67 Brocklesby Road,
Guisborough, Cleveland
TS14 7PX. (01287) 630649.
They do an annual 5 day group relations training laboratory using the T group method. This residential, includes food and accommodation.
They also hold an annual conference, normally held over 4 days late September, early October. The conference gives the opportunity to join in a range of activities, including the latest in personal growth and therapeutic techniques. They offer Group Oriented Therapy.

Guild of Vibrational Medicine
Waveney Lodge, Hoxne
Suffolk IP21 4AS.
They offer a training in Flower Essence Remedies

Haelan Centre
41 The Broadway, Crouch End
London N8. (0181) 340 1518.
Clinic above wholefood shop. They offer Acupuncture, Herbalism, Homoeopathy, Massage, Osteopathy, Shiatsu, Reflexology, Counselling.

Hahnemann College of Homoeopathy
243 The Broadway,
Southhall
Middlesex UB1 1NF.
(0181) 574 4281.
They run a training in Homoeopathy. They offer Homoeopathy.

Hahnemann College of Homoeopathy
342 Barking Road
Plaistow. London E13 8HI.
(0171) 476 7263.
Treatment by students of the college. They offer Homoeopathy.

Hale Clinic
7 Park Crescent, Regents Park
London W1N 3HE. (0171) 631 0156.
Also offer chiropody. They offer Acupuncture, Alexander Technique, Chiropody, Chiropractice, Herbalism, Massage, Naturopathy, Osteopathy.

Hampstead Healing Centre
9 Cannon Place
London NW3 1EH. (0171) 435 5432.
A centre established for 10 years approx. 8 mins walk from Hampstead tube. Ring for appointment. Flexible hours. No wheelchair access. Offer an experiential workshop "Living with Dying" 2 days duration. Not for the recently bereaved or under 14 years of age. The emphasis being on our own death and not the death of others. £40-£10 (For those on invalidity benefit). 'Living with Dying' workshop £60 varying with location. They offer Couple Therapy, Hand Healing, Massage, Reflexology, Counselling, Bereavement Counselling, Dream, Relaxation Training, Transpersonal therapy.

Hampton Holistic Centre for Homoeopathy and Autogenic Training
12 Wolsey Road
Hampton Hill
Middlesex TW12 1QW.
(0181) 998 2723.
Established for 7 years. Appointments only. They offer Autogenic Training, Counselling.

LIST OF CENTRES

Harry Edwards Spiritual Healing Sanctuary
Burrows Lea, Shere
Guildford
Surrey GU5 9QG.
(0148641) 2054.
Established in 1946, the Sanctuary covers 14 acres. Main work is distant or absent healing. Some books and cassettes available. They offer Hand Healing.

Hayes Hypnotherapy Centre
Suite 6
Grange Chambers
503 Uxbridge Road
Hayes, Middx UB4 8RL.
(0181) 561 5282.
The also provide sports improvement therapy. There is one therapist, fully qualified and experienced at the centre which, has been established for ten years and has treated over 3,000 clients. Many of the clients are by doctor's referrals. Their aims to enable clients to be in complete control of their lives. There is no wheelchair access. Free information pack available on request. Free initial consultation by mentioning Holistic London. They offer Anti-smoking Therapy, Assertion Therapy, Bereavement Counselling, Client-centred Therapy, Counselling, Diet Therapy, Eating Problem, Feminist Therapy, Hypnotherapy, Men's Therapy, Psychoanalysis, Psychoanalytic Therapy, Regression, Relaxation Training, Stress Management.

Healing Centre
Garden Flat
49 Cavenish St
London NW6 7XS.
They offer Hand Healing.

Healing Centre
91 Fortess Road
London NW5 1AG. (0171)
284 4143.
The centre has eight core practitioners, with many others involved in workshops and trainings. Individual sessions/weekend workshops and trainings offered. Their vision has personal, collective and planetary aspects. "It involves self-exploration to heal and empower ourselves, to release our creativity and spontaneity and to understand our relationships. It involves bringing together that which has been split apart, male-female, power-vulnerability, black-white, spirit-matter, child-adult, body-mind, love-hate. It involves discovering that we are both alone, responsible and have all within, but that we are also all one, responsible for each other and interdependent. And it involves the realisation that life is not a problem to be solved, but a mystery to be lived. The Healing Centre is unique - that all the therapists have spent many years travelling, searching and exploring different therapeutic processes and spiritual paths. We work together as a team but do not have a specific orientation because each of us has our own understanding and ways of working." In addition to the therapies below they also offer Deep Bodywork, Psychic Counselling and Womens Groups. £30 per individual session. £85 per weekend training. They run a training in Counselling. They offer Art Therapy, Bereavement Counselling, Bioenergetics, Child psychotherapy, Client-centred Therapy, Counselling, Couple Therapy, Encounter, Enlightenment Intensive, Family Therapy, Group Oriented Therapy, Massage, Men's Therapy, Primal Therapy, Psychodrama, Reichian Therapy, Sex Therapy, Tai Chi.

Healing Fields Practice
Garden Flat , 65 Anson Road
Tufnell Park, London N7 0AS. (0171) 607 1823.
Has been established for five years, and has two practitioners. There is no wheelchair access, and appointment should be made in advance. Their aim is to support clients in their 'journey towards wholeness of being, physically, emotionally, mentally, spiritually' and to improve the quality of life generally. Also practice Holistic Psychotherapy. £20 per session for flower remedies. £25 for therapy and massage. They offer Biodynamic Massage, Flower Essence Remedies, Psychosynthesis, Massage, Colour Therapy, Biodynamic Psychotherapy, Counselling.

Healing Shiatsu Education Centre
The Orchard
Lower Maescoed
Hereford HR2 0PH. (0187) 387 207.
They offer a training in Shiatsu

Healing Voice
Flat 3, 117 Church Road
Richmond, Surrey TW10 6LS. (0181) 948 5161.
Established for 20 years Jill Purce pioneered voice and Mongolian overtone chanting and has been inspired by the sonic yogas of India and Tibet, the use of mantra and shamanic use of sound and rhythm. Week long overtone and sacred chanting workshops, introductory weekends and one day 'Voice of Sha-

manism' workshops exploring sound for healing and transformation of consciousness using breathing. Her aim is to 're-enchant the world'. £45-£350. £75 per weekend workshop. Week long 'Healing Voice' course £350. They offer Voice Therapy, Dream, Meditation, Music therapy, Resonance Therapy.

Healing Workshops
PO BOX 1678
London, NW5 4EW.
(0171) 708 5721.
Not a centre, but an organisation offering a variety of courses and one-to-one therapies. Guided visualisation, attitudinal healing and positive thought techniques. Courses include study groups based on the best-selling book, You Can Heal Your Life by Louise Hay. Venues vary, but one to one healing sessions and weekly healing circle takes place in NW5. Also publishers and writers currently producing a range of books and audio tapes for mail order. Desk top publishing service available. They offer Counselling, Hand Healing, Meditation.

Health Connection
7 Hereward Rd
London SW17 7EY. (0181)
767 2935.
Eclectic approach includes humanistic therapy, gestalt, transpersonal psychology with an awareness of psychodymanic principles. They offer Integrative Psychotherapy.

Health in Action
9 St. Mark's Rise
London E8 2NJ. (0171)
249 5822.
Established Sept 1993. 2 full-time therapists and a pool of 6 who attend by arrangement. Appointments are needed, sometimes same day available. No wheelchair access but home visits always possible. Also will attend in-house at business premises. Their aim is to provide local affordable high quality treatments and courses in a variety of complementary therapies in a supportive and friendly environment. Offer courses in Shiatsu, Massage, Tai Chi and Parent-link. Their course fees are amongst the lowest in London. Courses average 10-12 weeks three times per year. Prices vary from £40 per ten week term for Tai Chi (three terms duration) to £120 per twelve week course for Shiatsu. They offer Counselling, Massage, Shiatsu, Tai Chi.

Health Management
90 Goldings Road, Loughton
Essex IG10 2QN. (0181)
502 4270.
Established 1982. Courses and holidays. Private lessons also given. They offer Stress Management, Massage, Yoga, Meditation.

Heath Health Care
5 Elm Terrace
Constantine Road
Hampstead
London NW3 2LL. (0171)
267 4222.
Situated in Hampstead, the centre has a modern appearance, and access for wheelchairs. There are twenty fully qualified practitioners, including doctors, dentists, homoeopaths and complimentary medicine practitioners. The aim of the centre is to co-ordinate traditional and complimentary medicine, and to foster understanding amongst the therapists. They also run Holistic Dentistry, Physiotherapy, Sports Injury Clinics, Post Natal Exercise, and Nutrition Clinics. They offer Acupuncture, Allergy Therapy, Anti-smoking Therapy, Autogenic Training, Bereavement Counselling, Child psychotherapy, Chiropody, Chiropractice, Client-centred Therapy, Counselling, Cranial Osteopathy, Diet Therapy, Eating Problem, Existential Psychotherapy, Family Therapy, Flower Essence Remedies, Herbalism, Homoeopathy, Hypnotherapy, Integrative Psychotherapy, Jungian Psychotherapy, Massage, Naturopathy, Osteopathy, Personal Construct Therapy, Psychoanalysis, Psychoanalytic Therapy, Reflexology, Relaxation Training, Shiatsu, Stress Management, Yoga.

Helios
61-71 Collier St
London N1 9BE. (0171)
713 7120.
Also specialises in services for those with HIV, phobias and stress. The Centre has been established for one and a half years and has 30 therapists. They aim to be spiritually based, setting up new approaches to illness. Treatment is by appointment only. £5 - £25 They offer Acupuncture, Aromatherapy, Client-centred Therapy, Co-counselling, Counselling, Enlightenment Intensive, Flower Essence Remedies, Hand Healing, Herbalism, Homoeopathy, Hypnotherapy, Iridology, Jungian Psychotherapy, Massage, Meditation, Men's Therapy, Mind Clearing, Naturopathy, Osteopathy, Polarity Therapy, Psychosynthesis, Rebirthing, Reflexology, Regression, Shiatsu, Spiritualism, Stress Management, Tai Chi, Voice Therapy, Yoga.

Herb Society
134 Buckingham Palace Road
London SW1W 9SA. (0171) 823 5583.
Disseminates information on herbs for all those interested. Members include professional growers, medical herbalists, beauticians, cooks and the merely curious, and receive quarterly Herbal Review, and use library. Also information on herb sources and local herb groups. Lectures for general public. They offer Herbalism.

Herts College of Art and Design
Division of Art and Psychology
7 Hatfield Road
St. Albans, Herts
They offer a training in Art Therapy and Dance therapy.

Heruka Buddhist Centre
13 Woodstock Road
London NW11 8ES. (0181) 455 7563.
Founded in 1991 by Geshe Kelsang Gyatso Rinpoche to provide a facility in London where people can experience pure Buddhist view, meditation and action. The centre offers three special study programmes providing a structured approach to the study and practice of Mahayana Buddhism. Phone for enquiries about weekly meditation classes and occasional one day and weekend courses in central London. They offer Buddhism, Meditation.

Hidden Strengths
97 Warren Rd, Whitton Middlesex TW2 7DG.
(0181) 755 0353.
Biodynamic psychotherapy workshops for women. Introductory days, weekend workshops and ongoing groups. Have been running groups for 4 years. They offer Feminist Therapy, Biodynamic Massage.

Highbury Centre
137 Grosvenor Avenue Highbury, London N5 2NH.
(0171) 226 5805.
Also self-presentation work. A small centre established for 9 years. The centre has a friendly atmosphere, with group and individual therapy rooms. There is no access to the public without prior appointment, and no wheelchair access. Alexander Technique £18 per session. Other individual sessions average around £15-30, weekend workshops £65-85. Concessions may be given by individual therapists. They offer Art Therapy, Counselling, Voice Therapy, Active Birth, Alexander Technique, Biodynamic Massage, Massage.

Hillside Practice
One Hillside, Highgate Road Dartmouth Park, London NW5. (0171) 482 3293.
The centre comprises three houses close together. Established 5 years. Overlooks the heath. Receptionist available for phone calls mornings 9-1. Wheelchair access by prior arrangement. They offer Counselling, Couple Therapy, Gestalt Therapy, Jungian Psychotherapy, Primal Therapy, Biodynamic Massage, Homoeopathy, Shiatsu, Yoga.

Hocroft Clinic
3 Hocroft Road, West Hampstead, London NW2 2BN. (0171) 435 9506.
They offer Naturopathy, Osteopathy.

Holistic Aromatherapy Practice
10 Bamborough Gardens London W12 8QN. (0181) 743 9485.
Offer deep healing techniques. They offer Aromatherapy, Cranial Osteopathy.

Holistic Health Consultancy
94 Grosvenor Road London SW1V 3LF. (0171) 834 3579.
The Consultancy, established in 1983, has an internationally renowned success rate and has expanded into a college for those who seek a similar or wider 'modus opporendi'. Wheelchair access. Bright, panoramic river view consulting room. Initial comprehensive consultations by appointment only, this comprises full Iris analysis, Homoeopathic medication, nutritional, naturopathic and herbal advice and instruction. Free phone-in times are offered to established patients, who can also order medicines mail order. The centre feels that the Holistic approach and the time taken to teach patients to understand their individualised problems and how to handle them achieves lasting results with independence. As the Holistic Health College they offer a training in Iridology, Naturopathy, Nutrition and Herbal Medicine with Homoeopathic Basics. They say that the consultancy is booked 3-4 weeks ahead, because their combination of therapies and analytical techniques is very successful, and that former patients and various colleagues have pressed them to pass on their knowledge in order to equip others across the country and worldwide. First con-

sultation is £73.00 incl. VAT for a full 2 1/2 hours. Colon cleanse, Homoeopathic or other single consultation £38 inc VAT. Concessions available to pensioners and children. They run a training in Naturopathy. They offer Diet Therapy, Herbalism, Homoeopathy, Iridology, Naturopathy, Colonic Irrigation.

Holistic Yoga Centre
The Old Manor House
The Green
Hanslope MK19 7LS.
(01908) 510548.
The centre is a large house set in one acre ground at the edge of a small village with open countryside at back. Strictly by appointment only. The centre has two practitioners, Jake and Eva Chapman, who each have twenty years of experience in the Psychotherapy field. Their aim is to teach individuals to discover the real truth about themselves, their relationships and the purpose of their lives. They run mostly residential courses. Enlightenment Intensives: three day fully residential cost £140. Two day couple therapy course for £160 per couple. They run a training in Mind Clearing. They offer Couple Therapy, Enlightenment Intensive, Mind Clearing, Yoga, Meditation.

Holwell Centre for Psychodrama and Sociodrama
East Down
Barnstaple
Devon EX31 3NZ. (01271) 850 267/597.
Sociodrama, playback theatre, journal process and dream workshops. Some workshops in the Greater London area, but see 'Residential Workshops' for bulk

of programme. Holwell is a farm dating back to 1244, with pond, lawns and a developing woodland. They run a training in Psychodrama. They offer Psychodrama.

Homoeopathic Centre
2 Amherst Road
Ealing, London W13 8ND.
(0181) 998 2723.
Established 1983. The centre is run in collaboration with a doctor/Homeopathy for additional medical opinions and investigations where necessary. They offer Autogenic Training, Counselling, Flower Essence Remedies, Homoeopathy, Hypnotherapy, Stress Management.

Homoeopathic Health Clinic
29 Streatfield Road
Kenton, Harrow
Middlesex HA3 9BP.
(0181) 907 4885.
The centre provides a well women's clinic and sports injury clinic. Established for 13 years. Medically qualified doctor. Four room centre with wheelchair access. Patients must make an appointment. They offer Counselling, Homoeopathy, Diet Therapy, Allergy Therapy, Child psychotherapy, Chiropody, Eating Problem, Massage, Meditation, Stress Management.

Hong Tao Acupuncture and Natural Health Clinic
21 St Thomas Drive
Hatch End, Pinner
Middlesex HA5 4SX. (0181) 421 2668.
They also provide Electro-Crystal Therapy and Chinese Herbal medicine. The clinic has been established for 20 years in total, 10 years at this address. They actively promote healing without drugs and prevent disease using a

holistic approach. They attempt to raise the consciousness of people towards a holistic and spiritual path. There is one practitioner and two staff. Wheelchair access can be arrange by appointment only. Consultation and first treatment £33, follow up £27. They offer Acupuncture, Herbalism, Allergy Therapy, Anti-smoking Therapy, Massage, Meditation.

House of the Goddess
33 Oldridge Road
London SW12 8PN. (0181) 673 6370.
Contact. Support, learning and celebration for the pagan community
For free contact list send SAE. Also counselling service, training courses (including initiation). Most important events are the Pagan Moon and Halloween. They offer Paganism.

Human Potential Resource Group
Dept of Educational Studies
University of Surrey,
Guildford
Surrey GU2 5XH. (01483) 259191.
Intensive Journal workshops, life work planning, exercises in expanding intelligence. Most workshops are held at the University of Surrey. Some are in London. Broad range of courses, often over the weekend, so it's possible if you're a Londoner for you to commute. They run a number of short (one week) training courses in gestalt, NLP, counselling, group work, stress management and birth trauma issues. They run a training in Group Oriented Therapy. They offer Bioenergetics, Co-counselling, Counselling, Creativity, Encounter, Feminist Therapy, Group Oriented

Therapy, Jungian Psychotherapy, Management, Neuro-linguistic Programming, Stress Management.

Hygeia College of Colour Therapy

Brook House, Avening Tetbury, Gloucestershire GL8 8NS. (0145383) 2150.
Large 14 bedroomed house, 29 rooms in all standing in 4 acres with pond and stream, orchard and field. They run a training in Colour Therapy. They offer Colour Therapy.

Hypnotherapy/ Psychotherapy Practice

37 Orbain Road. Fulham London SW6 7J2. (0171) 385 1166.
Large therapy room. They offer Counselling.

IBISS

17 Castle Road, Isleworth Middx TW7 6QR. (0181) 560 5436/9347.
Established for five years, there are about a dozen highly qualified tutors practising in the clinic at St John's Wood. They practice through art, form and theatre and are therapeutic as well as therapies. All work is practical with the emphasis on movement. Classes and workshops should be booked in advance. £24 per day, £50 per weekend. Weekly sessions are £29 for six weeks, £30 for 10 weeks, £45 for 12 weeks. They run a training in Aromatherapy. They offer Aromatherapy, Alexander Technique, Dance therapy, Yoga, Voice Therapy, Stress Management, Massage, Creativity, Feldenkrais, Feminist Therapy, Meditation, Natural Birth Control, Reflexology, Shamanism, Shiatsu, Tai Chi, Tibetan Medicine.

Identity Counselling Service

Marylebone Counselling Centre 17 Marylebone Road London NW1 5LT. (0171) 487 3797.
Are a counselling organisation for people with personal, relationship, sexual or identity difficulties. They offer Sex Therapy, Counselling, Couple Therapy.

Imprint

377 Wimbledon Park Road London SW19 6PE. (0181) 788 1500.
Based in the top floor of a private house with darkroom (photography), art and printing facilities. Fully equipped art studio. Established 1984. Appointment required. They offer Art Therapy, Dream, Jungian Psychotherapy.

Inner Track Learning

Forge House, Limes Road Kemble, Glos. GL7 6AD. (01285) 770635.
Courses on accelating learning skills. The inner track method is derived from Suggestopedia, accelerated learning, neuro linguistic programming and Yoga. It also incorporates study skills developed by Tony Buzan. Its aim is to help you develop your full learning potential. Books and cassettes available. They offer Integrative Psychotherapy.

Insight

37 Spring Street London W2 1JA. (0171) 706 2021.
Personal development seminars which aim to be gentle, nurturing and give participants an experience of their own value. Has been operating in London for 11 years. Address given is a small office, but visitors are very welcome, however their personal development seminars are held at another venue. Participants must be over 18 years of age. Insight has been operating world wide for 15 years. The course is extremely practical. Every concept is accompanied by exercises so participants can experience and evaluate new approaches for living for themselves. It allows participants to discover their lives the way they want, rather than being dependent on an outside agent. £350 per person for a six day course, but often special offers available for more than one person. Participants pay £75 registration fee before the course, then decide at the end of the course how much they would like to pay, using the £350 as a guideline. They offer Integrative Psychotherapy.

Insight Care

24 Chapel Market Islington, London N1 9EZ. (0171) 278 1212/4610.
Patients generally see the senior practitioner and are prescribed homoeopathic treatment. Other therapies are used to enhance homoeopathic treatment. Open Mon-Sat 8am-5pm. Established for five years. Linked to the College of Opthalmic Somatology. They offer Acupuncture, Homoeopathy, Iridology, Laser Therapy.

Institute For Arts In Therapy & Education

70 Cranwich Rd London N16 5JD. (0171) 704 2534.
Drama and sandplay. The institute holds it's courses at Regent's College, Regent's Park. They run a training in

Art Therapy. They offer Art Therapy, Music therapy, Dance therapy.

Institute for Complementary Medicine
PO Box 194
London SE16 1QZ. (0171)
237 5165.
Runs a referral service for the general public to complementary practitioners. Provides information on complementary medicine, campaigns and researches, and can give advice on trainings. Network of public information points around country run by people who are not practitioners (so that they can be independent). Library. Supporters' Club which meets and receives newsletter. Scientific journal. A very helpful and useful organisation.

Institute for Optimum Nutrition
5 Jerden Place, Fulham
London SW6 1BE. (0171)
385 7984.
ION was established in 1984, has 1,500 square feet. Educational, non-profit making organisation. Members can drop in a use library. Clinic and training. Register. Wheelchair access. Sell books, have space to hire, run annual conference and produce a quarterly magazine, 'Optimum Nutrition'. They run a training in Diet Therapy. They offer Diet Therapy.

Institute for Social Inventions
20 Heber Road
London NW2 6AA. (0181)
208 2853.
Promote social inventions (new and imaginative ideas and projects for improving the quality of life), they are the only organisation of their kind in the UK. Print a journal and a book called 'The Encyclopedia of Social Inventions'. Started in 1985, the institute is an educational charity which runs creativity workshops and counsels people on how to launch socially innovative projects. Creativity workshops are free in state schools in London. They offer Creativity, Counselling.

Institute of Clinical Aromatherapy
22 Bromley Road, Catford
London SE6 2TP. (0181)
690 2149.
Established 1970. They run a training in Aromatherapy. They offer Aromatherapy, Reflexology.

Institute of Family Therapy
43 New Cavendish St
Marylebone
London W1M 7RG. (0171)
935 1651.
Charity formed in 1977. They offer a clinical service to families with a wide range of behavioural and relationship problems. These problems may include difficulties with young children and adolescents or they may relate to marriage, bereavement or the care of elderly parents.
They practice a systems framework of Family Therapy. Some work with couples and individuals. Conciliation service. They hire out training videos, hold day workshops and organise conferences. Wheelchair access to some rooms. They run a training in Family Therapy. They offer Family Therapy.

Institute of Group Analysis
1 Daleham Gardens
Swiss Cottage
London NW3 5BY. (0171)
431 2693.
The institute is a teaching institution and has been responsible for the establishment of a widely recognised professional qualification in group-analytic psychotherapy. The Group Analytic Society is concerned with the development of group analysis as a treatment, prophylaxis and science, its advancement through study, research and teaching and the provision of library service, lectures and publications. Associate Membership £55, full membership £77. Also hold workshops, Think Tanks, Symposia, Conversation and large groups. Newsletter. They run a training in Group Oriented Therapy. They offer Group Oriented Therapy, Child psychotherapy, Family Therapy, Couple Therapy.

Institute of Holistic Massage
75 Dresden Road
London N19. (0171) 263
4994 or (0483) 426293.
Individual treatment in massage and body awareness. Introductory and advanced courses. They run a training in Massage. They offer Massage.

Institute of Psychosynthesis
65a Watford Way
Hendon NW4 3AQ. (0181)
202 4525.
Established 17 years, psychosynthesis psychotherapy for individuals, couples and groups. Group leaders will offer workshops and seminars. Counselling service with interview procedure. Mail order books. Wheelchair

access. They run a training in Psychosynthesis. They offer Psychosynthesis.

Institute of Pure Chiropractic
14 Park End Street
Oxford ONX 1HH. (01865)
246687.
They are a registered professional body for McTimony Chiropractic.
Send SAE for directory which lists practitioners throughout the UK, but also in London. They offer Chiropractice.

Institute of Structural Bodywork
15 Water Lane, Kings Langley
Herts WD4 8HP. (01923)
268795.
Cranio-sacral therapy and Traeger work is practised. This centre is an information service for the above services. Established in 1988. They advise on ergonomic products and sell books and products on tensional integrity models and books by Buckmaster Fuller. The 'Peak' is an exclusive health club on top of one of London's top hotels where Roger Golten practices Hellerwork. ISB is a mailing address for information about structural bodywork in general. They offer Astrological Psychotherapy, Aston Patterning, Hellerwork, Rebalancing.

Institute of Traditional Herbal Medicine and Aromatherapy
15 Coolhurst Road (Apt 5)
London N8 8EP. (0181)
348 3755.
They run a training in Aromatherapy. They offer Aromatherapy.

INTAPSY
7/9 Palace Gate,

Kensington, W8 5LS (0171)
581 4866
They run a training in Psychoanalytic Therapy. They offer Psychoanalytic Therapy.

International College of Oriental Medicine
Green Hedges House
Green Hedges Avenue
East Grinstead
West Sussex RH19 1DZ.
(01342) 313107.
They offer a training in Acupuncture and Massage

International Primal Association
79 Pembroke Road
London E17. (0181) 521 4764.
Will refer you to primal integration practitioners in the UK. They offer Primal Integration.

International School of Polarity Therapy
12-14 Dowell Street,
Honiton
Devon EX14 8LT. (01404) 44330.
They offer a training in Polarity Therapy

International School of the Golden Rosycross
45 Woodlands Road
Earlswood, Redhill
Surrey

International Sivananda Yoga Vedanta Centre
51 Felsham Road
London SW15 1AZ. (0181) 780 0160.
They offer a training in Yoga. Headquarters of Lectorium Rosicrucianum .

International Society for Krishna Consciousness (ISKON)
10 Soho Street
London W1. (0171) 437 3662.
Founded by Bhaktivendanta Swami Prabhupada, ISKON adheres closely to the Veda Scriptures, and chant the Hare Krisha Mantra. Practice Bhakti Yoga (the Yoga of devotion or love). They are Vaishnavas or worshippers of Vishnu, a Hindu deity. There's a residential community at centre and a vegetarian restaurant. They have a college for Vedic studies in Herts, 'Bhaktivedanta Manor'. The monastic followers wear the traditional saffron coloured robe and shaven head of Indian holy men, and lay followers wear white. They offer Hinduism.

Isis Counselling and Therapy Service
226 Links Road
London SW17 9ER. (0181) 769 0675 or (081) 656 9209.
Network of counsellors and psychotherapists working mainly in South London (though some in North and East London) trained in various approaches. All therapists have a minimum of 3 years training and 3 years' experience of working with individuals, and most have much more. All abide by the British Association for Counselling Code of Ethics and Practice. They offer Psychosynthesis, Counselling, Gestalt Therapy, Integrative Psychotherapy, Jungian Psychotherapy, Psychoanalytic Therapy, Stress Management.

Islington Green Centre of Alternative Medicine

33 Gaskin St
London N1 2RY. (0171)
704 6783.
Established four years ago. Open Mon-Fri 10am-6pm. Sat 11am-3pm. You are welcome to drop in. They encourage clients to get involved in their own treatment as much as possible and begin to take responsibility for their own health. They offer Counselling, Hypnotherapy, Acupuncture, Anti-smoking Therapy, Aromatherapy, Herbalism, Homoeopathy, Iridology, Massage, Men's Therapy, Neuro-linguistic Programming, Osteopathy, Psychosynthesis, Reflexology, Shiatsu, Touch For Health.

Iyengar Yoga Institute

223a Randolph Avenue
London W9 1NL. (0171)
624 3080.
The institute was established in 1979 and is a registered charity. They follow the method of B.K.S. yoga. Staff of about 20 teachers, all fully qualified. They run classes for children and adults from beginners to teaching level. Ordinary classes are open, enquire beforehand about therapy classes, also specialised classes for pranayama (breath control) and philosophy. Daytime, weekend and evening classes. Numbers are small. They also sell books, videos and yoga mats. Information is available about classes round the country. Yoga days, exhibitions, seminars and lectures. Have details of qualified yoga teachers countrywide. Their aim is to spread the knowledge and teaching of yoga. Ordinary classes £3.50. Yoga Therapy £7 per class. They run a training in Yoga. They offer Yoga.

Jamyang Meditation Centre

10 Finsbury Park Road
Finsbury, London N4 2JZ.
(0171) 359 1394.
Group following Gelug school of the Tibetan Buddhist tradition. Resident teachers are Geshe Namgyal Wangchen (who is resident in the UK) and Lama Thubten Zopa Rinpoche (who visits). Run evening and weekend groups on meditation and Buddhist philosophy. Have residential communities where members live. Many other visiting Lamas give teachings and initiations. Occasional retreats in the UK. Gompa (shrine room for meditation), bookshop, tea-room and library. Open for drop-in visits every day except Tues from 2pm. Regular pujas. Opening times weekdays 2-9.30pm, closed Friday; Sat and Sun 11-6pm. They offer Meditation.

Janice Ellicott School of Reflexology

42 Alder Lodge, Stevenage Road, London SW6 6NP.
(0171) 386 9914.
The school was established in 1984 and is the only intensive course available. They run a training in Reflexology. They offer Reflexology.

Jeyrani Health Centre

4-6 Glebelands Avenue
South Woodford
London E18 2AL. (0181)
530 1146.
Vega testing and courses for fertility gynaecological counselling. People are more than welcome to drop in or call for further information and an informal chat. The centre has five consulting rooms and a large reception area. Open six days a week, 9.30-9 and out of hours appointments are possible. Established for two

and half years. General evenings are on Tuesdays 7-9. Blended essential oils are sold. Creche facilities on Tuesdays. They run a training in Active Birth. They offer Gestalt Therapy, Stress Management, Acupuncture, Aromatherapy, Metamorphic Technique, Osteopathy, Polarity Therapy, Reflexology, Yoga.

John Seymour Associates

17 Boyce Drive
St Werburghs
Bristol BS2 9XQ. (0117)
9557827.
They offer a training in Neuro-linguistic Programming

Kando Studios

88 Victoria Road
London NW6 6QA. (0171)
625 6577.
The therapies above are incorporated in the Kando technique, a serious of movements for fitness, relaxation and releiving pain. It is based on the arts of Tai Chi, yoga and dance, using 'body furniture' to correct movement habits. There is a maximum of seven people per class in their bright studios. There is wheelchair access and classes especially for children. £75 for 15 classes (£5 each) of one and a half hours or £45 for a private class. They run a training in Dance therapy. They offer Dance therapy, Creativity, Relaxation Training.

Ken Eyerman School of Bodywork and Movement

17 Beechdale Road
London SW2 2BN. (0181)
674 9929.
Weekend workshops as well as training in the Eyerman technique. They run a training in Massage. They offer Massage.

LIST OF CENTRES

Kensington Consultation Centre
47 South Lambeth Rd
London SW8 1RH. (0171)
793 0148.
They offer Counselling, Couple Therapy, Family Therapy.

Ki Kai Shiatsu Centre
172 a Arlington Road
Camden NW1. (0181) 368
9050.
Qi Gong is also available. Established for five years, they offer a wide range courses and a low cost drop-in clinic on Wednesdays 10.30 am-1.30 pm. Their aim is to make shiatsu available to as wide a range of people as possible. £20 for treatments, with concessions available. Drop in centre £8. They run a training in Shiatsu. They offer Shiatsu, Meditation.

Kinesiology School
67 Muswell Hill
London N10 3PN. (0181)
883 3799
They run a training in Kineosotherapy. They offer Kineosotherapy, Touch for Health (Kinesiology), Touch For Health.

Kingston Natural Healing Centre
40 Eastbury Road
Kingston-Upon-Thames
Surrey . (0181) 546 5793.
Range of holistic therapies. They offer Acupuncture, Alexander Technique, Aromatherapy, Flower Essence Remedies, Biodynamic Psychotherapy, Colour Therapy, Diet Therapy, Hand Healing, Iridology, Hypnotherapy, Homoeopathy, Herbalism, Massage, Osteopathy, Reflexology, Reiki, Shiatsu, Stress Management, Yoga.

Laban Centre
Laurie Grove, New Cross
London SE14 6NH. (0181)
692 4070.
They offer a training in Dance therapy

Lavender Hill Homoeopathic Centre
33 Illminster Gardens
London SW11 1PJ. (0171)
978 4519.
Established May 1989. 5 Homoeopaths and 3 Osteopaths in residence. Appointments are necessary, reception between 9am and 2pm. £27-£50 for a first appointment of 1-1 1/2 hours; follow up appointments of between 40 mins and 1 hour £20-£34, depending on the type of therapy. Concessions available. They offer Cranial Osteopathy, Homoeopathy, Osteopathy, Psychoanalytic Therapy, Shiatsu.

Lever Clinic
25 Fyfield Road, Enfield
Middx EN1 3TT. (0181)
366 0666.
The clinic has been established since 1961. It is on the ground floor so there is easy access and there are three therapists in attendance. Approximately £25 per treatment. They offer Osteopathy, Acupuncture, Massage.

Life Directions
9 Cork St, Mayfair
London W1X 1PD. (0171)
439 3806.
Based in Cambridge, but some courses in London. Also in-house training for companies. Wheelchair access. They offer Assertion Therapy, Management, Stress Management.

Life Resources
50 Ramilles Road, Mill Hill
London NW7 4LX. (0181)
906 0346.
Established since 1989. They offer Allergy Therapy, Counselling, Diet Therapy, Massage, Meditation, Mind Clearing, Relaxation Training, Stress Management, Tai Chi.

Life Works
14 Saint George's Mews
London NW1 8XE. (0171)
722 7293 or (071) 586
5856.
Established 1985, a small successful clinic of six professional practitioners. A ground floor clinic situated in a mews with wheelchair access. They are happy to arrange appointments to suit patients waking hours. Taking the whole person into account, the treatments offered help to restore the body's health and vitality, through a programme of therapies and techniques for all age groups. 'The practitioners at Lifeworks work well together, offering a mix of therapies from East and West, that maintain an empowering holistic approach to healthcare. There is plenty of information available and patients are encouraged to work with their practitioners to overcome and avoid recurrence of, chronic conditions.' They offer Acupuncture, Counselling, Homoeopathy, Iridology, Massage, Naturopathy, Traditional Chinese Medicine.

Lifespace Associates
31 Ovington Street
London SW3 2JA. (0171)
584 8819.
Bodywork, eating disorders. Training in group work, individual and group therapy, weekend workshops, professional consultancy and train-

ing and non-managerial supervision. Summer workshop in Italy. They offer Client-centred Therapy, Gestalt Therapy, Transactional Analysis.

Lifespace Associates
31 Ovington Street
London SW3 2JA. (0171)
584 8819.
Summer workshops held in Motecoric They offer Client-centred Therapy, Gestalt Therapy, Transactional Analysis.

Living Art Training
14a Fore Street,
Buckfastleigh
Devon TQ11 0BT. (01364)
642793.
Personal and spiritual growth through painting and other creative work i.e. movement, chanting, music, meditation. Weekend workshops. Advance booking only. Living Art has been running for 15 years. They run a training in Integrative Psychotherapy. .

Living Centre
32 Durham Road, Raynes
Park, London SW20 OTW.
(0181) 946 2331.
The clinic which has been established seven years has twelve practitioners working there. Run meditation meetings led by monks and nuns from Chithurst Buddhist Monastery (free). The centre comprises fifteen rooms and large lecture room. Intensive courses on massage. Near to Raynes Park British Rail station. Near the A3. The vision of the centre is that there are many ways towards health and well being and the living centre exists to find those ways. They offer Acupuncture, Alexander Technique, Chiropody, Counselling, Ho-

moeopathy, Hypnotherapy, Massage, Osteopathy, Reflexology.

Living Centre
32 Durham Road
Raynes Park, London SW20
OTW. (0181) 946 2331.
Run meditation meetings led by monks and nuns from Chithurst Monastery. They offer Acupuncture, Alexander Technique, Chiropody, Counselling, Homoeopathy, Hypnotherapy, Massage, Osteopathy, Reflexology.

Living Colour
33 Lancaster Grove
Swiss Cottage, London NW3
4EX. (0171) 794 1371.
Established for 10 years, they were the first officially recognised colour therapy clinic in the UK. They have six practitioners and run courses on the effects of colour: colour counselling, colour reflection reading, colour crystal light therapy and Chakra balancing. They do talks and training at the clinic, to appointment only. Their aims are to provide colour related services products and training for the general public, and to establish the Living Colour Association as a way of linking people. £25-40 per hour. They run a training in Colour Therapy. They offer Colour Therapy, Counselling, Couple Therapy, Hand Healing, Meditation.

Living Colour
33 Lancaster Grove
Swiss Cottage, London NW3
4EX. (0171) 794 1371.
Run courses on body consciousness They run a training in Colour Therapy. They offer Colour Therapy, Counselling, Couple Therapy, Hand Healing, Meditation.

London Association of Primal Psychotherapists
18A Laurier Road
Tufnel Park
London NW5 1SH. (0171)
267 9616.
Primal therapy based on the work of Alice Miller and Arthur Janov. The centre has been established since 1986. They are four psychotherapists trained by Janov. Interviews on application. Therapy offered in German, French, Spanish, Italian and Norwegian. £35 per hour. £40 for intake interview. They run a training in Primal Therapy. They offer Primal Therapy, Group Oriented Therapy.

London Buddhist Centre
51 Roman Road
Bethnal Green, London E2
0HU. (0181) 981 1225.
Centre of the Friends of the Western Buddhist order, founded by the Venerable Sangharakshita, an Englishman who spent 20 years in India as a monk. Seek to synthesise elements from all Buddhist traditions. Day and evening classes, weekends in meditation and Buddhism. Own retreat centre in Suffolk, women's retreat centre in Shropshire and men's in Norfolk and Wales. The centre is a 19th century fire station, has two large meditation rooms, a bookshop and main reception room. The Cherry Orchard vegetarian restaurant is next door, and several other small 'right livelihood' businesses that are also run co-operatively by the Buddhists are in the vicinity, as is their natural health centre Bodywise. The London Buddhist Centre is at the hub of a Buddhist village in the East End. Their aim being to teach Buddhism and Meditation to all who wish to learn, Bud-

dhist or not. Introductory Meditation evening Weds £5, £3 concs. Introductory Meditation course £60, £40 concs. Residential weekend retreat £60, £40. They offer Buddhism, Meditation, Retreats.

London Centre for Psychodrama and Group Psychotherapy

15 Audley Road, Richmond Surrey TW10 6EY. (0181) 948 5595.
They offer a training in Psychodrama

London Centre for Psychotherapy

19 Fitzjohn's Avenue Swiss Cottage, London NW3 5JY. (0171) 435 0873.
They run a training in Psychoanalytic Therapy. They offer Psychoanalytic Therapy.

London Co-counselling Community

34 Albert Road, London N4 3RW. (0171) 272 3314.
You must do the training to become a member. In London there are about 700 members and more in the UK and worldwide. They do a newsletter which is now more a journal on co-counselling. Various workshops. They run a training in Co-counselling. They offer Co-counselling,

London College of Chinese and Oriental Medicine

129 Queens Crescent London NW5 4HE. (0171) 267 4561.
They offer a training in Acupuncture

London College of Classical Homoeopathy

c/o Morley College
61 Westminster Bridge Road London SE1 7HT. (0171) 928 6199.
Offices and classrooms in Morley College. Centrally located near Waterloo and Lambeth North Tube Station. Telephone or call for appointment for clinic. They run a training in Homoeopathy. They offer Homoeopathy.

National College of Hypnosis & Psychotherapy

12 Cross Street, Nelson Lancs BB9 7EN. (01282) 699378.
They offer a training in Hypnotherapy

London College of Massage

5-6 Newman Passage London W1P 3PF. (0171) 323 3574.
Established 1987 but moved recently. Central London location. They also visit businesses to provide relief for those aching muscles. They run a training in Massage. They offer Massage, Reflexology, Aromatherapy.

London College of Osteopathic Medicine

8-10 Boston Place, Marylebone London NW1 6QH. (0171) 262 5250.
Osteopathic association clinic, established 1927. Registered charity ostensibly to provide treatment for those who cannot afford usual private fees. Appointments always necessary. They run a training in Osteopathy. They offer Osteopathy.

London College of Shiatsu

Dugdale House, Santers Lane
Potters Bar, Herts (01707) 647351.
They run a training in Shiatsu. They offer Shiatsu.

London Focusing Centre

2 The Chase
London SW4 0HN. (0171) 498 7447.
Established May 1992. Peter Afford has been teaching Focusing, a body-centred technique for reaching beyond familiar thoughts and feelings to a 'felt sense' which lies beneath, for seven years and has been a psychotherapist for two years. The centre has wheelchair access. Appointments are necessary. The aim of the centre is to offer Focusing-Oriented Therapy by way of sessions, workshops and training programmes in Focusing and Listening Skills for self-help. Also offer a teacher training programme. £20-30 per individual session. £70 per weekend workshop. Teacher Training one year, part-time (mainly weekends), price on application. They offer Client-centred Therapy, Counselling, Creativity, Dream, Integrative Psychotherapy, Psychosynthesis, Relaxation Training, Stress Management, Transpersonal therapy.

London Institute for the Study of Human Sexuality

Flat C
Langham Mansions
Earls Court Square
London SW5 9UH. (0171) 373 0901.
Run weekend workshops, talks, women's sexuality groups, AIDS counselling courses, sex education courses. They run a training in Sex Therapy. They offer

Couple Therapy, Feminist Therapy, Feminist Therapy, Sex Therapy, Sex Therapy.

London Institute for the Study of Human Sexuality
Flat C
Langham Mansions
Earls Court Square
London SW5 9UH. (0171)
373 0901.
Runs weekend workshop They run a training in Sex Therapy. They offer Couple Therapy, Feminist Therapy, Feminist Therapy, Sex Therapy, Sex Therapy.

London Lighthouse
111/117 Lancaster Road
London W11 1QT. (0171)
792 1200.
Residential and support centre for those affected by AIDS/HIV, Established in 1986, the centre opened in 1988, they centre operates with a holistic approach to care and support. Their aim is to enable those affected by HIV/AIDS to live life to the full, and to relieve fears of AIDS and of death. Complementary therapies are very popular and are booked up quickly.
The therapies are free to those living with or affected by AIDS/HIV. They offer Bereavement Counselling, Massage, Acupuncture, Homoeopathy, Art Therapy, Music therapy, Aromatherapy, Client-centred Therapy, Couple Therapy, Dance therapy, Drama Therapy, Group Oriented Therapy, Hypnotherapy, Reflexology, Relaxation Training.

London Natural Health Clinic
Arnica House
170 Campden Hill Road
Notting Hill Gate
London W8 7AS. (0171)
938 3788.
A friendly, relaxed and caring environment where practitioners co-operate to the benefit of the patient. They offer Acupuncture, Aromatherapy, Homoeopathy, Massage, Osteopathy, Counselling.

London Personal Development Centre
2 Thayer St
London W1M 5LG. (0171)
935 8935.

London School of Acupuncture and Traditional Chinese Medicine
60 Bonhill Row
London EC1Y 8QD. (0171)
490 0513.
They have a teaching clinic as part of the school offering all aspects of Chinese Medicine. An appointment is required. Established eight years. Two supervisors, four students and four observers. Their aim is to broaden the availability of Chinese Medicine to the public. They have an established relationship with G.P.'s. They find that the joint goals of service to patients and the pursuit of knowledge is uplifting. The clinic is a charity. There is no set fee, £15 if possible, otherwise less. They run a training in Acupuncture. They offer Acupuncture, Herbalism, Massage.

London School of Acupuncture and Traditional Chinese Medicine (Clinic)
36 Featherstone St
London EC1Y 8QX. (0171)
490 0721.
They run a training in Acupuncture. They offer Acupuncture, Herbalism.

London School of Chinese Massage Therapy
49b Onslow Gardens
London N10 3JY. (0181)
856 8757.
Chinese Tui Na, physiotherapy. They run a training in Shiatsu. They offer Yoga, Shiatsu.

London School of Herbology and Aromatherapy
54a Gloucester Ave
London NW1 8JD.
They offer a training in Aromatherapy

London School of Macrobiotics
188 Old St
London EC1V 9BP. (0171)
251 4076.
Upstairs from the East-West centre macrobiotic restaurant, the Kushi institute runs courses on macrobiotic cooking and nutrition. They offer Macrobiotics.

London School of Osteopathy
8 Lanark Square
Glengall Bridge
London E14. (0171) 538
8334.
They offer a training in Osteopathy

London School of T'ai Chi Chuan (The)
45 Blenheim Road
London W4 1ET. (0142)
691 4540.
Incorporated in 1979 as an affiliate of the School of T'ai Chi Chuan Inc. in New York founded by Professor Patrick Watson. The London School now has nine teachers working together as a team. They teach the Yang style, short form, of T'ai Chi. They are also sponsors of Arica Trainings. They offer Tai Chi.

London Serene Reflection Meditation Group
23 Westbere Road,
Cricklewood
London NW2. (0171) 794
3109.
Private flat used on an occasional basis. They offer Buddhism, Meditation.

London Shambala Centre
27 Belmont Close, Clapham
London SW4. (0171) 720
3207.
Part of Vajradhatu, an international Buddhist organisation founded by the Tibetan teacher the Ven Chogyam Trungpa Rinpoche of the Kagyu School. His books such as Cutting Through Spiritual Materialism, and Shambhala are an excellent guide to the spirit of Buddhism framed in western terms. Provide Shambhala Training, a secular meditation programme of ten weekends. Retreats in Ireland. Study and meditation practice. Meditation practice free. Meditation instruction free. Introductory weekend courses from £35. They offer Meditation, Buddhism.

London Sufi Centre
21 Lancaster Road
Notting Hill, London W11
1QL. (0171) 266 3099.
The Centre was founded to offer genuine spiritual training for those interested in the Sufi path, and aims to be non-sectarian. Founded by Hazrat Inayar Khan. Present Head of Order Pir Vilayat Kahn, who visits the UK. Holds classes on their teachings and on traditional Sufi practices including meditation, dance, prayers, breath and sound, visualisation etc. Healing course and service. Classes are for participating in and enable one to understand and experience the teachings on a deeper level. Individual retreats at the London Centre, group retreats (meditation, sacred dance, chanting, etc.) and residential UK Sufi Summer Camp, both at Hourne Farm, Essex. They offer Meditation, Retreats, Sufism.

London Zen Society
10 Belmont Street, Camden
London NW1 8HH. (0171)
485 9576.
Rinzai sect Zen group, offshoot of Ryutaku-Jai monastery in Mishima, Japan, whose abbot is Kyudo Nakagawa Roshi. Sitting every day: Monday-Friday 6-8pm, Weds 7-9pm and Thurs 6-8am. 7 day retreats at centre, day sessions. Basic instruction given to beginners. Resident monk at centre. They offer Buddhism, Meditation, Retreats.

Lotus Healing Centre
7 Newcourt Street
St. John's Wood
London NW8 7AA.
(0171)722 5797.
Multi-disciplinary alternative therapy centre. Established 1989. Established the London Academy of Oriental Medicine 5 years ago. Specialise in Qi Kung Kundalini Yoga. 12 practitioners. Limited wheelchair access i.e. 3 stairs. Treatments by appointment. Classes are drop in. Their aim is to present a comprehensive preventative health care focus to empower people to make deep life changes. The Academy offers a comprehensive training course in Oriental Medicine. £15-£28 per session. Concessions by arrangement with practitioner. They run a training in Traditional Chinese Medicine. They offer Acupuncture, Herbalism, Aromatherapy, Meditation, Osteopathy, Astrological Psychotherapy, Cranial Osteopathy, Dance therapy, Massage, Reflexology, Shamanism, Tai Chi, Yoga.

Loving Relationships Training
Flat D
9 Claverton Street
London SW1V 3AY. (0171)
834 6641.
They offer a training in Rebirthing

Lucis Trust
Suite 54
3 Whitehall Court, Victoria
London SW1 2EF. (0171)
839 4512.
The Lucis Trust administers a number of programmes: The Arcane School, a meditation school run by correspondence; Triangles, which is a global network of individuals from different spiritual paths who use prayer and meditation to spread goodwill in the world; World Goodwill, which publishes material presenting a global spiritual perspectives on the issues facing humanity; and Lucis Press which publishes Alice Bailey's books. Established by Alice A Bailey, an

LIST OF CENTRES

author and lecturer in the first half of this century, the purpose was to act as an international agency in the raising of human consciousness. They run a training in Meditation. They offer Meditation.

Man To Man
17 Mackeson Road
London NW3 2LU. (0171)
267 0188.
Evening and weekend personal growth groups for men. Admission to evening groups by interview only. Open to men of any sexual orientation. The centre also runs residential men's groups in the country. They offer Men's Therapy.

Marigold Treatment Centre
134 Montrose Avenue
Edgware, Middlesex HA8
0DR. (0181) 959 5421.
They offer Herbalism.

Marigold Trust
PO Box 57
London WC1N 3NE.
(0171) 831 2962.
Registered charity providing Marigold therapy and homoeopathic chiropody. The trust furthers research into Marigold therapy and publishes the results for the public benefit and also provides training in homoeopathic podiatric medicine (chiropody). They offer Chiropody, Homoeopathy.

Martial Arts Commission
First Floor, Broadway House
15-16 Deptford Broadway
London SE8. (0181) 691
8711.
Contact for details of approved martial arts clubs in London. They offer Tai Chi.

Maskarray
14 Mornington Grove
Bow, London E3 4NS.
(0171) 980 4534.
Runs workshops using masks. Emotional expression using drama and play to have fun and gain insight. They offer Integrative Psychotherapy.

Massage Training Institute
24 Highbury Grove, London
N5 2EA. (0171) 226 5313.
They are a training organisation with registered massage tutors working for them in London and countrywide. Also have a register of qualified practitioners available for members of the public. Members of the British Massage Therapy Council and the British Complimentary Medicine Association. The aim of the organisation is dedicated to providing high standards of massage training, incorporating relevant practical anatomy and a holistic approach. Practitioners registered with them charge between £15 and £30. They run a training in Massage. They offer Massage.

Maudsley Hospital
Denmark Hill
London SE5 8AZ. (0171)
703 6333.
They offer a training in Family Therapy

McCarthy Westwood Consultants
25 Kite House, The
Falklands
Grant Road, London SW11
2NJ. (0171) 585 3445.
Management Courses in stress management and aromatherapy. They offer Stress Management, Aromatherapy.

Mehta Method of Therapeutic Head Massage
14 Stranraer Way
Freeling Street
Off Caledonian Road
London N1 0DR. (0171)
609 3590.
A home practice where Indian head, neck and scalp massage which has been practiced in India for over 1,000 years is offered. Also offer weekend training courses in head massage. They offer Massage, Osteopathy.

Metamorphic Association
67 Ritherdon Road, Tooting
London SW17 8QE. (0181)
672 5951.
Established since 1979. Meeting/session room, office and display for books and other material. £25 for a 50 minute session. They run a training in Metamorphic Technique. They offer Metamorphic Technique.

Metanoia
13 North Common Road
Ealing Common
London W5 2QB. (0181)
579 2505.
Large house near Ealing Common. Also offer assessment and referral service for counselling and psychotherapy, carried out by two senior clinical psychologists. Their aim is to enable people to manage changes in their lives. The centre was the vision of two women, which has grown to a larger network. No wheelchair access. £45 for initial consultation. They run a training in Counselling. They offer Couple Therapy, Gestalt Therapy, Transactional Analysis, Counselling, Client-centred Therapy, Integrative Psychotherapy, Rebirthing.

Micheline Arcier Aromatherapy

7 William Street
Knightsbridge
London SW1X 9HL. (0171)
235 3545.
Established 9 years. Mail order. They run a training in Aromatherapy. They offer Aromatherapy.

Mill Hill Health Care

3 Hankins Lane, Mill Hill
London NW7 3AA. (0181)
959 1752.
Small centre (private house). Established 10 years, no drop-in. They offer Counselling, Radiathesia, Reflexology.

Minster Centre

55-57 Minster Road
Cricklewood, London NW2
3SH. (0171) 435 9200.
The Minster Centre covers both traditional and humanistic psychotherapy, and offers Integrative psychotherapy and counselling, integrative group therapy and couples sessions. Appointments can be made over the phone for an assessment interview, where your needs and situation are clarified. You are then contacted directly by a therapist. The Centre also offers recognised training in Integrative Psychotherapy and Counselling, in which students develop a personal style. The emphasis is on the ability to facilitate rapport with clients and work in a flexible, accessible way. The Centre is unusual in its valuing of different approaches and the breadth of its training. This means that they can offer psychotherapeutic help to people with widely differing needs and backgrounds. Sessions cost from £6 to £30 on a sliding scale according to income. Reduced fee sessions are available when needed. They run a training in Integrative Psychotherapy. They offer Couple Therapy, Group Oriented Therapy, Integrative Psychotherapy, Counselling.

Monkton Wyld Court

Nr. Charmouth, Bridport
Dorset DT6 6DQ. (01297)
60342.
They offer a training in Integrative Psychotherapy

Moving Line Counselling and Therapy

c/o 13 Oldfield Mews
London N6.
Londonwide counselling and therapy network using the methods and perspective of psychosynthesis. Individual sessions, couples, workshops. South-East/Croydon (081) 656 9209, East/Central (071) 790 8146, South-West/West (071)733 7883, North/North West (081) 341 4413. They offer Counselling, Psychosynthesis.

Mu Sum Ba - Living Rhythm

Green Hedges, Nash Street
Near Hailsham, East Sussex
BN27 4AA. (01825)
872453.
Rhythm therapy in groups. Ring for details of workshops. Influenced by the rituals of Africa, Brazil and India. Workshops explore rhythm as inter-relation of stillness, sound, and movement. Vocal rhythm, various ways of clapping, stepping and chanting, utilise the body as the personal musical instrument and facilitate to find and trust the inner source of rhythm. They offer Music therapy.

Mushindokai

10 Camden Square
Camden Town
London NW1 9UY.
The centre is a small community of teachers and students which has been established for four years. Courses and talks on Buddhist meditation with occasional Chinese Yoga seminars which are held at the centre. They aim to promote Buddhist teachings and are unique in that the tradition of Buddhist practice (the Shingon School) includes dynamic physical training as well as a sitting meditation. Also practise Mushindo Kempo which is a Buddhist martial art. They offer Meditation, Yoga.

Muswell Healing Arts

169 Avenue Mews
London N10 3NN. (0181)
365 3545.
They offer Aromatherapy, Massage.

Nafsiyat Inter-Cultural Therapy Centre

278 Seven Sisters Road
Finsbury Park
London N4 2HY. (0171)
263 4130.
Specialises in offering help to people from ethnic and cultural minorities. Runs workshops and seminars for people in the helping professions to enable them to work across other cultures, including the Diploma in Intercultural Therapy (run in association with University College, London). Also in-service training for organisations. They offer Integrative Psychotherapy.

National Association of Counsellors, Hypnotherapists and Psychotherapists
145 Coleridge Road Cambridge CB1 3PN. (01223) 247893.
They offer Co-counselling, Hypnotherapy.

National Childbirth Trust (NCT)
Alexandra House, Oldhan Terrace, Acton London W3 6NH. (0181) 992 8637.
They offer a training in Active Birth

National Federation of Spiritual Healers
Old Manor Farm Studio Church Street Sunbury-On-Thames Middlesex TW16 6RG. (01932) 783164/5.
The head office of NFSH has been here for 12 years, looking after the needs of members and running a national referral register for those seeking a healer. Sell books and tapes, and publish 'Healing Review' quarterly (1, free to members). Courses and training in healing and its aspects. They offer Hand Healing.

National Institute of Medical Herbalists
9 Palace Gate Exeter EX1 1JA. (01392) 426022.
Established in 1864 , this is the oldest body of professional practitioners in the world. They have an annual conference for members. Maintain a register of qualified members, who must adhere to a code of ethics and practice. Members train on a four year

course at School of Herbal Medicine in Sussex. They offer Herbalism.

National School of Hypnosis and Psychotherapy
28 Finsbury Park Road London N4 2JX. (0171) 359 6991.
They offer a training in Hypnotherapy

Natural Death Centre
20 Heber Road London NW2 6AA. (0181) 208 2853.
The centre aims to improve the quality of dying; by helping people talk about death, encouraging people to prepare for dying well in advance and to help the family cope with bereavement. The centre is an educational charity, started in 1991, and run by 3 psychotherapists. They also run a 'living with dying' workshop. £6 for one-to-one session (one and a half hours), which can be reduced if necessary. They offer Bereavement Counselling, Counselling.

Natural Healing Centre
1A New Pond Parade West End Road Ruislip Gardens Middlesex HA4 6LR. (01895) 675464.
This small centre has been established for eight years. They offer Counselling, Acupuncture, Allergy Therapy, Herbalism, Homoeopathy, Radionics, Reflexology.

Natural Health Clinic
286 Preston Road, Harrow Middlesex HA3 0QA. (0181) 908 4272.
Two practitioners work there. Established for ten years. No wheelchair access. Appointment required. Aim to help

people who want to take responsibility in looking after themselves and they wish to promote an holistic approach. Caring and not too expensive. £12-£15 per session, plus cost of medicines. Concs to unemployed. They offer Allergy Therapy, Diet Therapy, Homoeopathy, Shiatsu, Massage, Autogenic Training, Chiropody.

Natural Medicine Centre
87 Beckenham Lane Shortlands, Bromley Kent BR2 ODN. (0181) 460 1117.
Established in 1989 the Natural Medicine Centre has 12 practitioners. Patients are seen by appointment (a free 15 minute chat with a practitioner can be booked). Sell a range of books on therapies and personal growth. Also sell a range of essential oils, aromatherapy products, homoeopathic medicines etc. Two steps for wheelchair. They aim to help people get in touch with their inner selves, to relate their physical pain to their emotional and mental selves and to grow through experience. Patients can be referred to another more suitable practitioner if necessary. 'All our therapists are fully trained, insured and experienced'. Reflexology £18 for one hour. Homoeopathy £38. Acupuncture £28, then £22. They offer Acupuncture, Aromatherapy, Homoeopathy, Massage, Reflexology, Shiatsu, Alexander Technique, Counselling, Hypnotherapy.

Nature Cure Clinic
15 Oldbury Place Marylebone, London W1M 3AL. (0171)935 2787.
Registered charity for those unable to afford private treatment. All patients see a quali-

fied doctor on their first visit who recommends an appropriate treatment. Four doctors and one massage therapist. Consultations by appointment only. Founded in 1928. Occasional lectures. Mailing list sent on request. Wheelchair access. Open Monday to Friday. Aim to provide alternative therapies to those unable to afford private treatment. £15 for first consultation. £10 for subsequent visits. £25 for massage. Concs. They offer Acupuncture, Diet Therapy, Massage, Homoeopathy.

Naturecare
16 Sunnyhill Road
Streatham, London SW16
2UH. (0181) 6646150.
They offer Aromatherapy, Reflexology, Flower Essence Remedies.

Naturemed Partnership
Silver Birches, Private Road
Rodborough Common
Stroud, Gloucs GL5 5BT.
(0145387) 3446.
Major centre in UK for Spagyrik therapy, also offer herbalism, AK, reflexology and Flyborg therapy. Register. Car parking facilities. Wheelchair access. They offer Complementary Medicine.

Natureworks
16 Balderton Street
London W1. (0171) 355
4036.
Based on the first floor of Danceworks, a dance and fitness centre. Houses a collection of therapists. Appointments necessary. In addition to the therapies listed below they also offer Beauty Therapy, Chivutti Thurimal (massage given with the feet), Indian Head massage, Kriya (yogic breathing), Aura Reading and Thai massage. The building also houses the Pilates Studio (body conditioning) and Phisioworks (specialists in Physiotherapy). Call for free brochure. Prices vary from £15 to £35. They offer Acupuncture, Aromatherapy, Flower Essence Remedies, Traditional Chinese Medicine, Chiropody, Chiropractice, Counselling, Diet Therapy, Colour Therapy, Cranial Osteopathy, Homoeopathy, Hypnotherapy, Iridology, Stress Management, Osteopathy, Psychoanalytic Therapy, Reflexology, Shiatsu, Kineosotherapy, Hand Healing, Yoga, Aikido, Alexander Technique, Naturopathy.

Neal's Yard Therapy Rooms
2 Neal's Yard, Covent Garden
London WC2H 9DP.
(0171) 379 7662.
Established 1982. Sixty practitioners work from here on a sessional basis. In addition to the therapies below they offer Past Life Therapy, Channel Healing, Lymphatic Drainage, Vedic/Tantric Astrology and Kanpo (Japanese) and Chinese herbalism. People can drop in for a chat and information. Free consultation sessions to help direct people to an appropriate therapy for their complaint. No wheelchair access. Appointments advisable. Toy box available for children. Gift vouchers available. Children's acupuncture clinic. Information pack can be sent countrywide. Advice freely given even to non residents of South East. Their aim is to increase awareness that health is each individual's responsibility and to show people they have a choice in their path to well being, and play an active role in the same. £20-45 First consultations often more expensive than follow ups (none greater than £45). Concs. They offer Autogenic Training, Sex Therapy, Acupuncture, Alexander Technique, Aromatherapy, Biodynamic Massage, Chiropractice, Colour Therapy, Cranial Osteopathy, Diet Therapy, Hand Healing, Herbalism, Iridology, Massage, Naturopathy, Osteopathy, Polarity Therapy, Reflexology, Shiatsu, Touch For Health, Allergy Therapy, Anti-smoking Therapy, Astrological Psychotherapy, Bereavement Counselling, Colonic Irrigation, Counselling, Eating Problem, Flower Essence Remedies, Homoeopathy, Hypnotherapy, Kineosotherapy, Reiki, Relaxation Training, Rolfing, Rosen Method, Stress Management, Voice Therapy.

New Cross Natural Therapy Centre
394 New Cross Road
London SE14. (0181) 469
0858.
Next to New Cross tube. Limited access and parking. Creche by arrangement. Established 1985. Run semi-collectively by approx. 18 practitioners. No wheelchair access, but some home visits can be arranged. People can ring or drop in to make an appointment. Also offer a therapy called Ortho-Bionomy. There is a room which can be rented by small groups. Waged: 1st visit £28, follow ups £23. Unwaged: 1st visit £19, follow ups £15. They offer Gestalt Therapy, Acupuncture, Alexander Technique, Cranial Osteopathy, Diet Therapy, Herbalism, Homoeopathy, Massage, Osteopathy, Postural Integration,

Reflexology, Aromatherapy, Chiropractice, Client-centred Therapy, Counselling, Feminist Therapy, Flower Essence Remedies, Group Oriented Therapy, Shiatsu.

Nichirin Shoshu of the United Kingdom

1 The Green, Richmond, Surrey (0181) 948 0381/2.
Founded on the teaching of Nichirin Daishonin who lived in 13th century Japan. Main practice is mantra chanting. They offer Buddhism.

Nimatullahi Sufi Order

41 Chepstow Place
Notting Hill Gate
London W2 4TS. (0171)
229 0769.
Centre of traditional Sufi order under the direction of the Master Dr Javad Hurbakush who is in residence. Order established in 700 A.D., London centres since 1976. Meditation takes place twice a week. Call or write for appointment. Books and journals about Sufism are available in English, French and Persian. Wheelchair access. Events free. Enquiries from seekers of Truth about their practice are welcome. They offer Sufism.

Nine Needles Health Care Centre

121 Sheen Road
Richmond upon Thames
Surrey TW9 1YJ. (0181)
940 8892.
Established in the UK since 1987, works on an appointments basis only. Practitioner trained in Japan, where he operated his own clinic for 7 years. Holds Japanese licences. The aim of the practice is to provide the highest quality oriental medicine as influenced by Japanese technique and approach. First

acupuncture session £35, thereafter £30. Shiatsu £28. They run a training in Shiatsu. They offer Acupuncture, Shiatsu.

Nordoff-Robbins Music Therapy Centre

2 Lissenden Gardens
London NW5 1PP. (0171)
267 4496.
The centre was established in the 1980's. 25 therapists trained in the Nordoff-Robbins technique. Mainly provides music therapy for children who have a wide range of disabilities/handicaps/behavioural and/or emotional problems. School term times are adhered to. Wheelchair access. Appointment necessary. Offer a post-graduate training course. Sessions are 1/2 hour once a week with one or two therapists according to need. The centre is funded 100% by charity and is unique in being both a music therapy clinic and training course for music therapists. £15 per session. Sliding scale. They run a training in Music therapy. They offer Music therapy.

North London Centre for Group Therapy

138 Bramley Rd, Oakwood
Southgate, London N14
4HU. (0181) 440 1451.
Established 12 years. Referrals are usually made through a GP. Other professionals in related fields may also refer, and individuals seeking psychotherapy can contact the centre direct. Individuals, couples and families are offered an initial consultation, at which the appropriate form of therapy is considered. They offer services to mental health professionals such as individual supervision, group supervision, consultations to

professionals and staff groups and work discussion groups. Lunch time seminars and an annual group-analytic workshop (with residential facility). They offer Couple Therapy, Family Therapy, Group Oriented Therapy.

North London Counselling Practice

5 Turner Drive
London NW11 6TX. (0181)
458 4036.
They are a group of trained counsellors and therapists, each working from home. Established four years. They offer Counselling, Couple Therapy, Sex Therapy, Bereavement Counselling.

North London Counselling Service

21 Northolme Road,
Highbury
London N5 2UZ. (0171)
359 2356 .
Established 1989. A network of approximately 2 dozen Psychosynthesis counsellors and therapists working from their homes in the North London area. Individuals, couples, courses and workshops for groups. No wheelchair access. Appointment only system for initial consultation and subsequent referral. £20-£35 per individual session. Some concessions based on a sliding scale. They offer Psychosynthesis, Counselling.

North London Teacher Training Centre

10 Elmcroft Avenue
London NW11 0RR. (0181)
455 3938.
They offer a training in Alexander Technique

Northwood Hills Acupuncture Clinic
163 Northwood Way Northwood, Middlesex HA6 1RA. (01923) 822972.
The clinic has been established for five years and specialises in Chinese Medicine. They also off Chinese Osteopathy. Their experienced practitioners use traditional Chinese techniques to diagnose and treat a wide variety of conditions within the local community. They work by appointment only. £25 for Chinese Herbal Medicine, £30 for a two hour acupuncture session, with a £5 discount for senior citizens. They offer Acupuncture, Herbalism.

Notting Hill Traditional Acupuncture Clinic
21 Ladbroke Grove London W11 3AY. (0171) 221 1326.
They offer Acupuncture, Alexander Technique, Homoeopathy, Herbalism, Shiatsu.

Open Centre
188 Old Street London EC1V 9FR. (0181) 549 9583.
Established in 1977, it is the UK's longest established independent growth centre. Run as a collective of six practitioners. Supply a wide range of group workshops and individual sessions, using different therapeutic approaches. Appointments are made by calling the answering service, open 8.30 am-11.00pm. They offer a variety of approaches within the field of Humanistic Psychology. Weekend workshops from £50. £25-£35 per individual session. Evening ongoing groups $30. They run a training in Postural Integration. They offer Bioenergetics, En-

counter, Psychodrama, Transactional Analysis, Feldenkrais, Massage, Postural Integration, Pulsing, Primal Integration, Biosynthesis, Gestalt Therapy, Group Oriented Therapy, Integrative Psychotherapy, Reichian Therapy.

Open Dance
East West Movement Centre 188 Old St, London EC1V 9PB. (0171) 250 3737.
Aim to: help 'non dancers' reconnect with their natural movement; help students self-explore through movement, sound etc; 'one to one' dance/movement therapy; foundation courses in running movement groups. They run a training in Dance therapy. They offer Dance therapy.

Open Gate
6 Goldney Road Clifton, Bristol (0117) 97345952.
Run a variety of workshops and residentials on shamanism. Courses on aspects of psychology and spirituality including Buddhism, dancing path workshops, myth, often with well known speakers and spiritual practitioners. They offer Creativity, Resonance Therapy, Retreats.

Oxford Psychodrama Group
10 Heyford Hill Lane Littlemore, Oxford OX4 4YG. (01865) 774731.
They offer a training in Psychodrama

Outreach Counselling
Sternberg Centre 80 East End Rd London N3 2SY. (0181) 346 2288.
They offer a training in Psychoanalytic Therapy

Pace Personal Development
86 South Hill Park London NW3 2SN. (0171) 794 0960.
They run a training in Neuro-linguistic Programming. They offer Neuro-linguistic Programming.

Pan Academy
PO Box 929, Wimbledon London SW19 2AX.
The P.A.N. Academy is the fist to conduct an all-encompassing, PanLife training programme especially for social and global pioneers. The PanLife course is designed to help you develop yourself and your project to the maximum potential. The training is rigorous, as each candidate is wholly prepared for leading and completing diverse projects on ever-expanding levels. For an interview, send a personal profile and SAE. They run a training in Integrative Psychotherapy.

Pearl Healing Centre
37 Carew Road, Thornton Heath, Surrey CR7 7RF. (0181) 689 1771.
The centre has been established for 7 years and all of the practitioners are fully trained and registered with the C.H.O. Their aim is to "work towards co-operation with others towards a world of peace through the cultivation of the beauty in you and the appreciation of each other."
Appointments by phone. £15-£25 They run a training in Colour Therapy. They offer Crystal Therapy, Colour Therapy, Hypnotherapy, Allergy Therapy, Art Therapy, Aston Patterning, Bates Eyesight Training, Bereavement Counselling, Biofeedback, Counselling, Couple

Therapy, Dream, Eating Problem, Family Therapy, Flower Essence Remedies, Group Oriented Therapy, Hand Healing, Hellerwork, Herbalism, Kabbalah, Magnetic Therapy, Massage, Meditation, Metamorphic Technique, Music therapy, Rebalancing, Regression, Relaxation Training, Sex Therapy, Shamanism, Stress Management, Yoga.

Pellin Centre
43 Killyon Road, Clapham
London SW8 2XS. (0171)
622 0148.
Adolescent counselling. They run a training in Gestalt Therapy. They offer Feminist Therapy, Gestalt Therapy, Couple Therapy.

Pellin Training Courses
15 Killyon Road
London SW8 2XS. (0171)
720 4499.
Short courses, workshops and individual therapy. They run a training in Gestalt Therapy. They offer Gestalt Therapy.

Person-Centred Art Therapy Centre
17 Cranbourne Gardens
London NW11 0HN.
(0181) 455 8570.
Person-centred counselling, using art therapy and gestalt therapy when appropriate. Mainly one to one. Supervision. Individual plus group consultancy. House in residential area. They run a training in Art Therapy. They offer Art Therapy.

Personal & Professional Development
19 Whittingstall Road
London SW6 4EA. (0171)
736 4911.
Deal with organisations and the effectiveness of workers in their workplace. .

Personal Development Centre
Lazenby House, 2 Thayer St
London W1M 5LG. (0171)
935 8935.
Offer a range of therapies for self discovery. .

Philadelphia Association
4 Marty's Yard
17 Hampstead High Street
London NW3 1PX. (0171)
794 2652.
Founded in 1965 as a Registered Charity and Limited Company in order to question the nature of mental illness and to open therapeutic communities for the severely distressed or ill for whom mental hospital is not appropriate. Since 1970 it has offered formal training in psychoanalytic psychotherapy and a psychotherapy referral service. This is an association which links together
1) A network of private psychotherapists (26 fully qualified and approx. 20 trainees) working from their own homes or practices. Some group therapy possible;
2) Low cost residential therapeutic community households. No drop-in. Monthly lectures. Individual therapy full fee £20-30 per session, £8-15 per session with trainee. The houses are according to local DHSS board and lodging (not expensive). They run a training in Psychoanalytic Therapy. They offer Psychoanalytic Therapy.

Photo-Language Workshop
PO Box 1328
London NW6. (0181) 961 6714.
Practise photo-language technique which involves subjects looking at photos and working with how the subjects construe the photos. They offer Integrative Psychotherapy.

Playspace
Short Course Unit
Polytechnic Of Central London
35 Marylebone Road
Marylebone
London NW1 5LS. (0171)
486 5811.
Runs a variety of part time courses in counselling and psychotherapy. They offer Art Therapy, Dream, Group Oriented Therapy, Psychodrama, Voice Therapy, Dance therapy, Feldenkrais.

Playworld
2 Melrose Gardens
New Malden
Surrey . (0181) 949 5498
Workshops and events around the theme of finding oneself: creativity, mask-making, movement and rhythm etc. Various venues in London. £12 per whole day workshop. Concessions. They offer Integrative Psychotherapy.

Portobello Green Fitness Centre
3-5 Thorpe Close
North Kensington
London W10 5XL. (0181)
960 2221.
They offer Acupuncture, Aromatherapy, Massage, Homoeopathy, Reflexology, Shiatsu.

Positive Health Centre
101 Harley Street
London W1. (0171) 935 1811.
Individual or group session, also in-house programmes for groups from one company or area can be arranged. They offer Autogenic Training.

Primal Integration Programme

36 Womersley Road Crouch End, London N8 9AN. (0181) 341 7226.

The centre was established in 1990. There are three practitioners each with 13 years experience. Contact by appointment only. No wheelchair access. Offer group and individual work in primal integration, on both a long and a short term basis; information and occasional publications on primal integration. Their aim is to promote the development of primal integration and to further the work of Bill Swartley's original vision of primal integration as a deep form of personal growth work. £70 per weekend group, £28 per hour individual sessions. Concessions in special cases. They offer Primal Integration.

Primrose Healing Centre

9 St George's Mews Primrose Hill, London NW1 8XE. (0171) 586 0148.

They run a training in Cranial Osteopathy. They offer Counselling, Rebirthing, Stress Management, Voice Therapy, Acupuncture, Alexander Technique, Aromatherapy, Flower Essence Remedies, Diet Therapy, Hand Healing, Herbalism, Massage, Naturopathy, Osteopathy, Polarity Therapy, Reflexology, Reiki, Shiatsu, Cranial Osteopathy.

Private Health Centre

37 Green Street, Forest Gate London E7 8DA. (0181) 472 0170.

Herbal teas, remedies and herbal shampoos are also sold here. X-ray department and pathology laboratory. They offer Acupuncture, Chiropody, Homoeopathy, Massage, Osteopathy, Reflexology.

Psychosynthesis and Education Trust

92/94 Tooley St London SE1 2TH. (0171) 403 2100.

Large centre set in a spacious South London building with easy access from London Bridge station. Have large group rooms, a kitchen, lifts and a disabled loo. Places must be booked in advance but they hold free open evenings throughout the year. Run public programme of courses on various topics from a psychosynthesis perspective (e.g. dreams, woman's identity, relationship with money, body etc). Also ongoing interpersonal groups, lectures. Courses available on psychosynthesis and education; personal growth; and professional development. Offer a youth programme for children 7-11 and young adults 16-18. Counselling service with 35 counsellors working from the Trust and from locations all over London. This has been established 12 years and all counsellors subscribe to a code of ethics. Clients are asked to complete a form and have an assessment session and are then referred to a selected counsellor. Professional training in Psychosynthesis. Mail order books and publications. Courses £80-£90 for 2 days. Youth programme £12 per day. Counselling assessment session £45, subsequent sessions £25-35. Concessions available. They run a training in Psychosynthesis. They offer Psychosynthesis, Client-centred Therapy, Counselling, Meditation.

Psychotherapy Centre

1 Wythburn Place London W1H 5WL. (0171) 723 6173.

Established 1960, seven practitioners all with at least 4 years of training and years of experience in practice. They and the training course occupy an entire building in Central London. Day and evening appointments available. Their aim is to provide the best psychotherapy service, using methods based on the outcome of experience and research into long term results, and free from theory, interpretation or drugs. Average £40 fee per 50 minute appointment. (Fees are stated in advance). They run a training in Psychoanalytic Therapy. They offer Allergy Therapy, Anti-smoking Therapy, Client-centred Therapy, Hypnotherapy, Psychoanalytic Therapy.

Psychotherapy Workshops for Women

97 Warren Road, Whitton Middlesex. (0181) 755 0353.

Groups for women: ongoing, weekend workshops, individual sessions in London and Brighton. They offer Feminist Therapy, Biodynamic Massage.

Putney Natural Therapy Clinic

11 Monserat Road, Putney London SW15. (0181) 789 2548.

Small friendly centre. Professional and confidential consultation. You can drop in (best between 9.30-3) for information. Leaflet available or ring for advice. Occasional workshops. Wheelchair access. They offer Acupuncture, Aromatherapy, Chiropody, Diet Therapy, Herbalism, Homoeopathy, Massage, Naturopathy, Osteopathy, Reflexology, Shiatsu.

Radiance Education Unlimited
24 Duncan House
7 Fellows Road
London NW3 3LS. (01536)
725292.
Established in England for 6 years. Introductory talks and seminars, books and tapes. Register. Reiki They offer Reiki.

Raphael Clinic
211 Sumatra Road
West Hampstead
London NW6 1PF. (0171)
794 0321.
Holistic healing centre. Also weekend courses including meditation, massage, dance, personal mythology, healing etc. Float room on the premises. They offer Hand Healing, Massage, Meditation, Acupuncture, Aromatherapy, Biodynamic Psychotherapy, Colonic Irrigation, Cranial Osteopathy, Diet Therapy, Homoeopathy, Naturopathy, Osteopathy, Polarity Therapy, Reflexology, Shiatsu, Flotation Tank Therapy, Neurolinguistic Programming.

Ravenscroft Centre
6 Ravenscroft Avenue
Golders Green
London NW11 0RY. (0181)
455 3743.
They offer Neuro-linguistic Programming, Assertion Therapy, Counselling, Couple Therapy, Creativity, Relaxation Training, Stress Management.

Raworth Centre
20-26 South St, Dorking
Surrey RH4 2HQ. (01306)
742150.
They offer a training in Aromatherapy

Reflexology Centre
8 Russell Court, London Lane
Bromley, Kent BR1 4HX.
(0181) 464 9401.
They offer a training in Reflexology

Re-Vision
8 Chatsworth Road
London NW2 4BN. (0181)
451 2165.
Re-Vision is a small organisation started in 1988 offering psychosynthesis training courses to practising counsellors, therapists and others in the caring professions who are wanting to widen their perspective of work. In addition, run self-development workshops in psychosynthesis, and some other therapies (e.g. gestalt, Jungian etc). Open evenings, network of therapists available for individual, couple or family therapy, supervision for professionals, inservice consultancy or training offered to organisations within the caring professions. Their aim is "to offer 1) a transpersonal approach to counsellors and therapy which has its roots in the ground as much as its branches in the sky and 2) that the organisation reflects the qualities of the therapeutic approach it teaches - that we 'walk our talk'." Low cost: working with student under supervision at £10 per hour. Qualified counsellors £15-£30. They run a training in Psychosynthesis. They offer Psychosynthesis, Gestalt Therapy, Integrative Psychotherapy, Psychoanalytic Therapy.

Rebirthing Centre
Flat B, 2 Wandsworth

Common West Side, Wandsworth
London SW18 2EL. (0181)
870 9284.
Dreamwork, the inner child, goal setting, balancing, the masculine/feminine polarities. Phone to make an appointment for a free introductory talk. Established for five years. Register of practitioners kept. They offer Rebirthing.

Redwood Women's Training Association
20 North Street, Middleton
Manchester
M24 6BD. (0161) 643
1986.
Founded in 1980 by Anne Dickson, this is the administrative office for a network of approximately 135 trainers. They can help to find a trainer for individuals, groups and organisations. Please contact them for information on courses available in your area. Training for trainers is also available for those women who wish to become Redwood members. Courses which lead to a Redwood Diploma, are available in several locations each year. They run a training in Assertion Therapy. They offer Assertion Therapy, Sex Therapy, Feminist Therapy.

Refuah Shelaymah Natural Health Centre
42c Braydon Road, London
N16 6QB. (0181) 800
2200.
Established 1987. This is a self-contained one-storey building with a consulting room for bodywork, small groups and colon hydrotherapy and a small consulting room for counselling and reflexology. They also specialise in Mother and Baby therapy and counselling.

Wheelchair accessible. Disability advice by disabled practitioner. Telephone advice line of the Natural Health Network. Ring for an appointment, 24 hour answerphone. £20 for most therapies, concessions £12. Colonic Irrigation £40. They offer Counselling, Colonic Irrigation, Herbalism, Polarity Therapy, Shiatsu, Assertion Therapy, Bereavement Counselling, Client-centred Therapy, Massage, Tai Chi, Music therapy.

Register of Qualified Aromatherapists
54a Gloucester Avenue
London NW1 8JD. (0171)
272 7403.
The register is a professional association. They offer membership to aromatherapists who have undergone a high level of training. They have a list of practitioners for public referral and supply a list of recognised trainings to prospective students. They offer Aromatherapy.

Register of Traditional Chinese Medicine
19 Trinity Road
London N2 8JJ. (0181) 883
8431.
Professional association for acupuncturists whose training and practice embody techniques of diagnosis and treatment used in the People's Republic of China. Directory of Practitioners £1.50.

Resonance
17 Station Terrace
Great Linford, Milton
Keynes
Bucks MK14 5AP. (01908)
605931.
This is not a drop-in centre. Located in large premises in annexe used exclusively for therapy which is also rented out the local therapists. Es-

tablished 12 years in the UK. Telephone or write for appointments in individual psychotherapy. Programme available (send SAE). They do training groups and talks etc for groups of people working together. Consultancy service available. Supervision for practising counsellors/therapists. Wheelchair access. £18-£20 per hour for individual sessions. £30-£40 per day for non residential groups. £8 per evening for ongoing encounter group. They offer Encounter, Gestalt Therapy, Client-centred Therapy.

RIGPA Fellowship
330 Caledonian Road
London N1 1BB. (0171)
700 0185.
Tibetan Buddhist group under the direction of Ven. Lama Sogyal Rinpoche who visits the centre and gives lectures and seminars and leads retreats in Britain, France and Germany. Courses are led by the Lama and eminent teachers of different traditions on topics such as meditation, developing compassion, healing, care for the dying and Buddhist view and philosophy. Bookshop. Centre open for meetings and by appointment. £3-£5 evening class. Concessions. They offer Buddhism, Meditation, Retreats.

Roehampton Institute of Higher Education
Senate House
Roehampton Lane
London SW15 5PS. (0181)
878 8117.
They offer a training in Dance therapy

Rolfing Centre
85 Judd St
London WC1. (0171) 388
6567 or (071) 834 1493.
They offer Rolfing.

Royal London Homoeopathic Hospital
Gt. Ormond St, Bloomsbury
London WC1.
NHS Hospital. They offer Homoeopathy.

Satyananda Yoga Centre
70 Thurleigh Road
London SW12. (0181) 673
4869.
Guru is Paramahamsa Satyananda who set up the Bihar School of Yoga in 1963 and has now gone into seclusion. Practice through yoga and teach asanas (postures), breathing practices, relaxation, meditation, yogic cleansing practices and Kirtan (chanting with music). Also Yoga teacher training courses. Classes, courses and seminars. Small centre established for 20 years with 7 trained teachers. Telephone first to check which level of class to join (beginners, 1st/2nd year, intermediate, advanced, pregnancy, HIV positive). Easy access. £3 per one and a half hour class. £10 for shat karmas. £15-£20 for residential weekends. Chanting classes free. They run a training in Yoga. They offer Yoga, Hinduism, Meditation, Relaxation Training.

Sayer Clinic
8 Sunningdale Gardens
Stratford Road
Kensington W8 6PX.
(0171) 937 8978.
Opened in 1983. Has X-Ray facilities. Quiet situation off Kensington High Street. Part of a chain of clinics across London. Opening times: Mon Wed Thurs 8-10, Tues Fri 8-6, Sat 8-2. Chiropractice £40 per consultation, £30 thereafter. X-Rays from £50-£100. They offer Chiropractice.

Sayer Clinic: Chelsea
The Harbour Club
Watermeadow Lane
London SW6 2RR. (0171)
371 7744.
Opened March 1993. Situated in an 'exclusive club' with limited membership. Part of a chain of clinics across London. Opening times: Weekdays 8-9, Sat 8-5, Sun 9-4. Also offer Physiotherapy. Prices are according to Therapy and are from £20-£60. Initial consultations are more. They offer Chiropractice, Chiropody, Traditional Chinese Medicine, Acupuncture, Homoeopathy, Hypnotherapy, Stress Management, Reflexology.

Sayer Clinic: City
The Broadgate Club (City)
1 Exchange Place
London EC2M 2QT. (0171)
375 0055.
Opened June 1990. Part of a chain of clinics across London. Opening times: Mon Wed Thur 8-6, Tues Fri 8-9, Sat 8-12. Situated in a very busy club in the heart of the city. Also offer Physiotherapy. £40 for an initial consultation, £30 session. They offer Chiropractice, Osteopathy.

Sayer Clinic: Covent Garden
Cannons Club, Endell Street
London WC2. (0171) 497
2741.
Opened in June 1990. Situated in a club in the centre of Covent Garden. Opening times: Mon 12-8, Tues Wed Thur 8-8, Fri 12-7, Sat 1-4. One of a chain of clinics across London. Chiropractice £40/£30, Reflexology £25. They offer Chiropractice, Reflexology.

Sayer Clinic: Croydon
The Surrey Tennis and
Country Club, Hannibal way
Off Stafford Road
Croydon CR0 4RW. (0181)
686 9265.
Opened August 1989. Situated in a busy club. Opening times Weekdays 8-9, Sat 8-3. One of a chain of clinics across London. Also offer Physiotherapy. According to therapy, £20-£30. Initial consultations more. They offer Chiropractice, Aromatherapy, Massage, Acupuncture.

Sayer Clinic: Marble Arch
22 Seymour Street
London W1H 5WD. (0171)
723 2725.
There are seven Sayer Clinics in London and three outside London. This is the Head Office as well as a practising clinic. Centrally located behind Marble Arch, established in 1987. Opening times: Weekdays 8-6, sat 9-12. Their overall aim is to "combine alternative and orthodox medicine to offer patients the widest choice leading to the best of health." All practitioners are highly qualified. Chiropractice £40 consultation, £30 thereafter, (£80 and £40 with MD). Chiropody £20. Shiatsu £35 per hour. Massage £35 ph. They offer Chiropractice, Chiropody, Shiatsu, Massage.

School for Living Yoga
90 Goldings Road, Loughton
Essex IG10 2QN. (0181)
502 4270.

School of Electro-Crystal Therapy
117 Long Drive, South
Ruislip
Middlesex HA4 0HL.
(0181) 841 1716.
Electro-crystal therapy only. This is a method of diagnostic assessment and treatment of energy imbalances, whereby crystals are stimulated by pulsed, high frequency electro-magnetic waves, generated by a battery operated unit. Established for 14 years. Lectures throughout UK and abroad. Books. Wheelchair access. Easy parking. Appointments only. Clinic days are Mon Tues Weds only. Offer the only training for Electro-crystal therapy in the country. £30 initial consultation. £15 per hour for treatments. Concessions available. They run a training in Crystal Therapy. They offer Crystal Therapy.

School of Holistic Systems Therapy
Admin. Office, 178 High
Street
Acton, London W3 9NN.
(0181) 993 6351.
Run courses in Holistic Massage and modular training in Psychodynamic Bodywork and Counselling at their training venue: IATE, The Windsor Centre, 15-29 Windsor Street, London N1 8QG. Course: £600 for ten weeks. They run a training in Biodynamic Psychotherapy. .

School of Meditation
158 Holland Park Avenue
London W11 4UH. (0171)
603 6116.
Frequent public meetings. Ring office for details and they will send you a booklet. They offer Meditation.

LIST OF CENTRES

School of Psychotherapy and Counselling
Regents College, Inner Circle
Regents Park
London NW1 4NS. (0171)
487 7406.
They run a training in Counselling.

School of T'ai-chi Ch'uan - Centre for Healing
5 Tavistock Place, St.
Pancras
London WC1H 9HH.
(0181) 444 6445.
Intuitive foot massage, personal guidance, talks, workshops. Founded by Beverley Milne, director Ghislaine Picchio. Spiritual school providing complete studies for inner unfoldment. Lending library of books and cassettes. Sell monographs, lecture cassettes, study papers. Workshops and Lectures. They run a training in Tai Chi. They offer Tai Chi, Meditation.

Serpent Institute
18 Mark Mansions,
Westville Rd, London W12
9PS. (0181) 743 8124.
Psychotherapy for individuals and couples. Some talks and workshops. They run a training in Integrative Psychotherapy. They offer Counselling, Feminist Therapy.

Shanti Sadan
29 Chepstow Villas
Notting Hill Gate
London W11 3DR. (0171)
727 7846.
'Shanti Sadan' is Sanskrit for 'Temple of Inner Peace', and it was founded in 1933 by Dr Hari Prasad Shastri, who died in 1956. It is his teachings which are carried on by his followers. These are on the philosophy and practice of Adhyatma Yoga, the yoga of self-knowledge, as taught in the ancient Indian classical texts, the Upanishads and Bhagahvad Gita, and adapted to modern life. Lectures on Weds and Frios at 8pm during term time. Publish over 30 books on yoga and related subjects. Also lectures at other venues in central London. They offer Yoga, Hinduism, Meditation.

Shiatsu Clinic
Unit 62, Pall Mall Deposit
126-128 Barlby Road
Ladbroke Grove, London
W10. (01923) 220860.
They offer Shiatsu.

Shiatsu College
20a Lower Goat Lane
Norwich NR2 1EL. (01603)
632555.
Established 1985. Beginners classes held in London. They run a training in Shiatsu. They offer Shiatsu.

Shiatsu College
The Pall Mall Deposit
126-8 Barlby Road
London W10. (0181) 964
1449.
They offer Shiatsu.

Shiatsu Society
5 Foxcote
Wokingham
Berks RG11 3PG. (0181)
299 2152.
Register of practitioners. Network organisation for everyone interested in Shiatsu. Quarterly newsletter. They offer Shiatsu.

Shirley Goldstein
30 Gloucester Crescent
Camden Town, London
NW1. (0171) 267 2552.
American essences diagnosis. Also sell massage tables and angel cards. Various courses. They run a training in Massage. They offer Counselling, Aromatherapy, Flower Essence Remedies, Hand Healing, Massage, Polarity Therapy.

Shirley Price Aromatherapy Ltd.
Essentia House, Upper Bond Street, Hinckley
Leicestershire LE10 1RS.
(01455) 615466.
They offer a training in Aromatherapy

Silver Birch Centre
29 Chambers Lane,
Willesden
London NW10 2RJ. (0181)
459 3028.
A centre for alternative medicine, healing and self development. Small and friendly, run from a private house. Run talks given by residential and visiting therapists and therefore extend beyond the therapies offered at the centre. Sessions vary from one to one and half hours and cost £25. They offer Aromatherapy, Astrological Psychotherapy, Flower Essence Remedies, Counselling, Feldenkrais, Herbalism, Hand Healing, Massage, Reflexology, Stress Management, Voice Therapy, Acupuncture, Yoga.

Skills with People
15 Liberia Road, Islington
London N5 1JP. (0171)
359 2370.
Skills With People is an association of practitioners across London offering individual and/or group personal and professional training in a wide variety of therapies. They offer training in all the areas necessary to improve the communication and inter-personal skills of employees or individuals. Varying degrees of access. £25+ for individual sessions. £300 per day for organisational training. They offer Counselling, Group Ori-

ented Therapy, Stress Management, Assertion Therapy, Client-centred Therapy, Bereavement Counselling, Co-counselling, Couple Therapy, Gestalt Therapy, Massage, Men's Therapy, Neuro-linguistic Programming, Relaxation Training, Transactional Analysis, Voice Therapy.

Social Effectiveness Training
37 Layfield Road, Hendon
London NW4 3UH. (0181)
202 3373.
They offer Integrative Psychotherapy.

Society for Existential Analysis
Regents College
Inner Circle, Regents Park
London NW1 4NS. (0171)
487 7556.
They offer a training in Existential Psychotherapy

Society of Analytical Psychology
1 Daleham Gardens
Swiss Cottage
London NW3 5BY. (0171)
435 7696.
Register. They run a training in Jungian Psychotherapy. They offer Jungian Psychotherapy.

Somatics
PO Box 1207, Hove
East Sussex BN3 2GG.
(0181) 549 9583.
They offer a training in Feldenkrais

Sound Health
261 Grove Street
London SE8 3PZ. (0181)
691 7519.
Five people work at this address and at 24 Knoll Road, London SW18 2DF. Established 5 years. Appointments need to be made to see indi-

vidual therapists. Not suitable for wheelchairs and it's a no smoking zone. Their vision is to enable change, growth and healing in a safe, orderly and beautiful environment. Some people using the centre have commented that it is 'a garden of the unconscious'. Individual sessions £30 per hour. Concessions occasionally. They offer Voice Therapy, Bereavement Counselling, Biodynamic Massage, Biodynamic Psychotherapy, Counselling, Couple Therapy, Group Oriented Therapy, Integrative Psychotherapy, Postural Integration, Psychoanalytic Therapy, Stress Management.

Sound Moves
10 Jasmine Grove, Anerley
London SE20 8JW. (0181)
960 6612.
Inner creativity through sound and movement. They offer Voice Therapy.

South London Natural Health Centre
7A Clapham Common South Side, Clapham Common
London SW4 7AA. (0171)
720 9506/8817
Open to personal visits 9.30-9.30 Mon-Fri, 9.30-5.30 Sats. Established 8 years. 25 practitioners. Drop in any time to browse, plenty of information on everything at the centre and other interesting connected local events, workshops etc. Half hour consultations available for people to find out about what it available and which therapy might be appropriate for them. No wheelchair access, but will carry people and chairs upstairs. Friendly, peaceful waiting room. They still run the multi-floatation room. Free 15 minute consultation with any practitioner to discuss op-

tions. Just next to Clapham Common tube station. £20-30 for a session. They run a training in Massage. They offer Acupuncture, Alexander Technique, Allergy Therapy, Anti-smoking Therapy, Aromatherapy, Bereavement Counselling, Chiropractice, Colonic Irrigation, Colour Therapy, Counselling, Cranial Osteopathy, Diet Therapy, Eating Problem, Flotation Tank Therapy, Flower Essence Remedies, Herbalism, Homoeopathy, Hypnotherapy, Kineosotherapy, Massage, Meditation, Naturopathy, Osteopathy, Polarity Therapy, Radionics, Reflexology, Regression, Relaxation Training, Sex Therapy, Shamanism, Shiatsu, Touch For Health, Yoga.

South London Psychotherapy Centre
6 Owen Walk, Sycamore Grove
Anerley, London SE20 8BY.

Southfields Clinic
41 Southfields Road
London SW18 1QW. (0181)
874 4125.
They offer Acupuncture, Counselling.

Spectrum
7 Endymion Road
London N4 1EE. (0181)
341 2277.
Established for 13 year, Spectrum offer a humanistic, eclectic approach to psychotherapy. There are 17 rooms and 25 therapists are involved. Drop-in evenings and seminars. Run an incest project which has charitable status, a sexual abuse and dysfunction programme. Run a standing conference on incest. Wheelchair access. They run a training in Integrative Psychotherapy. They offer

LIST OF CENTRES

Bioenergetics, Couple Therapy, Encounter, Feminist Therapy, Gestalt Therapy, Psychodrama, Sex Therapy, Homoeopathy.

Spiral
93 Percy Road
Shepherds Bush, London
W12 9QH. (0181) 743
7246.
Spira aims to empower the individual by applying the ancient arts of Chi Kung and Tai Chi, using breathing and movement meditations. They also are intended to help you discover the source of your inner strength (Chi) and find ways to express and direct the unified power of body mind and spirit. These methods can help deal with stress and increase assertiveness. All women are welcome regardless of age or abilities. Day workshops, intensives and six to twelve week courses. Runs workshops on empowerment for women. They offer Tai Chi, Assertion Therapy, Counselling, Stress Management.

Spiritualist Association of Great Britain
33 Belgrave Square
London SW1X 8QL. (0171)
235 3351.
Seminars, workshops, lectures and demonstrations of clairvoyance. Individual sessions with mediums, which the SAGB state are 'to provide evidence of survival (after death) and NOT to predict the future'. They offer Hand Healing, Spiritualism.

Splashdown Birth Pools
17 Wellington Terrace
Harrow-on-the-Hill
Middlesex HA1 3EP.
(0181) 904 0202.
Free information, advice and workshops on water birth. Hire waterbirth pools which can be used at NHS hospitals or home and can be sent anywhere in the UK. Run regular workshops and show videos of underwater birth. Carry a small stock of books. Their service is run from home where their baby was born underwater on 20th Jan 1989. Give talks and demonstrations to the public and to midwives, not only at above address, but also in central London They offer Active Birth.

St James Centre for Health and Healing
197 Piccadilly
London W1V 9LF. (0171)
734 4511.
Psychotherapy, self-care, therapies and support groups. Cancer support. They offer Art Therapy, Counselling, Relaxation Training, Stress Management, Acupuncture, Hand Healing, Herbalism, Osteopathy, Meditation.

St. Marylebone Healing and Counselling Centre
St. Marylebone Parish Church
17 Marylebone Road
London NW1 5LT. (0171)
935 6374.
There is both a pastoral centre here and a medical centre. The pastoral centre was opened in 1987 and has a drop-in and referral system for counselling and befriending. It is situated in the restored crypt of St. Marylebone church and has six counselling rooms, a small hall and a teaching room.

The medical centre is an NHS general practice which also provides osteopathy, acupuncture, massage, homoeopathy etc. for NHS patients registered with the practice. Sadly for those not living with the catchment area, this is only for locals. Let's hope however that this is the shape of things to come, and that more people will be able to be referred for complementary treatments on the premises by their GP. They offer Counselling.

Stress Centre
60 Downside Road
Sutton, Surrey SM2 5HP.
(0181) 642 7064.

Studio 8
10 Wycliffe Row,
Totterdown
Bristol BS3 4RU. (0117)
9713488.
Not so much therapeutic in orientation, more an exploration of creativity and imagination through art in weekend and residential format. They offer Art Therapy.

Studio E
49 The Avenue, London
NW6 7NR. (0181) 459
5442.
Weekend workshops on myth, expression painting, inner dance etc. Tai chi weekly classes. Individual psychotherapy sessions. They offer Transpersonal therapy, Tai Chi, Meditation.

Subud Central London
50 Shirland Road
London W9 2JA. (0171)
286 3137.

Sunra
26 Balham Hill
Clapham South
London SW12 9EB. (0181)
675 9224.
Large centre in South London established in February 1990. Thirty practitioners work out of the centre offering a wide variety of therapies. Also offer classes and a training in Massage. Have sauna and jacuzzi (with electronincally purified water) on the premises, day membership available for these. Classes and therapies do not require membership. Also offer cystitis clinic, oriental medicine, reiki healing, Chinese herbal medicine, mind clearing, tarot, compulsive eating, and floatation therapy. They run a training in Massage. They offer Counselling, Rebirthing, Acupuncture, Aromatherapy, Homoeopathy, Massage, Osteopathy, Reflexology, Shiatsu, Yoga, Meditation, Alexander Technique, Hand Healing, Traditional Chinese Medicine, Cranial Osteopathy, Client-centred Therapy, Couple Therapy, Family Therapy, Feminist Therapy, Gestalt Therapy, Hypnotherapy, Men's Therapy, Relaxation Training.

Synthesis of Light Holidays (SOL)
112 Wood Vue, Spennymoor
Co Durham DL16 6RZ.
(01388) 818151.
They offer a training in Yoga

Swedenborg Movement
Melilot, Well Hill Lane
Chelsfield, Kent BR6 7QJ.
(01959) 534220.
Promotes the work of Emanuel Swedenborg. Produce a full colour quarterly journal 'Outlook' which is sent free and without obligation. They offer Integrative Psychotherapy.

Tavistock Clinic
120 Belsize Lane Swiss Cottage
London NW3 5BA. (0171)
435 7111.
They run a training in Family Therapy. They offer Family Therapy, Group Oriented Therapy, Kleinian Analysis, Psychoanalytic Therapy.

Technologies for Creating
13 Poets Road
London N5 2SL. (0171)
226 1004.
They do not offer a therapy. Affiliated with the arts rather than the human potential movement. They offer a variety of courses for learning the skill of creating. The organisation was formed in 1985. Hold regular introductory evenings. They offer Creativity.

Thames & Ganges Trading Co
94 Leonard Road
London SE20. (0181)
6590641.
Treatment with herbs (often Indian and Pakinstan herbs). Appointment necessary. Open 5-8pm Mon ,Tues, Wed and Sat. They offer Herbalism.

Theosophical Society
50 Gloucester Place
London W1H 3HJ. (0171)
935 9261.
Public lectures on spirituality.

Therapy Made Unique
21 Primrose Road
South Woodford
London E18 1DD. (0181)
989 3510.
Aromatherapy for arthritic ailments and sports injuries. Specialists in homoeopathy for children's illnesses. Workshops on how to use Bach flower remedies, nutrition, and on the last Saturday of every month, pendulum dowsing to help maintain good health. They offer Aromatherapy, Flower Essence Remedies, Diet Therapy, Homoeopathy, Reflexology.

Tibet Foundation
10 Bloomsbury Way
London WC1A 2SH. (0171)
404 2889.
Registered charity aiming to increase understanding of Tibetan Buddhism and culture, including language and history. Information on Tibetan medicine. The Foundation runs seminars with Tibetan physicians who visit four times a year, with whom consultations are also available. Promotes Tibetan culture and events in the UK. They offer Tibetan Medicine.

Tisserand Institute
65 Church Road, Hove
East Sussex BN3 2BD.
(01273) 206640.
Weekend courses. Introductory courses held at Kensington Park Hotel in London. They run a training in Aromatherapy. They offer Aromatherapy.

Tobias School of Art
Coombe Hill Road
East Grinstead
Sussex RH19 4LZ. (01342)
313655.
The centre is on a rural campus with student accommodation. Summer courses (July/August). Weekend courses during school year. Lectures. They run a training in Art Therapy. They offer Art Therapy, Creativity.

Traditional Acupuncture Centre
75 Roupell Street, Waterloo
London SE1 8SS. (0171)
928 8333.
Established February 1983. Single storey Victorian building, converted to provide 7 treatment rooms. 25 practitioners. Wheelchair access. Appointment system. Aim to foster the practice of Classical Acupuncture, based on the promotion of health. The practitioners have all had a similar training and the centre aims to provide a supportive learning environment for them. Aim to meet the guidelines suggested in the recent BMA report for 'Centre of Excellence'. Diagnosis £40. Treatment £25. Practitioners are willing to reduce fees in certain circumstances by negotiation. They offer Acupuncture.

Traditional Chinese Medicine Clinic
10 Sandown Way, Northolt
Middx UB5 4HY. (0181)
743 0706.
Specialise in treating gynaecological problems and cancer patients that cannot be treated by orthodox medicine. Appointment only. Patients are seen by Dr Hsu who also tries to prevent the side effects of western drugs on cancer patients. Children's

problems also treated. They run a training in Acupuncture. They offer Acupuncture, Diet Therapy, Herbalism.

Transcendental Meditation
Freepost, London SW1P
4YY. (01800) 269303.
Centres countrywide. Three residential and seventy non-residential. One community. They offer Meditation.

Transcendental Meditation Baker Street Centre
24 Linhope Street,
Marylebone
London NW1 6TH. (0171)
402 3451.
Run courses on transcendental meditation. Free introductory presentations, phone for details. They offer Meditation.

Transcendental Meditation National Office
Mentmore Towers, Mentmore
Leighton Buzzard
LU7 0QH.
Can put you in touch with your local TM centre. They offer Meditation.

Transformational Trainings
23 Albany Terrace
Leamington Spa
Warks CV32 5LP. (01926)
882494.
They offer a training in Rebirthing

Trinity Hospice
30 Clapham North Side
London SW4 0RN. (0171)
622 9481.
Has cared for those suffering from advanced cancer and other illnesses for the last 100 years. If you cannot get bereavement counselling from your present community then this hospice will see you for bereavement counselling free of charge. They offer Bereavement Counselling.

United Kingdom Council for Psychotherapy
Regents College
Inner Circle
Regents Park
London nw1 4ns
(0171) 487 7554
A federation of psychotherapy organisations representing the profession of psychotherapy in the UK. The aims of the Conference are to protect the public by the promotion of high standards of training, research and education; to foster the dissemination of knowledge about psychotherapy; and to increase its availability. The Conference has set up a register of psychotherapists and can refer a psychotherapist to you, by providing a list of therapists who live in your area.

Universal Training
Keepers Cottage
Mynthurst Farm
Leigh, nr Reigate
Surrey RH2 8QD. (01293)
862828.
Courses in personal development which include meditation, body language training, affirmations plus own brand of self exploration. Format for core course, Turning Points, is one weekend plus three evening. They offer Integrative Psychotherapy.

Universitas Associates
5 Cedar Road, Sutton
Surrey SM2 5DA. (0181)
643 4898.
Soul directed astrology, soul directed therapy. Are a group of professionals who help people to discover their full potential and purpose in life. Individual consultation, training and seminars are offered. They offer Stress Management, Hand Healing, Creativity, Art Therapy.

Violet Hill Studios
5-7 Violet Hill
St John's Wood
London NW8 9EB. (0171)
624 0101 or (081) 458
5368.
The centre opened in January 1993 and already has 35 practitioners working either with weekly practices or running workshops. They have a diverse range of weekly and weekend workshops and training courses. All practitioners are highly qualified and experienced, they work as a team and regular meetings for practitioners are held at the centre. The vision has been to create an environment whereby healing and art exist together. The atmosphere is one of peace and beauty. The ethos of the centre has been to provide a very wide range of therapies, workshops and training courses and to become a useful and integral part of the local community. The range of therapies is regularly increasing. The studios have been sensitively restored from an 18th Century barn. Although the centre is situated in the heart of London it has the feel of the country. Open Afternoons are held throughout the year, combined with Art Exhibitions which also include Children's Art. The Studios are also equipped for Art Workshops, and Children's Workshops are also held at the centre. In addition to the therapies below they also offer Psychic Counselling, Aura Soma Colour Therapy, National Childbirth Trust groups, Geopathic Stress, Anti-Drug therapy and Manual Lymphatic Drainage. It is necessary to make an appointment. Offer a training in Aromatherapy through the Mother Earth Aromatherapy School. £20-£25 per hour for one to one consultations. They run a training in Aromatherapy. They offer Art Therapy, Colour Therapy, Counselling, Crystal Therapy, Homoeopathy, Hand Healing, Massage, Kineosotherapy, Osteopathy, Reflexology, Rebirthing, Shiatsu, Tai Chi, Yoga, Alexander Technique, Aromatherapy, Acupuncture, Anti-smoking Therapy, Bereavement Counselling, Biodynamic Massage, Biodynamic Psychotherapy, Client-centred Therapy, Colonic Irrigation, Couple Therapy, Cranial Osteopathy, Creativity, Diet Therapy, Eating Problem, Family Therapy, Flower Essence Remedies, Group Oriented Therapy, Hypnotherapy, Integrative Psychotherapy, Meditation, Metamorphic Technique, Naturopathy, Radionics, Rebalancing, Reiki, Relaxation Training, Rolfing, Stress Management, Touch For Health, Transpersonal therapy.

Welbeck Counselling Service
5 Clarkes Mews, Marylebone
London W1N 1RR. (0171)
935 3073.
Humanistic counselling encompassing Rogerian, Egan, Gestalt and Transactional Analysis, as well as behavioural therapy and career counselling 2 consulting rooms. A number of the staff are chartered psychologists. Run open training events programme. Space to rent occasionally. They offer Counselling, Sex Therapy, Stress Management.

Welcome Home Birth Practice
42 Elder Avenue, Crouch End
London N8 8PS. (0181)
347 9609.
They offer Active Birth.

Wendy Rigby School of Natural Therapies
3 Ellerdale Road,
Hampstead
London NW3 6BA. (0171)
435 5407.

West London School of Therapeutic Massage
41A St Luke's Road
London W11 1DD. (0171)
229 7411.
They run a training in Massage. They offer Aromatherapy, Massage, Reflexology, Shiatsu.

Westminster Natural Health Centre
34-36a Warwick Way
London SW1V 1RY. (0171)
834 0861.
A fully modernised therapy centre in Victoria/Pimlico area. Close to tubes and bus routes. Ten practitioners, three treatment rooms. Established in 1987, this natural health centre won the Journal of Alternative and Complementary Medicine's 'Practice of the Year' award in 1988 and 1989. Small reading room. No wheelchair access. Information centre. Appointment only by phone 9-5pm Mon to Fri. Their aim is to create a centre that has information available to local people on alternative therapies, and to make these available to a wider range of patients through concessions and awareness campaigns. Range £20-35. Concessions. They offer Counselling, Acupuncture, Alexander Technique,

Aromatherapy, Naturopathy, Osteopathy, Reflexology, Shiatsu, Colour Therapy, Diet Therapy, Homoeopathy, Hypnotherapy, Rolfing.

Westminster Pastoral Foundation
23 Kensington Square Kensington, London W8 5HN. (0171) 937 6956.
A national organisation with headquarters at Kensington, affiliated centres in different parts of the country. Short courses on aspects of counselling and spirituality. Individual and group sessions. They run a training in Counselling. They offer Bereavement Counselling, Counselling, Family Therapy.

White Eagle Lodge
9 St. Mary Abbots Place Kensington High Street London W8 6LS. (0171) 603 7914.
They have a large voluntary team of helpers who offer spiritual healing. Services of worship, healing, meditation and prayer for 'sending out the light'. Meetings at above address, at set times Mon &Tues 3.15pm, Wed and Thurs 6.45 pm. No appointment necessary. Bookshop, library, chapel for meditation. Their aim is the" quiet unfoldment of the Christ Light in the individual human heart. The White Eagle Lodge is an open community of service for the light stretching around the world. It's centre in London acts as a focus for the practice and teaching of meditation and healing." They hold classes in Meditation: Thursday 1.15-2pm and every 4th Wednesday at 7.45pm. The Lodge also offers opportunities for service through absent healing. Training in contact healing within the Lodge

is only given after two years absent healing service. Healing is free, £2 per class for Meditation. They offer Hand Healing, Meditation.

Whole Health Clinic
31 Eton Hall Eton College Road London NW3 2DE. (0171) 722 9270.
There is one practitioner, aiming to practice truely holistic health and help people realise their full potential. The clinic is close to Chalk Farm tube station, with lifts. £30-£40 They offer Aromatherapy, Colonic Irrigation, Kineosotherapy, Massage, Counselling, Client-centred Therapy.

Wholeness
26 Mulberry Way South Woodford London E18 1ED. (0181) 530 8804.
Husband and wife team established since 1986 at this address and they now also have a clinic at 140 Harley Street (Tel: 0171 2726). The provide colonic irrigation with hypnosis. They charge £30-60 for colonic irrigation and £25 for hypnotherapy. They offer Neuro-linguistic Programming, Colonic Irrigation, Hypnotherapy, Pulsing, Reflexology, Stress Management.

Wholistic Health and Life Extension
Four Winds Church Hill Arnside, Cumbria LA5 0DQ. (01524) 762526.
Workshops on use of crystals and gems in healing. Also electronic gem therapy, dowsing and assemblance point shifting. They offer Crystal Therapy, Aromatherapy.

Wild Dance
5 Clanricarde Gardens London W2 4JJ. (0171) 221 7399.
Organise day and weekend events, mainly for men, based on the work of Robert Bly and James Hillman who annually come to lead them. They offer Men's Therapy.

Wild Goose Company
65 Roderick Road London NW3 2NP. (0171) 482 5502.
Provide a place in which people can experience energy work and other meditations. Most of the work is in groups; £2 per evening, £10 per day (apart from larger workshops). Videos and talks on energy work. They offer Massage, Meditation.

Will (Workshop Institute for Living Learning)
218 Randolph Avenue London W9. (0171) 328 8955.
They practice 'theme-centred interaction' which is a group dynamic method based on the belief that thought and feeling should not be separated and that every group member has equal rights. They offer Group Oriented Therapy.

Wimbledon Clinic of Natural Medicine
1 Evelyn Road, Wimbledon London SW19 8NU. (0181) 540 3389.
A large centre with up to date equipment for diagnosis and treatment, which has been established since 1981. Six practitioners. They also offer Medigen, a full health screen, ozone therapy, an obesity and cellulite programme and biological medicine. Open days, mail order water filters, equipment. Wheelchair access. By

appointment only. Their aim is to combine some of the most up to date systems of diagnostics with conventional laboratory analysis in order to arrive at an objective health evaluation and subsequent treatments by wholistic natural therapies. From £15-50. They offer Acupuncture, Alexander Technique, Allergy Therapy, Colonic Irrigation, Laser Therapy, Osteopathy, Bioenergetic Medicine, Chiropody, Herbalism, Homoeopathy, Magnetic Therapy, Naturopathy.

Women and Health
4 Carol St
London NW1 0HU. (0171)
482 2786.
The organisation is a charity and a voluntary sector community centre which was primarily set up for women who live or work in Camden as a result of a survey whose results suggested that women felt their health needs were not being adequately addressed by their GPs and other health care sources. Sliding scale of £5-£16 according to ability to pay. They offer Counselling, Alexander Technique, Acupuncture, Aromatherapy, Herbalism, Homoeopathy, Massage, Osteopathy, Shiatsu, Reflexology, Aikido, Allergy Therapy, Anti-smoking Therapy, Art Therapy, Assertion Therapy, Bereavement Counselling, Biofeedback, Child psychotherapy, Co-counselling, Colour Therapy, Diet Therapy, Drama Therapy, Eating Problem, Family Therapy, Flotation Tank Therapy, Iridology, Kabbalah, Rebirthing, Relaxation Training, Sex Therapy, Shamanism, Spiritualism, Tai Chi.

Women Unlimited
79 Pathfield Road
London SW16 5PA. (0181)
677 7503.
Also Counselling from Conception, Conflict Resolution, Time Management and Team Building Sessions. Consultancy work and group work offered to organisations. Founded in 1989, Women Unlimited offers a wide variety of services for women to improve their personal and working lives by offering counselling and development workshops for women that empower the individual. £70 for a two day workshop, Sliding Scale for individual sessions. 'In House' consultations by negotiation. They offer Assertion Therapy, Feminist Therapy, Stress Management, Bereavement Counselling, Client-centred Therapy, Counselling, Couple Therapy.

Women's Therapy Centre
6-9 Manor Gardens
Holloway
London N7 6LA. (0171)
263 6200.
Established since 1976 the centre now has a total of 17 therapists. They aim to provide help to women in emotional distress by means of individual and group psychotherapy in a safe, women only environment. Their aim is to provide psychotherapy to emotionally distressed women regardless of income, age, socio-economic background or ethnic origin. They also provide educational/training programmes for mental health workers. They specialise in eating problems. Sell books. Sliding scale for workshops and therapy £0.00 minimum, £25 maximum. They run a training in Psychoanalytic Therapy. They

offer Eating Problem, Feminist Therapy, Psychoanalytic Therapy.

Wood Street Clinic
133 Wood Street, Barnet
Herts EN5 4BX. (0181)
441 0231/449 7656.
Marriage guidance, psychotherapy, chiropody. Owned and run by Mr Mervyn D Cole. Consultation service for those unsure of which therapy to choose (for a fee). Appointments always needed. Established 1984. They offer Counselling, Acupuncture, Alexander Technique, Aromatherapy, Chiropractice, Herbalism, Homoeopathy, Massage, Osteopathy, Reflexology.

Working With Men
St. Giles Hospital
St Giles Road
London SE5 7RN. (0171)
703 0898 x6019 & (071)
703 8780.
They run a training in Men's Therapy. They offer Men's Therapy.

Workshops with a Difference
19 Fourth Cross Road
Twickenham
London TW2 5EL. (0181)
894 5980.
Motivational workshops in groups and one to one work with individuals wishing to move into their vision through accessing their higher consciousness. Workshops take place in different venues - health clubs and centres mostly. One to one work in Twickenham or the client's own homes. Lending library of Lazaris material for clients and rental service for the general public. Wheelchair access. They offer Integrative Psychotherapy.

INDEX

A

Abraxas 269
Abshot Holistic Centre 239, 269
Acca and Adda 269
Achilles Heel 212, 53
Active Birth 172
Active Birth Centre 258
Acumedic Centre 269
Acupressure 163
Acupuncture 100
Acupuncture and Osteopathy Clinic 270
Adlerian 79
Aetherius Society 197
Affirmations 70
Agency (The) 259
Aikido 104
Ainsworths Homoeopathic Pharmacy 200, 262
Air Improvement Centre 200, 255
Air purifiers 255
Alexander Technique 105
All Hallows House 246
Allchurch's Investment Management Service 222
Allergy Therapy 107
Alternative Centre 253
Alternative Sitting 257
Alternatives 250
Amadeus Centre 225
Analytical psychology 50, 77
Andrew Still College of Osteopathy 271
Angel Gate 233
Anima 51
Animal Aid 251
Animus 51
Anthroposophical Association 195
Anti-smoking Therapy 79
Applied Kinesiology / Touch for Health 109
Arkana 209
Aromatherapy 110
Aromatherapy oils 255
Aromatique 255
Arrow Books 209
Art Therapy 15
Ashgrove Distribution 209
Assagioli, Robert 67
Assertion Training 18
Association for Analystic and Bodymind Therapy 225
Association for Therapeutic Healers 218
Aston Patterning 172
Astrological birth control 150
Astrological Counselling 19
Astrology Products 257
Astrology Shop 202
Atlantis Bookshop 200
Aura Soma 240
Aurora 200, 259, 263, 265, 266, 267
Autogenic Training 21
Ayurvedic Medicine 115

B

Bach Flower Remedies 130
Bach Flower Remedies Ltd 262
Back Products 257
Back Shop 201, 257, 264
Back Store Ltd 201, 257
Baha'i Faith 197
Baldwin and Co 256
Banana Chair Company 257
Bandler, Richard 56
Barry Long Foundation 195
Basal Body Temperature 150

Bates, Carrie 226
Bates Eyesight Training 116
Beacon Centre 240, 244
Bennett & Luck 201
Bereavement Counselling 79
Berne, Eric 76
Beshara Trust 198
Bethany Vegetarian and Vegan Nursing Homes 238
Bhagwan Shree Rajneesh 184
Biodynamic Massage and Psychology 116
Bioenergetics 22
Biofeedback 24
Biofeedback Machines 257
Biomonitors 258
Bion, W. 45
Biosun 260
Biosynthesis 79
Birkbeck College - Centre for Extra-Mural Studies 220
Birthing Pools 258
Birthing Tub Company 258
Bloomsbury Alexander Centre 89
Bodywise 225
Books Etc 201
Books For A Change 202
Books for Cooks 202
Bookshops 200
Botton Camphill 237
Brainwave 226
Breakspear Hospital 239
Breakthrough Centre 218, 217, 227, 229
British Association for Counselling 212
British Holistic Medical Association 99
British School of Oriental Therapy and Movement 91
British School of Osteopathy 219
Buddhism 186
Bumblebee Natural Foods 232
Bumblebees Natural Remedies 202
Bunjie's Coffee House 233
Bushwacker 232
Business Network 2000 218

C

C W Daniel Ltd 209
Cabala 191
Caduceus 212
CAER 240
Calendar method 150
Campus 247
Cancer Help Centre 253
Candles 258
Carl Rogers 25, 37
Centre for Complementary Health Studies 220
Centre for Creation Spirituality 250
Centre of Light 241
Ceremonial products 259
Chanting 180
Charlie's Rock Shop 202, 260
Cherry Orchard 233
CHI Centre 253, 262
Child psychotherapy 79
Chiropractic 119
Chlorella Health 261
Choosing a Particular Therapy 91
Christian Community 195
Christianity 187
Church Street Library 217
Churchill Centre 248
City University 219
Client-centred therapy 25
Cloud Nine Music 266
Co-counselling 26

INDEX

H

I

J

K

L

M

INDEX